☐ DRUG ABUSE AND THE ELDERLY:

An Annotated Bibliography

by
DOUGLAS H. RUBEN

The Scarecrow Press, Inc.
Metuchen, N.J., & London
1984

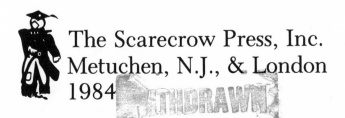

Library of Congress Cataloging in Publication Data

Ruben, Douglas H.
  Drug abuse and the elderly.

   Includes indexes.
   1. Aged--United States--Drug use--Bibliography.
2. Aged--United States--Alcohol use--Bibliography.
3. Epidemiology--Bibliography. 4. Drug abuse--United
States--Bibliography. I. Title. [DNLM: 1. Substance
dependence--In old age--Bibliography. 2. Substance abuse
--In old age--Bibliography. ZWM 270 R895d]
Z7164.N17R82 1984   016.3622'92'0880565   83-20463
[HV5801]
ISBN 0-8108-1677-6

To

CEILA RUBEN

Her unshakable pride breathes through the heart
of future generations.

CONTENTS

ACKNOWLEDGMENTS

The need for assistance abounds during each stage of preparation of a book. Inasmuch as I owe several debts of appreciation to friends and students, certain persons in particular truly dedicated their time and deserve special recognition. C. Dennis Simpson, Director of the Specialty Program in Alcohol and Drug Abuse, and Ellen-Page Robin, Director of the Gerontology Program, both offered many suggestions on interpretation and were generous with resource materials. Their insights into the problems of elderly and substance abuse greatly guided my analysis in each annotation. Shaghil Husain and Rosamond Robbert, both from the Department of Sociology, Western Michigan University, brought to my attention several current demographic facts about the elderly population. And responsible for my efficiency as she, too, shared excitement over the book was my wife, Marilyn J. Ruben. Perhaps more than others, I am grateful to Marilyn for being patient, enthusiastic, and involved in this scholarly venture.

LIBERATION

Now and then I'd start to fret
And to change things I'd never get
And to endure with needless pain
Things I dreamed of went down the drain.
So had to change my mode of life
To do some good I'll only strive
Will try and bring some cheer
To sick and aged who live in fear.
If I'll be lucky and succeed
Will such an act my poor soul feed.
When all seems wrong a heart is torn
In anguish, self-pity--a rhyme is born.

--Helen Lasser, 1966

PREFACE

Specialty populations vary in our society by how we define
minority or underprivileged subgroups and whether, culturally, these definitions fit into programs and other service
agencies developed to aid specialty populations.   During the
last three decades a trend in cultural definitions of specialty
groups has shifted from those groups experiencing oppression
and discrimination to those groups that are demanding better,
more relevant services.   The elderly continue to represent
one such specialty population for whom social services have
been weak.   Older Americans constitute a minority in constant growth because of improved medical technology and
hence prolongation of life.   Aging, of course, is a "natural"
process during an individual's lifetime that evolves through
the transition of cultural changes.   Some cultural changes
within this century in which elderly have become deeply in-
tertwined have been the introduction and mass dissemination
of prescriptive medications.   Elderly persons who seek the
relief of "physical" and "mental" ailments through the attainment of chemical preparations make up a large proportion of
today's drug abusers.

With this revolutionary introduction of "medical" drugs
and drug therapy there has emerged an obvious pitfall.   Elderly people taking medications for prescriptive or nonprescriptive reasons are subject to fluctuations in their compliance or regimen and eventually this disrupts the medication
schedule.   So, too, are the elderly physically susceptible to
the need for increments in medication dosage as their tolerance and absorption rates change in reaction to continual usage.   Incremental amounts of medication are predictably precipitant to "drug dependency" or "drug addiction," a physiological and psychological response acquired over a period of
drug-taking history.   Just as adolescent drug users can become physically or psychologically dependent on substances,
so, too, might the elderly develop a psychological or physiological dependency or addiction.   Addicted or potentially

ix

addictive elderly make up an ever increasing population in our current society, especially as the accessibility of "over-the-counter" (OTC) medications increases and chemical substances in the highest risk categories become more easily obtainable. Addicted elderly not only represent a shift in the epidemiology of drug use in America today, but also account for a minority of persons from all different strata of society who depend on the culture either to sustain their addictive habits or bring about their rehabilitation.

The prevalence of elderly substance abuse is thus a topic in demand of greater consideration. This annotated bibliography attempts to reach those audiences familiar with elderly populations for whom substance abuse problems are potential realities. In this volume there are publications which range over a long period of time (some as early as 1932) and which reflect the period of greatest documented concentration of this problem (1960's to present). Publications reported here do vary in terms of local and national circulation, but for the most part they consist of periodicals (serials) and books on the subject of elderly and drug abuse or addiction. Projects, grants, and federal and state documents on elderly and substance abuse studies are, in large part, a difficult category to represent since many selections copyrighted by government agencies, although in the public domain, entail many obstacles in acquiring them. Consequently, documents of this type will not have an exhaustive representation in this volume. Moreover, articles appearing in serials of "general human interest" or which identify as their philosophy a certain dimension in society indirectly related to gerontology and substance abuse (e.g., clothing styles, automobiles, etc.) may not be cited in this volume. By contrast, book publications on this topic are not entirely "scholarly" or "research-oriented," since books in this field are fairly scarce and only have been increasing in demand over the past five years.

Because the topic of "elderly and substance abuse" is, by dint of certain implications, a widely diverse subject in which many different types of drugs and issues are raised, a preferable approach to organization was for sections to include major categorical areas rather than specific drug interactions. Except for section 1 on Alcohol, every other part assumes a single or polydrug addiction and highlights representative areas of interest related to the addiction (e.g., pharmacology, pathology, illegality, compliance, epidemiology, etc.). Moreover, references to certain topics are even more accessible by using the Subject Index. Users of this book also have the Journal Index and Author Index in which to locate information.

One last definitional aspect of this volume concerns the descriptor "elderly." Who is the elderly person? Somebody over 60, over 65, over 70 years of age? Or, moreover, is there a more subtle connotation of the term which defines it based on something else besides chronology? For the purposes of this work the term "elderly" is a generic referent to all individuals over the age of 60, but not excluding middle-aged adults over 55 years. Our reason for this inclusion is simple: Chronology is an insufficient line of demarcation. Conventional linguistic practices in society make it easy to speak of 55-year-olds as "not" being an elderly "type" because most rules, regulations, and public talk revolve around this middle-age versus 65-year-old dichotomy. However, the body's physiological changes are not suddenly more "pronounced" at age 60 or 65 any more than they are at age 55, and in several reported cases of "older age substance abuse" the person described is 50 years old. We therefore feel a rational compromise is to speak of old age as including anywhere from 55 years of age and beyond.

Toward this end, readers from all disciplines are encouraged to extract information presented in this bibliography for whatever relevant use it serves in their professions. Mental health service providers, administrators, and even "nonprofessionals" who come in daily contact with elderly family members or friends and need a quick guide for locating articles on the topic of substance abuse will find this volume helpful. Elderly people who either suspect being addicted or fear it may occur to them under certain circumstances may also wish further information. Readership in this area is especially diverse because the topic has become a paragon for recent interest in the elderly in general.

INTRODUCTION

Known etiologies of elderly drug abuse have been in the research literature as far back as recorded history dates ine-
briation and drug addiction.   That this etiologic knowledge
has gradually aroused national interest and research endeav-
ors is a sign that elderly abusers are, themselves, increasing.   State and national demographics showing the statistics
for medication and alcohol abuse over the past decade reveal
staggering upward numbers as the routes of access to medication and alcohol multiply. Skid-row alcoholics no longer
dominate this lot.   Many middle-aged persons of upper socioeconomic status, employed, or even with full educational
backgrounds are vulnerable by the fact that they know very
little about medicine or drug interactions.   Mismedication or
medication noncompliance is a fairly easy channel to addiction, developing from poor physician-patient communication.
The same holds true for alcohol--except here, more than
with other drugs, the knowledge base is more circulated.

Here we review important considerations about the
elderly community that are pronounced in alcohol abuse,
clinical and administrative aspects of drug misuse, the aging process and psychoactive drug misuse, and casefinding.

Alcohol and Old Age

There is no shortage of opinions about alcohol and
old age.   Theories abound that alcohol use is dangerous at
any age, in any amount--and even more dangerous in old
age.   Opposing theories suggest that alcohol has therapeutic
potential for older people, is part of the good and satisfying
life, and therefore is prescriptive.   Relatively few people
have carefully examined the abuse side of alcohol in old age
until recently.

Portions of this discussion are co-authored by Shaghil Husain.

Popular surveys suggest the elderly tend to drink alone or in family groups more than younger people do. Thus, elderly drinkers are less noticeable than are their younger counterparts who drink in public places. Several epidemiologic burdens are responsible for the older alcoholic's relative obscurity. First, elders suffer more health and social problems in general. Those who live on fixed retirement incomes or social security benefits may develop a habit they can ill afford; liquor then becomes a financial burden. Secondly, elderly widows and widowers may drink to overcome their loneliness and bereavement; for them, liquor becomes a psychological burden. Third, a relatively small portion of elderly hold jobs and experience boredom; drinking thus becomes a vocational burden.

Older individuals who are not diagnosed or treated as problem drinkers are also known to (a) avoid contact with agencies who could provide care, (b) terminate contact with a care-providing system before the drinking problem is detected, or (c) manage to receive treatment for "other" symptoms while the alcohol-related problems remain undiagnosed and untreated.

There have been a number of hospital studies that give some indication of elderly alcoholics who receive treatment. Statistical data tabulated by the U.S. National Institute of Mental Health (NIMH) (1971a, 1971b) supply reports on the diagnoses of patients admitted for treatment in various facilities. Data collected in 1969, for instance, indicate that 6 percent of people over age 65 admitted to state and county mental hospitals suffer from alcoholism. This same age group constitutes 2 to 4 percent of all outpatient psychiatric services. Among this percentage, 12 percent are diagnosed as having alcohol-related problems.

Alcoholism in the elderly is not an isolated phenomenon. Case surveys show there is a behavioral pattern or some attitudinal problem associated with drinking. Essentially, the many reasons for chronic drinking are similar to those given for younger alcoholics. Most frequent ones include the deterioration of physical, mental, or social conditions, followed by self-neglect, falls, excessive incontinence, aggravation of confusion, paranoia, and family quarrels or estrangement. Marital separation and, in particular, alienation from the family and children are both highly volatile forms of distress accountable for high rates of alcohol recidivism.

Clinical and Administrative Aspects of Drug Misuse

In the forefront of medication abuse problems is the elderly's expenditures per annum on preparations for personal health and hygiene. According to Reference on Statistics on the Aging Population, drugs and medical sundries occupy much of the elderly's budgetary income and, in some cases, represent as high as 5.1 billion dollars (per total population) and $192 (per capita) during a single year (1980). Physician services ($589 per capita) rank as the highest expenditure overall, with 15.6 billion dollars spent in 1980. With so much money being spent on medication and medical services, it would seem these commodities are understood by their consumers. However, studies on communication between physician and patient clearly show this is not the case. Rather, elderly consumers who spend way beyond their affordable budgets for medication refills are very uncertain about potential hazards and contraindications of drugs to their health. Consequently, the growing incidence of drug abuse has become a rampant epidemic.

Prescriptive medicaments are potentially abusable in several different ways. One way is to administer them not for therapy, but rather to subdue patients so they create a minimum of disturbance for the staff. Drugs have thus become a tool for administrative efficiency. Drug abuse and misuse in hospitalized settings are an offense against patient rights and can be summarized by some of the findings of the Subcommittee on Long-term Care (cf. Williams, Carruth and Hyman, 1973):

1. The average nursing home patient receives seven different drugs a day, with many being taken up to four times daily. Although physicians are required by law to review the skilled nursing facility patients' medications every 30 days, physicians frequently re-order medications month after month without ever seeing or examining the patient.

2. Approximately 40% of the drugs prescribed are for analgesics, sedatives, and tranquilizers. Of this number, half are for tranquilizers. Given normal clinical need for tranquilizers, this suggests a vast overuse of this class of drugs. The use of tranquilizers as "chemical straightjackets" can render an alert and ambulatory resident helpless, undemanding, and confined to his or her bed or wheelchair.

3. Drug distribution systems are ineffective and inefficient. The lack of an adequate professional nursing staff often results in aides or orderlies administering medications. This brings about several possible medication errors. Medication errors are defined as (a) the wrong drug, (b) the wrong dose, (c) the wrong patient, (d) the wrong route, (e) missed dose, or (f) wrong time. Such errors average 30 percent of all drug administrations in nursing homes. Definitions of medication error apply only to those who administer the medications; it does not include the physician who may prescribe the wrong drug or pharmacist who can dispense in error.

4. Inadequate drug control encourages theft for personal use or sale. Medication orders are sometimes not terminated when the patient dies or is discharged or transferred. When such drugs are permitted to accumulate, they often become the property of employees. Furthermore, medications are often charged as being administered when, in fact, they are diverted by unscrupulous employees.

5. Most nursing homes do not employ the services of an in-house pharmacist. Some homes get their medications from several pharmacists; others use a single community pharmacist. Competition among pharmacists to provide medicine and service to a nursing home gives the home the opportunity to shop around for the greatest benefits to the patient, or, in some cases, the greatest kickback for itself. Latest estimates show that 35 percent of the cost of each prescription is paid back to the nursing home operator. Further indicated is that 65 percent of all pharmacists working for nursing homes use this method of extortion.

Physicians, too, play a significant role in the drug problems of older people. Many are unaware of the sensitivity of older people to powerful drugs. Toward addictive drugs, they frequently adopt the attitude that it is acceptable for an older person to become addicted if it will relieve some discomfort. While their intentions may be honest, iatrogenic addiction and reactions to chemical side-effects are just as probable for older persons as for addicts on the street. At best, the legitimacy for prescribing addictive drugs when the older patient is in terminal stages of illness should be approached with skepticism. This is because prescribing drugs for the elderly is both complicated and hazardous. Age-associated decrements in physiologic function as with the effects of illness or trauma erase the reliability of the "average" dose for the "average" patient. These decrements also require that physicians weigh benefits and risks using a different set of parameters than are considered for younger patients. Above all, physicians must approach the treatment of geriatric patients with a sense of caution, accomplished by an awareness of available treatment regimens.

The Aging Process and Psychoactive Drug Misuse

Deplorably, the elderly consume over 25 percent of all prescription drugs. An increasing proportion of these prescriptions are psychoactive drugs, defined as major or minor tranquilizers, antidepressants, stimulants, sedatives, and hypnotics. However, there is growing, though limited, evidence of intentional and nonintentional misuse of psychoactive drugs by the aged that often results in physical and social harm. Frequently, faulty diagnosis or application by the physician is the causal factor, whereas in other cases the individual's misuse of drugs is owing to a "mistake."

Elderly patients frequently suffer from general morbid conditions or diseases at a time in life when reserve functional capacity, energy metabolism, and enzymatic processes are all greatly reduced. Impaired capacities to absorb, distribute, metabolize, and excrete drugs will often result in an increase of adverse drug effects. Persons aged 70 to 79 experience adverse drug reactions at a rate seven times greater than those 20 to 29 years old, and the rate for those 60 to 70 years is twice that for persons age 30 to 40 years. Age-related reduction in gastric juice acidity (a slowed stomach emptying rate) and reduction in intestinal blood flow can lead to delays or reduction in drug absorption. Moreover, drug distribution is affected by circulatory disturbances while the decreasing activity of several enzymes can hamper drug metabolism. Decreases in kidney size, glomeruli, tubule cells, glomerular filtration rate, and renal flow all rapidly accompany the aging process. Renal pathology and especially diminished renal functions are the norm in elderly persons, while water imbalance and general metabolism imbalances are frequently disruptive. Reduced peristaltic activity, leading to constipation and diarrhea can also alter the elimination of drugs, especially those which exhibit enterhepatic circulation. In short, the pharmacokinetic reactions include the following:

MAJOR IRREVERSIBLE DEMENTIAS

Alzheimer's Disease	The most frequently observed type of dementia. Clinical appearance is one of consistent mental deterioration beginning with marked mental deficits as well as tendencies toward agitation. It proceeds to more severe symptoms such as rigidity, inability to stand, walk, talk, and incontinence.
Pick's Disease	Pick's disease is clinically very similar to Alzheimer's disease. Usually an earlier onset. Genetic factors may be relevant. Prognosis is always fatal.
Binswanger's Disease	Slowly progressing dementia. Apparently resulting from arteriosclerosis of the arteries supplying the grey matter. Occurs only between the ages of 50 and 65.
Creutzfeldt-Jakob Disease	A rare progressive and rapidly fatal type of dementia. Etiology has been attributed to a virus which is transmissable.
Huntington's Disease	A hereditary disease that usually begins in middle age, but can occur in children and octogenarians. Steady progress to death some 10 to 20 years after inception. Each child of an affected family has a 50% chance of developing it, but there is no diagnostic test prior to inception.
Korsakoff's Disease	Associated with dementia secondary to nutritional deficiency most frequently observed in alcoholics. Usually develops after 20 to 30 years of alcohol abuse.

1. Absorption of some substances is reduced or delayed.

2. Changes in drug activity are the result of impaired circulation and membrane permeability.

3. The rate at which drugs are metabolized and eliminated is decreased.

4. Changes in the number of receptors and concentration of substrate occur, thus reducing the action of stimulants and enhancing the action of depressants.

Because the aging process increases physical illness, older people are exposed to and consume more drugs than they legitimately need to. There is no better indication of overconsumption than with psychiatric disorders. The incidence of geropsychiatric illness dramatically increases with age and is largely treatable through psychotropic medication. For example, there is a decade-by-decade rise in depression including the peaking of suicide among men in their eighties. Twenty-five percent of all suicides occur in persons over 65 years of age. While the abuse of drugs does not automatically correlate with psychiatric illness, a strong tendency exists at all age-levels for the chronically depressed to turn to drugs as a way to numb emotional suffering and escape the painful environment with which they cannot deal.

Prescription drugs are implements in one of three suicides in the United States. The elderly are prone to suicides because of failing health and diminished life satisfaction. The older white male, in particular, is called upon to adjust to income and status loss at the time when he is least able to adapt. The suicide rate for this group exceeds that for all other combinations of age, sex, and race. Compounded by this late onset of depression are the manifestations of "irreversible dementias." Diagnosed symptoms of dementia tend to overlap between the six most common categories shown in the chart on page xviii.

To combat this depression, prescriptions for hypnotics and psychotherapeutic drugs are used. Barbiturate hypnotics accounted for over 20 million prescriptions filled in America during 1973; half of these were ordered for hypnotic purposes. However, barbiturate drugs may also intensify any existing tendencies toward depression or suicide and are particularly dangerous when mixed with alcohol. Prescribing physicians

thus sit uncomfortably on the horns of a dilemma. In one
sense, provisions of psychotropic drugs enable an easy means
of suicide. But to do without these drugs, however, leaves
the patient alone in his or her struggle with depression (and
withdrawal). For these reasons, medical diagnosis should
conform to the practice of prescribing drugs based on each
elderly person's own mental and physical status.

Apart from physician errors, problems with prescriptions are also due to patient compliance or regimen errors.
One frequent kind of error is omission or "forgetting" to take
medication. Omission errors also arise through communication errors. This is when patients misunderstand or never
understand the physician's instructions. Finally, immediate
patterns in one's life situation may also cause medication
omission. Patients who are too sick to remember to take
medicine or lack both the money and transportation for obtaining prescriptions are prone to noncompliant schedules.

The next most frequent problem associated with medication error is not knowing "why" a certain drug has been
prescribed. Although this is not immediately dangerous,
more remote repercussions are that biological systems could
be thrown out of alignment. Take, for example, the patient
who is simply told to increase his heart medicine to twice a
day. If he forgets or never learns about the purposes for
correct medication, a potential hazard may arise in the near
future.

Lastly, most elderly reactions to drug consumption
also depend upon idiosyncrasies relative to "environment-
behavioral" influences. These are quite different from
biological or iatrogenic dependency, in which aging persons
on a specific dosage must receive medicine to avoid a withdrawal syndrome. Rather, when sensory deterioration accompanies economic, psychologic or social pressures as part of
the aging process, these factors combined can determine how
elderly perceive their physical changes. Frequently these
perceptions are distorted. Underlying most perceptions is
the identification of physical decay as a "sign" or "cue" for
seeking medical attention. This is a problem best described
as pharmopathy. Pharmopathy simply means there may or
may not be organic pathology caused by circulatory, respiratory, digestive, excretory, or some other internal system,
but the elderly person will still seek medication simply because it is the customary or culturally-indoctrinated action
to take.

Casefinding

More problematic than many think is trying to find out who needs a service in the community. Consumer advocacy programs set up outreach and casefinding strategies to reduce this burden, although the struggle is not entirely resolved. Alcoholism and drug abuse are very different diagnostic symptoms than a cold or virus and are less accessible to detection (covered up) by the public. Primarily the fault of social indoctrination, the degree of social acceptance of substance abuse in aging persons is still at its infantile stages. This makes early intervention nearly impossible. Patients who do receive primary prevention, such as from hospitals or intake outpatient units (clinics, etc.) greatly benefit from the early start. Only a handful of elderly knowledgeable of benefits and services really understand their potential for addiction and the reason why early intervention can reduce this potential.

Worst yet, casefinding is further retarded by uncooperative physicians or medical workers afraid to refer alcoholics or drug users, fearing that it may be a reflection of iatrogenic addiction and hence grounds for malpractice. Ethical restraints add to the already strong social logistics in trying to find elderly users. Social service agencies prepared to educate elderly users or potential users recognize this drug abuse epidemic. They realize there is no sense in formalizing or financing "treatment" programs (secondary and tertiary prevention) when the preponderance of drug misinformation or absence of information more properly requires "educational" programs.

Educational materials and a structure in general outlining the basic needs for a course on drugs and the elderly must take into account many considerations. Two considerations are especially noteworthy. First, what types of information are most effective for prevention? And second, are there personnel available who can collect or teach this information? Actual lecture presentations or a combination of lecture with practicum are two popular methods frequently adopted into program curricula. Lectures stress the vulnerability of elderly in social or physical situations and then also review certain contraindications of drugs or drugs combined with physical habits (overeating, drinking, smoking, etc.). The applied practica provide opportunities for the elderly participants to learn and employ self-control strategies to better cope with a medication regimen.

By contrast, less is known about how local or volunteer staff are recruited for these sometimes voluminous programs. Time commitments affect the work load and severely eat into competing schedules and responsibilities. Staff who do get assigned to instruction, then, are at a great disadvantage. But their disadvantage goes beyond simple schedule conflicts. They also may or may not know enough about dynamics of drugs or geropharmacology to lecture on the topic. When agencies have to look beyond their house staff into the community for hiring instructors, contract costs become prohibitive and this consequently buries the goals of drug prevention deeper into the morass of integrated social networks.

REFERENCES

Reference on Statistics on the Aging Population. Washington, DC: U. S. Department of Commerce, Bureau of the Census, 1982.

U. S. NIMH, Statistical note No. 48-49. Washington, DC: U. S. Government Printing Office, 1971a, 1971b.

Williams, E. P.; Carruth, B.; and Hyman, M. M. Alcohol and Problem Drinking Among Older Persons. Springfield, VA: National Technical Information Service, 1973.

THE BIBLIOGRAPHY

1. ALCOHOL USE AND ABUSE

1. Adams, James T. Cecostomy effectively relieves adynamic
   ileus of the colon. Archives of Surgery, 1974, 109, 503-507.
   Twenty patients aged 41 to 95 are treated for adynamic ileus
of the colon. Reasons for hospitalization range from extra-abdominal
trauma, respiratory or urinary infection, and cardiac disease to alcoholism. Medical management alone is used on six patients while
for patients with increased abdominal distension, a cecostomy is
performed. Post-operative recovery rates in relation to types of
morbidity are discussed.
   Descriptors: Alcoholism, surgery, alcohol-related pathology.

2. Alcoholism and the Elderly. (Report no. NCAI-027757).
   Rockville, MD: National Institute on Alcohol Abuse and Alcoholism, 1976.
   Analyses are presented on the prevalence and severity of alcoholic elderly in the state of Iowa. Data on available services and
treatment programs indicate a growing concentration of clients aged
55 and over. Survey results also suggest a need for continual program expansion.
   Descriptors: Drinking patterns, alcoholism.

3. Alcoholism and the elderly. Advances in Alcoholism, 1980, 1,
   1-3.
   Alcohol-related pathologies in the elderly are reported with
respect to natural history and treatment. Factors affecting prevalence are assessed for interpretation of treatment goals.
   Descriptors: Alcoholism, treatment goals.

4. Alterman, A.I.; Gottheil, E.; and Crawford, H.D. Mood
   changes in an alcoholism treatment program based on drinking decisions. American Journal of Psychiatry, 1975, 132,
   1032-1037.
   Comparisons appear on the amount of discomfort experienced
by drinking and nondrinking alcoholics during a treatment and research program. An increase in discomfort for drinkers is attributed more to decisions about drinking (i.e., mood alterations) than
to actual amounts of alcohol consumption. Differences in mood
states for both drinkers and abstainers are hypothesized to vary as
the environment changes.
   Descriptors: Alcoholism, drinking patterns, emotional states.

1

5. American Attitudes Toward Alcohol and Alcoholics: A Survey
   of Public Opinion Prepared for the National Institute on Alcohol
   Abuse and Alcoholism. (Report no. NCAI-002525). Rockville,
   MD: National Institute on Alcohol Abuse and Alcoholism, 1971.
   Attitudinal survey is done on 2,131 Americans regarding their
position on alcohol and alcoholic persons. Key concerns addressed
by the field interviews include the extent of the drinking problems,
awareness of alcohol education, and perceptions of drinking habits.
Among the results reported, confusion and misconceptions of the
middle-aged and elderly alcoholic are equally as pervasive as the
failure to understand the extent to which social and economic problems enter into early stages of addiction.
   Descriptors: Alcoholism, attitudes, racial and ethnic groups.

6. Aminoff, M.J., and Simon, R.P. Status epilepticus. Causes,
   clinical features and consequences in 98 patients. American
   Journal of Medicine, 1980, 69, 657-666.
   The etiology, clinical features, and outcome of generalized
major motor status epilepticus in patients over the age of 14 are
reviewed. Identified causes are largely from noncompliance to anti-
convulsant drug regimens and alcohol withdrawal. Motoric manifestations (convulsions, etc.) do not necessarily indicate there is lo-
calized structural pathology, but rather that the symptoms are multi-
factorial and should be screened carefully even when the cause is
readily apparent.
   Descriptors: Alcoholism, epilepsy, head injury.

7. Anderson, G.M. Alcoholism and the aging. America, 1980,
   143, 139-142.
   Fear, isolation, and diminished physical strength are identified as underlying precursors to alcohol abuse. The article discusses the diminishing social contacts elderly have with family and
friends in relation to previous studies that examine factors of susceptibility in older men and women who use barbiturates and stimulants. Also shown is the correlation between aging and tendency
toward alcoholism, and preventive and therapeutic programs available in most elderly communities.
   Descriptors: Alcoholism, psychological factors.

8. Angel, R.W. Analysis of Normal and Abnormal Motor Behavior
   in Man. (Report no. ZO-30706 7). Washington, DC: U.S.
   Veterans Administration, Department of Medicine and Surgery, 1977.
   Neural tracking test is administered to subjects with Korsakoff syndrome, as well as to subjects with different neurological
diseases. While normal subjects are able to reverse false moves
without feedback from a display, removal of the display for elderly
Korsakoff patients is not much different. Induced to make false
movements, subjects still achieve a frequency of error-correcting
responses above the chance level.
   Descriptors: Neurological diseases, alcholism.

9. Apfeldorf, M.; Franks, G.; and Porges, S.W. Respiratory

Feedback and Modification of Attention. (Report no. ZO-33369 2). Washington, DC: U.S. Veterans Administration, 1975.

Using an A-B-A design, respiratory feedback techniques are applied in a small population of chronic alcoholics to improve attentional deficits. Training consists of teaching clients to breathe with respiratory patterns exhibited by normal attentional performance. Relationships between respiratory activity, heart rate variability, and reaction time performance are explored for different age groups.

Descriptors: Attention, alcoholism, respiration.

10. Apfeldorf, M., and Hunley, P.J. Application of MMPI alcoholism scales to older alcoholics and problem drinkers. Quarterly Journal of Studies on Alcohol, 1975, 36, 645-653.

This study determines whether four alcoholism scales from the MMPI are sufficiently sensitive to differentiate between older persons with disciplinary problems and older domiciled alcoholics from domiciled nonalcoholics with no disciplinary problems. Diagnostic superiority of one scale over another is not evident, but scales could identify older problem drinkers along those dimensions commonly interpreted for diagnosed alcholics.

Descriptors: Differential diagnosis, alcoholism, MMPI.

11. Apfeldorf, M.; Hunley, P.J.; and Cooper, G.D. Disciplinary problems in a home for older veterans: Some psychological aspects in relation to drinking behavior. Gerontologist, 1972, 12, 143-147.

Study compares domiciliary residents with histories of disciplinary offenses to residents without such histories in relation to alcohol diagnosis, hostility and control scales of the MMPI, and scales from the Adjective Check List. Disciplinary offenses are shown to be possible for diagnosed older alcoholics and nonalcoholics with hostile attitudes about drinking problems.

Descriptors: Alcoholism, military veterans, MMPI.

12. Asander, H. A field investigation of homeless men in Stockholm. Acta Psychiatrica Scandinavica, 1980, 281, 1-125.

Exploratory analysis of etiologic and treatment factors involved in homeless elderly men in Sweden. Comparisons are made along dimensions of life change events, marital status, morbidity, resident characteristics, socioeconomic factors, employment, and severity of alcoholism.

Descriptors: Alcoholism, socioeconomic factors, Sweden.

13. Atkinson, J.H. Alcoholism and geriatric problems. Part I. Advances in Alcoholism, 1981, 2 (2 pages)

Risk factors associated with vulnerability in older substance abusers, especially alcoholics, are examined closely. Identified factors include the normal aging process, diseases, bereavement, social devaluation, poverty, and a multiplicity of unresolved physical and psychological problems. These factors are put in perspective

in terms of comparative differences to younger populations.
Descriptors: Alcoholism, stress, retirement, environmental stress.

14. Atkinson, J. H. Alcoholism and geriatric problems. Part II. Advances in Alcoholism, 1981 (3 pages).
Characterization of elderly alcoholic is placed into two categories. First, early onset alcoholics who experience problems before age 40 and survive beyond age 65 usually become abstinent by their late 50's. Second, late onset alcoholics continue drinking past age 65. Geriatric problems interpreted for both alcoholic types are discussed in regards to prevalence and treatment.
Descriptors: Alcoholism, patient management, alcoholic typology.

15. Bahr, H. M. Lifetime affiliation patterns of early- and late-onset heavy drinkers on skid row. Quarterly Journal of Studies on Alcohol, 1969, 30, 645-656.
Difference reported between life-history interviews given to men living in the New York City Bowery and also in a rehabilitation center for aged and infirm alcoholics. Late-onset heavy drinkers (after age 30) show more affiliations to familial, employment, and voluntary activities, ranking higher on occupational levels.
Descriptors: Alcoholism, interpersonal skills, skid row.

16. Barnes, G. M. Alcohol use among older persons: Findings from a western New York State general population survey. Journal of the American Geriatrics Society, 1979, 27, 244-250.
Epidemiologic factors for the drinking patterns of older persons are discussed based on a sample of adults living in two New York counties. Also presented are implications for prevention and treatment strategies.
Descriptors: Alcoholism, New York.

17. Barnes, G. M.; Abel, E. L.; and Ernst, C. A. Alcohol and the Elderly: A Comprehensive Bibliography. Westport, CT: Greenwood Press, 1980.
An alphabetical listing of 1,228 items dealing with alcoholism, the elderly, and related topics concerned with both experimental (infrahuman) and clinical applications in various settings. Bibliography does not include abstracts but has a subject index with cross-references.
Descriptors: Alcoholism, bibliography.

18. Bartholomew, A. A. Alcoholism and crime. Australian and New Zealand Journal of Criminology, 1968, 1, 70-99.
Prisoners sentenced for being "drunk and disorderly" are found to be middle-aged to elderly. In over 50 percent of the cases, elderly alcoholic criminals are chronically disabled and have few, if any, social contacts.
Descriptors: Alcoholism, crime.

19. Beck, E. C.; Dustman, R. E.; Ajax, E. T.; and Grundvig, J. L.
    Clinical and Evaluative Applications of the Sensory-Percep-
    tual Examination. (Report no. ZO-31521 5). Washington,
    DC: U. S. Veterans Administration, 1976.
    Use of the Sensory-Perceptual Examination is to compare
the effects of aging versus chronic alcoholism on test performance
for determining if heavy alcohol ingestion results in premature aging.
Three basic purposes of the study are (1) to investigate symptomatic
patterns of test performance related to certain pathologies; (2) to
provide indices of sensory, perceptual and motor function in the elderly; and (3) to evaluate effects of sustained alcohol ingestion on the
central nervous system.
    Descriptors: Alcoholism, Sensory-Perceptual Examination,
    perceptual-motor function.

20. Beck, E. C.; Snyder, E. W.; Dustman, R. E.; Schenkenberg, T.;
    and Ajax, E. T. Clinical and Evaluative Applications of the
    Sensory-Perceptual Examination (SPE). (Report no. ZO-31521
    6). Washington, DC: U. S. Veterans Administration, Depart-
    ment of Medicine and Surgery, 1976.
    Continual investigation and standardization of SPE norms on
elderly chronic alcoholics. Emphasis, here, is upon examining test
results of several hundred "brain-damaged" patients.
    Descriptors: Alcoholism, Sensory-Perceptual Examination,
    perceptual-motor function.

21. Beck, E. C.; Snyder, E. W.; Dustman, R. E.; Schenkenberg, T.;
    and Ajax, E. T. Clinical and Evaluative Applications of the
    Sensory-Perceptual Examination (SPE). (Report no. ZO-31521
    7). Washington, DC: U. S. Veterans Administration, Depart-
    ment of Medicine and Surgery, 1977.
    Standardized tests on perceptual-motor performance are more
thoroughly examined regarding norms for older patients and consis-
tency of effects across alcohol ingestion and other commonly abused
drugs.
    Descriptors: Alcoholism, Sensory-Perceptual Examination,
    perceptual-motor function.

22. Becker, P. W., and Cesar, J. A. Use of beer in geriatric
    psychiatric patient groups. Psychological Reports, 1973, 33,
    182.
    Experimental study showing the increased sociable partici-
pation of geriatric patients when given beer during daily group sessions. Hospital staff ratings of patients on orientation, self-care,
mood, ward adjustment, and social activity indicate less medical
sedation is necessary. Suggestions are offered on combining psychotropic medication with beer in subsequent therapeutic interventions.
    Descriptors: Beer, psychotropic medication

23. Becker, P. W., and Conn, S. H. Beer and social therapy treat-
    ment with geriatric psychiatric patient groups. Addictive
    Diseases, 1978, 3, 429-436.
    Elderly psychiatric patients offered either beer or social
therapy are rated for general ward behavior and sociability on dif-

ferent measurement instruments. Increases in social activity ratings during the beer group, over sociability ratings for both fruit juice and social therapy groups, closely resembled the improvements also achieved by psychotropic drugs.

Descriptors: Beer, social therapy, psychotropic medication.

24. Beregi, E.; Lengyel, E.; and Bird, J. Autoantibodies in aged individuals. Aktuelle Gerontologie, 1978, 8, 77-80.

A study of autoantibody concentration in 282 volunteers (159 of them from 64 to 74 years of age) shows it to be most significant in elderly individuals who drink alcohol and smoke.

Descriptors: Alcoholism, autoantibodies.

25. Biener, K. Health problems as well as stimulant and drug consumption of prisoners. Studies on 258 prisoners in eastern Switzerland. Sozial- und Präventivmedizin, 1980, 25, 186.

Investigation of middle-aged and elderly alcoholic prisoners in Switzerland whose addiction is interactive with high recurrences of health problems.

Descriptors: Alcoholism, prisoners, Switzerland.

26. Bissell, L.; Fewell, C. H.; and Jones, R. W. The alcoholic social worker: A survey. Social Work and Health Care, 1980, 5, 421-432.

Survey data presented on alcoholic social workers whose eventual recoveries follow visibly frequent arrests, inpatient admissions, suicide attempts, and a high reported incidence of polydrug addiction. Despite these actions, social workers from whom they sought treatment are reluctant to identify and treat alcoholism. Authors urge a more systematic method of detection for colleague patients than is currently available.

Descriptors: Alcoholism, professional competence, social worker.

27. Black, A. L. Altering behavior of geriatric patients with beer. Northwest Medicine, 1969, 68, 453-456.

A controlled study of geriatric patients showing differences in social behavior following availability of beer. Cooperation and congeniality increase as the need for psychotropic medication is significantly reduced over baseline levels.

Descriptors: Beer, social behavior, medication.

28. Blusewicz, M. J.; Dustman, R. E.; and Schenkenberg, T. Neuropsychological correlates of chronic alcoholism and aging. Journal of Nervous and Mental Diseases, 1977, 165, 348-355.

Examined closely, neuropsychological correlates to both chronic alcoholism and premature aging in elderly populations are measured on the Tactual Performance Test and Category Test. Authors acknowledge the potential for confounding age and generational effects and suggest that differences may reflect cultural conditions.

Descriptors: Alcoholism, Tactual Performance Test, Catgory Test, neuropsychology.

29. Blusewicz, M. J.; Schenkenberg, T.; and Dustman, R. E. WAIS
    performance in young normal, young alcoholic, and elderly
    normal groups: An evaluation of organicity and mental ag-
    ing indices. Journal of Clinical Psychology, 1977, 33,
    1149-1153.
    Results of a comparison study lend relative support to the
validity for "organicity" and "mental aging" indices of the Wechsler
Adult Intelligence Scale. Scores of the young normal group are
superior on both verbal and performance subtests to alcoholic and
elderly groups, with the two latter groups sharing similar score
patterns. Moreover, similarities between alcoholic and elderly group
scores are consistent with the hypothesis of "premature aging" in
alcoholics.
    Descriptors: Alcoholism, WAIS.

30. Bort, I. L. The relationship of alcohol to aging and the elder-
    ly. Alcoholism: Clinical and Experimental Research, 1978,
    2, 17-21.
    Discussion on alcohol's relation to both diminution of function
in tissues and organ systems and also individual personality. Concepts explored are the cellular aging process during incipient stages
of alcoholism and how these changes conflict with traditional myths
about drinking.
    Descriptors: Alcoholism, personality.

31. Bort, R. Ambulatory management in alcoholism. American
    Family Physician, 1977, 16, 131-234.
    A model is presented for ambulatory treatment of alcoholics
based on the University of Michigan's alcoholism and drug abuse
clinic. This twofold process involves (a) responsibility of physician
to advise patient of symptoms that might require hospitalization, and
(b) follow-up appointments scheduled intermittently to monitor clinical
and medication adjustment. Ultimately the goal is to limit drinking
rather than abstain, a goal recognized as incompatible with many
medical treatments for elderly.
    Descriptors: Alcoholism, treatment model.

32. Brezinova, V.; Hort, V.; Vojtechovsky, M. Sleep deprivation
    with respect to age: An EEG study. Activitas Nervosa
    Superior, 1969, 11, 182-187.
    Study of short-term sleep deprivation tolerance and pro-
longed sleep deprivation in abstaining middle-aged alcoholics. EEG
sleep patterns recorded during different stages of sleep and without
sleep were indicative of better tolerance by younger, nonalcoholic
men.
    Descriptors: Alcoholism, EEG, sleep deprivation.

33. Brickner, P. W., and Kaufman, A. Case finding of heart dis-
    ease in homeless men. Bulletin of the New York Academy
    of Medicine, 1973, 49-475-484.
    A program for medical care for homeless men is conducted
in a hotel of substandard quality with 1,200 residents, 35 percent
of whom are chronic and elderly alcoholics. Symptoms of cardiomyopathy in only two of the 160 persons diagnosed challenge the

belief that cardiac disease is frequent in alcoholic men.
Descriptors: Alcoholism, cardiomyopathy.

34. Brody, J. A. Aging and alcohol abuse. Journal of the Amer-
     ican Geriatrics Society, 1982, 30, 123-126.
     Demographics of alcohol abuse among elderly are presented
among four factors: (a) retirement, (b) deaths among relatives and
friends, (c) poor health and discomfort, and (d) loneliness. Surveys
conducted in older age groups, especially elderly women, suggest a
proportional increase in alcoholism in relation to population growth.
Also, 10 to 15 percent of elderly seeking medical attention are alcoholic, fairly easy to treat, and rank among a group of unhealthy
elderly for whom more effective prevention strategies can be developed.
     Descriptors: Alcoholism, drinking patterns, prevention.

35. Burrill, R. H.; McCourt, J. F.; and Cutter, H. S. Beer: A
     social facilitator for PMI patients? The Gerontologist, 1974,
     14, 430-431.
     This experimental study is designed to test comparisons of
drinking beer and soft drinks on the social responsivity and drinking
behavior of psychiatric infirm patients. Explored are the ramifications of alternatives to medication.
     Descriptors: Beer, social behavior.

36. Cameron, D. D. The elderly alcoholic. In Second Symposium
     on the Clinical Problems of Advancing Years. Philadelphia,
     PA: Smith, Kline, and French Laboratories, 1951.
     Identified reasons for increasing alcohol addiction in the
elderly include (a) progressive disorganization of life due to decom-
pensating neurotic adjustment, (b) progressive reduction in effectiveness, (c) retirement, (d) disruption of cosmetic appearance, and (e)
disruption of lifelong relations or dependent situations, such as a
spouse dying.
     Descriptors: Alcoholism, personality.

37. Cannon, W. G. Cortical evoked responses of young normal,
     young alcoholic and elderly normal individuals. Dissertation
     Abstracts International, 1974, 35, 6-B.
     Critically shown that visual evoked potentials as measured
by EEG rates are comparatively different for younger alcoholics over
normal elderly. As with somatosensory evoked responses, changes
in rate vary by health problems rather than by age alone.
     Descriptors: Alcoholism, EEG, evoked potentials.

38. Carruth, B. Alcoholism and Problem Drinking Among Older
     Persons: Life-styles, Drinking Practices and Drinking
     Problems of Older Alcoholics. Paper presented at the
     National Council on Alcoholism Annual Meetings, Denver,
     April 1974.
     Male elderly alcoholics complete a precoded questionnaire
on different symptoms. Unsupported evidence for the belief that
subjects are social isolates lacking environmental interaction is

challenged. However, significantly more subjects did show psychological problems than common literature reports. One conclusion, then, is that more physical problems foster maladaptive social tendencies.
Descriptors: Alcoholism, personality.

39. Carruth, B.; Williams, E. P.; and Nysak, P. Alcoholism and Problem Drinking Among Older Persons. (Report no. NCAI-018869). Rockville, MD: National Institute on Alcohol Abuse and Alcoholism, 1973.
Findings of a final report on alcoholism among elderly people in the United States are presented. Confirming that a substantial problem exists, authors recommend the establishment of community task forces to develop care-providing systems and early detection programs.
Descriptors: Alcoholism, drinking patterns, community programs.

40. Carruth, B.; Williams, E. P.; Nysak, P.; and Boudreaux, L. Alcoholism and problem drinking among older persons. Community Care Providers and the Older Problem Drinker. A Policy and Planning Statement. Presented at the Twenty-fourth Annual Meeting of the Alcohol and Drug Problems Association of North America, Minneapolis, September 1973.
Analyses made from agency data, attitudinal scales, and prior research all point to the barriers in obtaining special treatment for elderly alcoholics. Attitudes toward problem elderly drinkers are more relevant than attitudes toward older persons in general.
Descriptors: Alcoholism, attitudes.

41. Cermak, L. S., and Ryback, R. S. Recovery of verbal short-term memory in alcoholics. Quarterly Journal of Studies on Alcohol, 1976, 37, 46-52.
Study showing that patients over 50 years of age perform better on short-term memory distractor test than both younger patients and alcoholic Korsakoff patients. Questioned by these results is the hypothesis that alcoholic persons suffer a temporary impairment of ability to memorize new material, especially those of older ages. Comparative results after a one-month testing period show that older patients improving over initial tests clearly exceed scores by other subjects, but to what extent this effect is produced by length of counseling is uncertain.
Descriptors: Memory, dependence and withdrawal syndromes, neurology.

42. Chalmers, D. M.; Chanarin, I.; and Levi, A. J. Alcohol and the blood. British Medical Journal, 1978, 2, 203.
Comments cover a recently published paper on blood disorders that reported characteristic differences in the "Skid Row" subjects seen in the United Kingdom. Authors explain that British physicians rarely contact alcoholics with sideroblastic anemia, thrombocytopenia, or Zieve's syndrome, at the same frequency as mormoblastic bone marrow, normal hemoglobin, cyanocoblamin

and folate levels, and a raised mean cell volume that fluctuates after abstinence.

Descriptors: Alcohol-related pathologies, organic.

43. Ciale, J.; Csank, C. Z.; Lella, J.; Irving, R. W.; and Bayne, J. R. Classification of Chronic Alcoholics in a Veterans Treatment Center According to Response to Treatment and Outcome. Research conducted at Ste-Anne's Veterans Hospital, Ste-Anne-De-Bellevue, Quebec, 1967.

Observational study on categories that are applicable to describe types of patient responsiveness under different treatments. Classifications schemes attempt to provide, prognostically, outcome projections for treated patients after hospitalization.

Descriptors: Alcoholic typology, treatment outcome.

44. Ciompi, L., and Eisert, M. Long-term catamnestic studies on the aging of alcoholics. Social Psychiatry, 1971, 6, 129-151.

Review study investigates the evolutional trends of alcoholism in the aged. In addition, results of interviews with 197 former alcoholics over 65 indicate that improvement in later ages is frequent, as alcohol consumption is reportedly decreased by nearly two-thirds of the subjects along with diagnosed psychiatric disorders such as depression, mania, and aggressiveness either on physical or behavioral levels. Statistically noted are correlations to age, physical health, and social and employment status, but not historical data, onset of alcoholism, or age at the time of first diagnosis. Social status, in particular, appears more stabilized and dependent than during alcoholic period.

Descriptors: Aggressive behavior, depression, interpersonal interaction, consumption.

45. Clark, W. B. Loss of control, heavy drinking and drinking problems in a longitudinal study. Quarterly Journal of Studies on Alcohol, 1976, 37, 1256-1290.

Reported here are longitudinal data from a four-year study of 582 white male alcoholics that question the concept of alcoholism as a typically progressive disease process with regular, predictable stages. Self-reports (during intake) regarding "loss of control" apparently had equally as much predictive power of future problems as such concurrent variables as interpersonal and organic deterioration. Explored to this extent are data on associations among drinking-related problems, remission and continuity over time, and predictions of past and multiple pathologies as uniquely related to intrinsic and external consequences of drinking. Recommendations are then given for examining closer the "loss of control" phenomenon.

Descriptors: Self-control, longitudinal studies, loss of control.

46. Cohen, S. Geriatric drug abuse. In S. Cohen (ed.), The Substance Abuse Problems. New York: Haworth Press, 1981.

Chapter focuses on drug abuse problems involving older people as indicated by studies conducted in San Francisco and New York. Geriatric alcoholics typically display lifelong histories of excessive and destructive drinking that begins later in life in response to situational episodes of depression or chronic illness. Prognostically, elderly alcoholism is ameliorative by creating opportunities for close interpersonal contact and also, the author suggests, through antidepressant medication.

Descriptors: Personality, drug therapy, drinking patterns.

47. Conner, C. S. Beneficial effects of alcohol. Drug Intelligence and Clinical Pharmacy, 1981, 15, 703.

Critical literature analysis of article by Turner, et al. (Johns Hopkins Medical Journal, 1981, 148, 53-63) concerning published data on alcoholism and risk of coronary heart disease, including the potential benefits of alcohol with regard to relieving stress, improving quality of life, and nutritional benefits. The author's conclusions are threefold. First, that beneficial effects of alcohol contradict existing evidence that drinking is harmful to health. Second, that elderly alcoholics should avoid drinking at all costs. And third, that the association between moderate alcohol intake and traffic accidents (and also fetal alcohol syndrome) are insufficiently clear. However, benefits from moderate ingestion of alcohol are considered possible, in concurrence with the analysis by Turner, et al.

Descriptors: Cardiovascular system, drinking patterns, stress.

48. Coppin, V. E. Life styles and social services on skid row: A study of aging homeless men. Dissertation Abstracts International, 1974, 35, 6-A.

Sociological analysis is provided on factors of race, occupation, drinking habits, available social services, and attitudes of service givers as they affect aging homeless males on Skid Row. Confirming similar research, results show that service delivery systems are resistant to adopt optimistic treatment attitudes and this discourages alcoholics from seeking assistance.

Descriptors: Drinking patterns, social delivery systems.

49. Crandall, R. C. Aged alcohol abuser. The Catalyst, 1980, 1, 56-63.

Article presents an overview of elderly alcoholics in society and the conditions frequently relevant to etiology. Early developmental stages of alcoholism are attributed to contemporary society, special problems confronting abusers, positive effects of limited alcohol consumption and inadequacies in social services. Familial relationships and the medical profession are identified as major contributors to effectively replacing reliance upon alcohol for social or psychological adjustment. Community awareness of this problem among elders ranks second in the author's prevention strategies.

Descriptors: Alcoholism, etiologic factors.

50. Csank, C. Z.; Lella, J.; Irving, R. W.; Bayne, J. R. D.; and Ciale, J. Objective Rorschach Test Correlates of Response to Treatment Outcome in Chronic Alcoholic Veterans. Research conducted at Ste-Anne's Veterans Hospital, Ste-Anne-De-Bellevue, Quebec, 1967.

A projective diagnostic instrument is used in determining the level of outcome success in alcoholic elderly patients. Responses ("free associations") taken shortly before hospital discharge, and purportedly reflective of abstinence patterns, correlate significantly with the treatment goals.

Descriptors: Alcoholism, Rorschach test.

51. De Lutterotti, A. L'àlcool nella vecchiàia: Aspetti clìnici, con particolare riguardo alla miocardiopatia alcoòlica. Giornale Gerontologia, 1974, 22, 1010-1013.

Clinical aspects of alcoholic cardiomyopathy are examined relative to the susceptibility of old people to this and other sequelae of prolonged alcohol consumption. Because of frequent coronary sclerosis, alcoholic diagnosis can be made through statistical or "exiuvantibus" criteria to show that alcohol-induced damage to the myocardium and other organ systems is attributed to the concentration, duration, and frequency of alcohol contact with the body cells. Regarding these observations, the author further notes that enzyme contact is reducible either by earlier alcoholism with liver damage or by general impairment due to "old age".

Descriptors: Alcohol-related pathologies, cardiomyopathy.

52. Ditman, K. S. Newer Concepts in the Psychopharmacological Treatment of Alcoholic Patients. Conference paper available through Alcoholism Research Clinic, Department of Psychiatry, UCLA, Center for the Health Sciences, Los Angeles, CA, 1963.

Evaluation of relatively recent psychopharmacological treatment concepts in alcoholism. Psychopharmacology is an integration of pharmacology, psychology, and psychiatry applied to treating characteristics of emotional disturbance manifested by consumption of chemical compounds. Interest in and enthusiasm for using such psychotropic drugs as tranquilizers, ataractics, antidepressants, disulfiram, and the hallucinogens are limited to certain symptoms common to schizophrenia and alcohol withdrawal states. Application of drugs can shorten recovery time from depression but, the author notes, will be misapplied unless proper forms of psychotherapy accompany treatment.

Descriptors: Psychopharmacology, therapy, medicine.

53. Drahn, T. L. Alcohol and working Americans. Industrial Gerontology, 1974, 1, 1-19.

Extensive review on methods commonly employed in industry to deal with aging alcoholic workers. Prevalence of this problem in factories and private industry anathematizes the controversy regarding coerced early retirement and whether company policies and referral services are designed for internal or external treatment conditions.

Descriptors: Alcoholism, industry.

54. Drew, L. R. H. Alcoholism as a self-limiting disease. Quarterly Journal of Studies on Alcohol, 1968, 29, 956-967.

Survey reporting that alcoholism increasingly disappears with increasing age as shown in Victoria (Australia), where the number of alcoholics in treatment decreases after the age of 40 years, from about 260 per 100,000 men at age 40 to about 200 at age 50. Mortality and chronic morbidity account for some of the diminution, but a large part the author attributes to spontaneous recovery, that prognosis in alcoholism improves after age 40 and criminality and psychopathy mutually decrease. Such factors as developmental maturity, social withdrawal, decreasing drive, and changing social pressures are all speculated to resolve with age as well.

Descriptors: Alcoholism, Australia, spontaneous recovery.

55. Droller, H. Some aspects of alcoholism in the elderly. Lancet, 1964, 2, 137-139.

Reported case histories on seven alcoholics who in receiving different modes of psychological therapy produce dissimilar outcome resistance to drinking. Evidence the author provides indicates that conditioning therapies (aversion, social learning, etc.) may be less effective in the long run than psychotherapy, which takes as its major focus the development of family relationships.

Descriptors: Conditioning therapy, alcoholism.

56. Duckworth, G., and Rosenblatt, A. Helping the elderly alcoholic. Social Casework, 1976, 57, 296-301.

Article describes a 15-week seminar in which workers in an adult protective service agency learn how to deal with elderly alcoholism. Educational methods of instruction include transactional analysis, role-playing, and meetings with actual alcoholics to experience nonantagonistic interventions. Article provides a practical pedagogy for in-service training.

Descriptors: Alcoholism, social casework.

57. Duckworth, G.S., and Ross, H. Diagnostic differences in psychogeriatric patients in Toronto, New York and London. Canadian Medical Association Journal, 1975, 11, 217-222.

Article provides national statistics in psychogeriatric illness of elderly patients in Canada, United States, and United Kingdom. Comparisons run on types of illness, available treatment facilities, and outcome results show more alcoholics residing in Canada and that, regarding national differences, diagnostic practices in each country conceptualize alcoholism with emphasis upon different symptoms.

Descriptors: Canada, United States, United Kingdom, geropsychiatric illness.

58. Dunham, R.G. Aging and changing patterns of alcohol use. Journal of Psychoactive Drugs, 1981, 13, 143-151.

Summarizes comparisons between studies on drinking patterns among elderly. Interviews are taken from 310 persons 60 years of age and older, living in government-funded, low-income housing in Florida. Subjects' responses largely fall into seven life drinking patterns including (1) lifelong abstainers, (2) rise and fall, (3) rise and sustain, (4) light throughout life, (5) light with late rise, (6) late starters, and (7) highly variable. Transitional movement between each of these seven patterns is considerable and affects

levels of alcohol consumption (e. g. , heavy, moderate, light, infrequent, and nondrinker).   More importantly, author notes that these
results are not to be generalized beyond the sample of individuals
studied (elderly residents of Miami).
    Descriptors: Drinking characteristics, ethnicity, socioeco-
    nomic status.

59.   Dunlop, J.   Alcohol Problems Among the Elderly: Implications
         for the Nurse. (Report no. NCAI-056209). Rockville, MD:
         National Institute on Alcohol Abuse and Alcoholism, 1980).
    Partial results of a three-year project to determine implica-
tions for nurses of elderly alcohol abuse indicate that there is a
special need for closer unity between physical and mental health,
social and family relationships, and economic security. Demonstrated
needs also include a better assessment of total client readiness for
referral and counseling resources.   Nurses actively employed in
health care agencies for the aged are recommended for educational
training so they can develop awareness to subtle, nondisclosed
problems possibly elicited while recording a case history.
    Descriptors: Nurses, health care agencies.

60.   Durand, D.   Effects of drinking on the power and affiliation
         needs of middle-aged females.   Journal of Clinical Psychol-
         ogy, 1975, 31, 549-553.
    Article describes results of administering TAT to middle-
aged females before and after alcohol consumption.   Needs for power
and personal power motives decline significantly under alcohol influence.   Affiliation needs also decrease, being contrary to experimental expectations and results reported on similar tests with middle-
aged males.   Authors admit their reliance on the predictability of
the TAT.
    Descriptors: Affiliation, motivation, TAT.

61.   Elderly alcoholism--a special problem. Newsletter of Wisconsin
         Association on Alcoholism and Other Drug Abuse, Inc. ,
         October-November 1977, 1-2.
    Leading story of a newsletter apprises members of Madison,
Wisconsin Association on Alcoholism and Other Drugs of increasing
problems with elderly alcoholism.   Studies, different intervention
models, and case histories attesting to local and national statistics
on elderly consumption rates and why this condition largely begins
after retirement (e. g. , 15 percent) are briefly reviewed.   Discussion
is given on steps taken in Madison to introduce new programs and
other prevention strategies.
    Descriptors: Local and national news, alcoholism.

62.   Encel, S. , and Kotowicz, K.   Heavy drinking and alcoholism:
         Preliminary report.   Medical Journal of Australia, 1970, 1,
         607-612.
    A survey of drinking practices and attitudes is drawn from
a random sample of 823 persons of different ages in Sydney, Australia.   Indicated results of the study show that, regarding age and
sex characteristics, female drinking patterns relate more to education, occupation, and income, whereas heavy drinking is charac-

teristic for every demographic factor in males. Authors conclude
that alcoholism is a major health problem and will persist regard-
less of changing cultural practices, as compared to results by
Knupfer and Room whose similar findings are from a study in metropolitan communities in the United States.
Descriptors: Drinking patterns, attitudes, Australia.

63. Epstein, L. J.; Mills, C.; and Simon, A. Antisocial behavior
    of the elderly. California Mental Health Research Digest,
    1970, 8, 78-79.
    Brief look at national trends reporting that the majority of
arrests of people over 60, especially in San Francisco, is for
drunkenness. Treatment alternatives and medical-psychological
aspects of aging endemic to social alienation make up the framework
within which geriatric alcoholism is currently perceived.
Descriptors: Criminality, San Francisco, sociopathy.

64. Epstein, L. J., and Simon, A. Organic brain syndrome in the
    elderly. Geriatrics, 1967, 22, 145-150.
    Investigation of 534 persons, 60 years and over, admitted to
a psychiatric screening ward of a metropolitan general hospital.
Social history and interview instruments serve as indices in determining that 65 percent of the sample are abstainers or social drinkers, 12 percent are excessive drinkers, and 23 percent start drinking before age 60. Alcoholic patients are also found to have diagnosable organic brain disorders (chronic, acute, etc.) and to be
experiencing recent social or interpersonal loss.
Descriptors: General hospital, organic disorders.

65. Estes, N. J.; Smith-DiJulio, K.; and Heinemann, M. E. Alco-
    hol problems in special groups: Women, the elderly, nurses.
    In N. J. Estes, (ed.), Nursing Diagnosis of the Alcoholic
    Person. St. Louis, MO: C. V. Mosby, 1980.
    Chapter presents information about elderly women and nurses
with alcohol problems and classificatory systems in their assessment.
Attitudes toward these two groups are matched against factors of
depression, precipitating parental or familial factors, polydrug use,
biological factors, and psychosocial factors. Discussion pursues
causative factors beyond these five and how they interface with
symptomatology both before and after treatment intervention.
Descriptors: Nurses, alcoholic females, polydrug abuse.

66. Etemad, B. Alcoholism and aging. In J. H. Masserman (ed.),
    Current Psychiatric Therapies. New York: Grune and
    Stratton, 1980.
    This chapter outlines primary features in the moral, med-
ical, and psychological models of elderly alcoholism, with implications for behavior and drug therapy. Carefully examined are three
common assumptions made within the etiologic and subsequent treatment phases. First, experimentally, alcoholism in the elderly tends
to accompany boredom, loneliness, and feelings of rejection or
alienation caused by retirement or perceived loss. Second, incidences of elderly alcohol abuse, according to certain studies, range

from 18 to 24. 8 percent with the ratio of male to female being 5:1.
And last, normal drinking early in life is often accompanied by heavy
drinking in later years. Caution in following these assumptions is
advised through the development of new therapeutic techniques and
educational programs for health professionals.
Descriptors: Psychiatric diagnosis, theories of addiction,
etiology.

67. Examination of Problems and Solutions Related to the Chronic
    "Revolving Door" Alcohol Abuser. (Report no. NCAI-06357).
    Rockville, MD: National Institute on Alcohol Abuse and
    Alcoholism, 1981.
    Report on the planning guidelines proposed to assist Wis-
consin elderly residents who are chronically or severly disabled.
Underlying this proposal is an alternative solution to revolving-door
alcohol abusers and the problematic system that serves and funds
them (via detoxification and treatment facilities). Noted failures in
traditional treatment methods are costing Wisconsin taxpayers about
$5. 8 million annually, with as little as only 5 percent of the patients
being motivated toward recovery within the current medical system.
Authors petition 26 recommendations toward reconstructing agency
(residential) diagnosis and treatment programs, in particular toward
community placement programs.
    Descriptors: Wisconsin, social casework.

68. Favre, A. , and de Meuron, B. Aspect psychosocial de l'al-
    coolisme du 3e âgé. Praxis, 1963, 52, 711-716.
    Exploratory analysis concerns the special difficulties in
treating long-term alcoholism in the elderly. The damage caused
by "alcohol" itself compounds the psychological state of a patient
approaching the end of life, loss of adaptability, and endless im-
possibility of obtaining gainful employment. Author urges an observation of multiple causative factors involved in alcoholism before
treatment decisions are made.
    Descriptors: Alcoholism, psychotherapy, psychosocial.

69. Fillmore, K.M. Relationships between specific drinking prob-
    lems in early adulthood and middle age: An exploratory
    20-year follow-up study. Quarterly Journal of Studies on
    Alcohol, 1975, 36, 882-907.
    Drinking problems originally measured 20 years ago on men
and women who were students are re-measured in the current survey.
Time-ordered comparisons indicate that some form of intoxication
or psychological dependence on alcohol prevailed for most women.
For middle-aged men, early symptomatic drinking behavior (reported
as either frequent intoxication or binge drinking) was clearly predictive of later alcohol abuse. Longitudinal measures on related
variables to alcohol (arrests, hospitalization, etc.) confirm these two
results.
    Descriptors: Drinking patterns, follow-up studies, drug
    dependency.

70. Fowler, N. , and Gueron, M. Primary myocardial disease in
    the elderly. Geriatrics, 1964, 19, 110.

Considers the potential inflictive effects on cardial enlargement, congestive heart failure, and a high incidence of pulmonary
and systemic arterial embolism.   Symptoms of primary myocardial
disease caused by heredity, infectious disease, cirrhosis of the
liver, vitamin deficiencies, abnormal myocardial metabolism and,
especially, alcoholism, are viewed in reference to treatment direction.   Prescriptive treatments by the author include (a) ordinary
management of congestive heart failure, (b) adrenal steroid therapy,
(c) prolonged bed rest, (d) anticoagulants, and (e) surgical management.   Implications for each advised procedure are discussed.
Descriptors: Myocardial disease and treatment, alcoholism.

71. Foy, D. W.; Miller, P. M.; Eisler, R. M.; and O'Toole, D. H.
     Social-skills training to teach alcoholics to refuse drinks
     effectively. Quarterly Journal of Studies on Alcohol, 1976,
     37, 1340-1345.
     Experimental study on teaching alcoholic inpatients (ages
from 48 and over) to refuse drinks when they return to their natural
environment.   A social skills training model based largely on assertiveness programs breaks down into five components, each evaluated
using a multiple-baseline design (single-case design).   In short,
subjects role-play three scenes depicting social situations resembling
those they are familiar with.   Target behaviors selected for change
through each component include (a) requests for change, (b) offer of
alternative, (c) change of subject, (d) duration of looking (at liquor),
and (e) affect.   Modeling techniques plus "focused instruction" are
superior methods over modeling alone.
     Descriptors: Social skills, behavior therapy.

72. Fresneau, M. L'alcoolisme des vieillards à Angers. Revue
     de l'Alcoolisme, 1969, 15, 58-60.
     Randomly sampled group of infirm, elderly men are inter-
viewed on information regarding their drinking habits.   Nearly half
of the group drink regularly, serving alcoholic beverages either at
every meal or through customary and traditional practices.   A much
smaller proportion drink to the point of intoxication, in contrast to
recent statistics on elderly residents in Paris.   Conclusions for this
disparity offer, among other points, the argument against stereotyping
European drinking patterns.
     Descriptors: Drinking patterns, France, alcoholism.

73. Funkhouser, M. J. Identifying alcohol problems among elderly
     hospital patients. Alcohol Health and Research World, 1977,
     2, 27-34.
     Investigated in this study are the physiological and psycho-
logical problems that obscure accurate detection of elderly alcoholism and its prevalence in society.   Out of 47 patients (aged 55-89),
26 scored 4 or above on the Michigan Alcoholism Screening Test,
and 55 percent of the hospitalized veterans are alcoholics.   A symptom index and corrobative laboratory indices demonstrate signs of
physiological disturbance in most patients, extending the belief that
alcoholic sequelae reach significant levels before appropriate treatment begins.   Alternatively, the author stresses the obligation of
health professionals to improve diagnostic procedures.

Descriptors: Alcoholism diagnosis, hospitalization, Michigan Alcohol Screening Test.

74. Gabelic, I.   Geriatric service and geriatric club.   Anali Bolnice Dr. M. Stojanovic, 1971, 10, 221-226.
Theoretical discussion urging that scientific research establish the relationship between alcoholism and the "involutive" age, along with the psychopathology that develops.   Research is apparently inept in tying together sociocultural inducements to illness with the medical problem of alcohol abuse.   Author encourages an examination of the prophylactic effect on the process of aging and on work productivity during and after alcohol recovery.
Descriptors: Sociocultural factors, scientific research.

75. Gaillard, A., and Perrin, P.   L'alcoolisme des personnes âgées.   Revue de l'Alcoolisme, 1969, 15, 5-32.
Surveys a small sample of elderly pensioners residing in a rest home in Lille.   Interview data reveal that 90 percent of the men and 80 percent of the women suffer from known (or remembered) alcoholism.   Diagnostic verification is available for few of the subjects, while in large part their past or current diagnosis coincide with observable behavioral symptoms of potential alcohol abuse (feelings of rejection; isolated social interaction, etc.).
Descriptors: Nursing homes.

76. Gaitz, C. M. and Baer, P. E.   Characteristics of elderly patients with alcoholism.   Archives of General Psychiatry, 1971, 24, 372-78.
Study examines a high rate of alcoholism in 100 consecutive admissions of persons, aged 60 and older, to a county psychiatric screening ward.   Data are collected on groups arranged into three categories--alcoholic without organic brain syndrome, alcoholic with organic brain syndrome, and nonalcoholic with organic brain syndrome.   Sociodemographic, physical, psychiatric, and cognitive variables measured on subjects in each category suggest that alcoholics with organic brain syndromes, though younger than their nonalcoholic counterparts, are less impaired cognitively, show fewer signs of psychosis, but feel more animosity toward family memories.   Mortality rates and physical status for both groups are similar.
Descriptors: Cognition, organicity, psychiatry.

77. Galdi, Z., and Vertes, L.   Alkoholismus im Alter.   Aktuelle Gerontologie, 1980, 10, 305-307.
This includes survey results of 860 new admissions to an alcoholism treatment unit in Budapest screened between 1972 and 1975 (64 of whom are between 60 and 74 years).   Aversion therapy using low-dosage disulfiram (0.25-0.50 tablet daily) is administered to only 25 mentally sound and sufficiently motivated patients.   Abstinence and improved physical health in these patients directly challenge the frequent contraindication of aversion therapy for geriatrics in medical rehabilitation.   Authors thus advise a cautionary low dose as a supplement to group therapy.
Descriptors: Budapest, aversion therapy, group therapy.

78. Giacinto, J. P.; O'Neil, P. M.; and Waid, L. R.   Comparison of
    early-onset versus late-onset elderly alcoholic males.   Alco-
    holism : Clinical and Experimental Research, 1981, 5, 150.
    The hypothesis that early-onset elderly alcholics are usually
men whose condition exacerbates with age is tested using two experimental groups--early- and late-onset alcoholics.   Sociodemographics
for both groups are similar, whereas differences on the MacAndrew
scale of the MMPI are significant for early-onset alcoholics.   This
same group reports significantly longer periods of drinking abstinence, more legal problems and surprisingly, more brothers in
their families.   Score differences on other psychological measures
(Profile of Mood States, SC L-90, Strait-Trait Anxiety Inventory) are,
however, not significant.
    Descriptors: Alcoholic men, MMPI, onset of alcoholism.

79. Gibson, W. G. , and Reimer, K. A.   Multiple coronary artery
    dissections in old age: A unique case.   Archives of Pathol-
    ogy and Laboratory Medicine.   1980, 104, 419-421.
    This case study presents a coronary artery dissection with
clinical and pathologic features in a 71-year-old man dying of alcoholic cirrhosis and pulmonary emphysema.   Older than previously
reported victims of this dissection, the patient's disorders are similar morphologically to those predisposed to pregnant women.   Like
pregnant women, cirrhotic men show stigmata of hypoerestrinism.
Implications of sociopsychological influences on this pathology and its
manifestation from alcoholism are explored by the author.
    Descriptors: Alcohol-related pathology, cardiovascular sys-
    tem.

80. Glatt, M. M.   Distraneurin therapy in old age cerebral sclerosis
    and in alcohol withdrawal syndrome.   Possibilities and lim-
    itations.   Fortschritte der Medicine, 1980, 29, 784-786.
    Critical evaluation explores the risk of sedative drugs to
elderly alcoholics.   Misuse, abuse, and dependence on drugs such as
clomethiazole is remediable when treatment is applied only to the
withdrawal period (not longer than six to seven days).   Tendencies by
alcoholic versus nonalcoholic elderly to abuse sedatives beyond withdrawal periods, may also be due to increased cerebral sclerosis.
By contrast, nonalcoholic elderly not suffering from cerebral sclerosis are in no risk of developing dependence.
    Descriptors: Alcohol withdrawal, sedatives, physical depend-
    ence.

81. Goby, M. J.   Follow-up study of patients over 60 treated at the
    alcoholism treatment center for Lutheran General Hospital.
    In M. J. Goby and J. E. Keller (eds.), Perspectives on
    Treatment of Alcoholism.   Park Ridge, IL: Lutheran Gen-
    eral Hospital, 1978.
    Discusses a study of 37 patients over 60 years of age after
6 to 18 months following release from a residential alcoholism treatment program.   Recidivism rates are low, with 62 percent reporting
sobriety.   Those patients who, during follow-up, still drink alcohol
have reduced the daily consumption amount to less than prior to

hospitalization. Alcoholics Anonymous meetings are identified as the primary follow-up session attended and nearly 89 percent consider their lives to have improved since discharge.
Descriptors: Follow-up therapy, hospitalization.

82. Gomberg, E. Alcohol use and alcohol problems among the elderly. In Alcohol and Health Monography No. 4: Special Population Issues. Washington, DC: U. S. Government Printing Office, 1982.
    Chapter reviews alcohol use and abuse in the elderly's social drinking patterns. Incidence and prevalence issues are traced with respect to major roadblocks in the casefinding process. Prevention activities for this population are also reviewed, contrasting the current aging service network with projected priorities in research and program development.
    Descriptors: Epidemiology, drinking patterns.

83. Gomberg, E. Alcohol and the old folks. Digest of Alcoholism Theory and Application, 1982, 1, 49-51.
    Proposed is that a philosophical distinction be made between the study of "aging" and study of "old age". This distinction clearly enables the collection of available data on alcohol and the aging process and, at the opposite extreme, on alcohol and the elderly. Issues raised by this distinction with the existing literature are enumerated.
    Descriptors: Process of aging, alcoholism, research.

84. Goodrich, C. H. , and Johnson, L. A. Study of Effects of Alcohol and Old Age (Phase I). City University of New York School of Medicine, 1973.
    Outlines the results of surveying men and women 70 years of age (and older) via questionnaires to determine their drinking habits, use of other drugs (including prescriptions), and adaptability in the community as perceived by significant others. In this first phase, population characteristics are interpreted against a criterion defined by the New York School of Medicine and are later compared to norms reported in the literature.
    Descriptors: Demographic survey, drinking patterns.

85. Gordon, J. J. ; Kirchoff, K. L. ; and Philipps, B. K. Alcoholism and the Elderly: A Study of Problems and Prospects. Iowa City, IA: Elderly Program Development Center, 1976.
    Describes a survey to determine percentage of alcohol abusers (55 years and older) and assesses number and content of programs as well as attitudes of treatment personnel. Five hundred agencies chosen at random from the 1973-1974 ADPA directory (ten from each state) are sent questionnaires, with a 45 percent return rate. Estimated percentage of alcoholic clientele in agencies is 18. 4 percent and 10. 7 percent report having special programs designed for elderly abusers.
    Descriptors: Agency services, national survey.

86. Graux, P. L'alcoolisme des vieillards. Revue de l'Alcoolisme, 1969, 15, 46-48.

Cumulated analysis of surveys conducted in France is presented. The incidence of "acute" and "chronic" alcoholism in 161 rest homes is high. Author speculates that alcoholism is due to low educational levels, familial discordance, inactivity, and "boredom." Conceptual alternatives to increase activity levels in rest homes is part of the author's model for rehabilitation.
Descriptors: France, rest homes.

87. Guillemant, S.; Vitoux, J. F.; Desgrez, P.; Saigot, T.; and Sarazin, A. Dosage radio-immunologique de l'arginine-vasopressine plasmatique chez le cirrhotique: Quinze malades. Nouvelle Presse Medicale, 1978, 7, 3048-3049.
Condition of plasma arginine vasopressin in eight patients with alcohol cirrhosis is presented in case study form. Patients without ascites show twice as high plasma arginine vasopressin levels, and with it show four times the amount over eight control groups. Significant correlations between plasma (plasma arginine vasopressin) and sodium are observed only in the group with ascites. Indications for medical treatment with alcoholic patients are provided in relation to polymorbidity.
Descriptors: Plasma arginine vasopressin, cirrhosis, alcohol-related pathologies.

88. Gunderson, E. K., and Schuckit, M. A. Prognostic indicators in young alcoholics. U. S. Naval Health Research Center Report, 1975, January (No. 75-15).
Predictive studies are conducted on 2,865 young and old enlisted male alcoholics admitted to the U. S. Navy medical programs during two different time periods. Statistical relations are correlated across diagnosis, pay grade, length of service, and days hospitalized, in predicting dispositional success at the medical facility. Standardized and actuarial tables developed in the process aid in the assessment and prognostic procedure.
Descriptors: Hospitalization, prognosis, navy personnel.

89. Happy-hour therapy. Human Behavior, 1974, 3, 31-32.
Study reports the efficacy of using beer in social therapy with elderly psychiatric patients. Enhancements in social activity, physical status and adjustment to ward appear as hypothetically possible consequences from the beer, as opposed to drinking fruit juices. Sociability in the fruit-drinking group is commensurable to that of the control group. Authors explore additional therapeutic advantages small doses of alcohol provide for the psychiatric treatment plan.
Descriptors: Beer, social therapy, psychiatry.

90. Harris, C. S. Aging and alcohol use: A pilot project. Perspective on Aging, 1978, 7, 4-8.
Findings of a study by the National Council on Aging on normal drinking patterns in the older populations are briefly provided. The direct proportion between increasing age and increasing consumption levels corresponds with statewide surveys on sampling groups of different ethnic, racial, and educational backgrounds.

Medical recovery or participation in some transitionary phase between physical and psychological illness and rehabilitation are also clear predictors of drinking patterns.

Descriptors: Cultural trends, drinking patterns.

91. Hartford, J. T. , and Samorajski, T. Alcoholism in the geriatric population. Journal of the American Geriatrics Society, 1982, 30, 18-24.

Theoretical study contends that physiological effects of alcohol in the elderly population affect the aging process and cognitive performance. Deterioration rates of liver and organ performance influenced by alcohol are especially an impediment to cognitive abilities due to four basic reasons. First, blood levels of ethanol are higher in elderly, causing brain neurons to be more sensitive to the drug. Second, ethanol ingestion can greatly disturb sleep and sexual activity. Third, cognitive reasoning and adaptation is slower. And last, drug-drug interactions mixed with ethanol pose hazards to physiology in general. Symptomatic signs for physicians to observe include intellectual dysfunction and short-term memory loss.

Descriptors: Cognitive ability, alcohol-related pathology.

92. Hasenbush, L. L. Successful brief therapy of a retired elderly man with intractable pain, depression, and drug and alcohol dependence. Journal of Geriatric Psychiatry, 1977, 10, 71-88.

Discusses case history of successful psychoanalytic therapy performed on a geriatric patient with depression complicated by (a) self-injurious foot pain, (b) drug and alcohol dependence, and (c) progressive invalidism. Accompanying psychotherapy stressed compatible personality styles of patient and his wife. Indicated by therapy was that post-retirement depression can be effectively relieved even when severe emotional and somatic symptoms persist from neurotic character problems.

Descriptors: Psychoanalysis, depression.

93. Hobson, G. N. Ethanol and conditioning Quarterly Journal of Studies on Alcohol, 1966, 27, 612-619.

Results reported of a study of university recruited nonabstaining volunteers (aged 21 and over) who went through different phases of conditioned responding (CR-eyelid). Using an apparatus, the subjects' eyelid conditioning is apparently retarded by a depressant drug in support of Eysenck's predictions. Partially supported is the hypothesis that the action of ethanol upon the formation of CR's depends on dosage, stimulus intensity, and the manner of response acquisition.

Descriptors: Conditioned response, drug effects.

94. Hochla, N. A. Premature aging in female alcoholics. A neuropsychological study. Journal of Nervous and Mental Diseases, 1982, 170, 241-245.

Neuropsychological battery performed on 35 alcoholic and 35 nonalcoholic women (27 elderly) is examined regarding problem-solving and other cognitive-oriented abilities. Demonstrated differences are due to vast inequalities of drinking patterns among the

subjects' cultural and ethnic backgrounds.
Descriptors: Neuropsychology, cognitive ability.

95. Hochrein, M., and Schleicher, I. Herz-kreislaufbeeinflussung durch alkohol. Medizinische Klinik, 1965, 60, 41-46.
Evaluates physical benefits of moderate drinking habits in 1,300 persons over 80 years old. Wine-drinking elderly in countries accustomed to moderate daily consumption are physically and mentally more vigorous and live an average of ten years longer than their counterpart beer drinkers. Cross-cultural implications are noted for future sociological comparisons.
Descriptors: Wine-drinking, beer.

96. Horwitz, L. D. Alcohol and heart disease. Journal of the American Medical Association, 1975, 232, 959-960.
Heart disease and susceptibility to myocardial depression are reported to correlate highly with alcoholic beverages. Cardiac patients, in particular, are at risk when the adverse effects of alcohol on myocardium are direct, rather than mediated through the autonomic nervous system. The mechanisms by which rapid administration of alcohol alters myocardial function are detailed in reference to recent laboratory research.
Descriptors: Myocardial (cardiac) function, alcohol-related pathology.

97. Huang, C. Y. Peripheral neuropathy in the elderly: A clinical and electrophysiologic study. Journal of the American Geriatrics Society, 1981, 29, 49-54.
Explains preponderance of peripheral neuropathy in 59 elderly patients. Heavy alcohol consumption and sensorimotor impediments observed in clinical trials prior to treatment are reduced after vitamin therapy began. The extent of neuropathic alteration in Wernicke-Korsakoff syndrome is also discussed.
Descriptors: Alcohol-related pathology, peripheral neuropathy.

98. Hubbard, R. W.; Santos, J. F.; and Santos, M. A. Alcohol and older adults: Overt and covert influence. Social Casework, 1979, 60, 166-170.
Case analyses are presented of older adults referred to the Mental Health Outreach Program for the Elderly. Four types of alcohol-related problems indicated are (a) chronic long-term alcoholism, (2) onset of alcoholism in later years, (3) debilitating interactive effects of alcohol use, and (4) victimization of older adults by alcoholics. Case reviews also show that service providers and family members need more awareness of multiple effects of alcohol abuse on elderly.
Descriptors: Social casework, mental health programs.

99. Hunter, K.; Linn, M. W.; and Harris, R. Dietary patterns and cancer of the digestive tract in older patients. Journal of the American Geriatrics Society, 1980, 28, 405-409.
Study shows that alcohol, smoking, sugar, and fat (multiplied together) are fairly accurate predictors of upper digestive-tract cancer.

Veterans (45-65 years) interviewed about their lifetime dietary patterns and alcohol and smoking behaviors reveal few differences in terms of age, physical activity in childhood or adulthood, or incidence of obesity. Colon, rectal and upper digestive tract cancers predicted by these data are even more significant when dietary "fiber" is considered.

Descriptors: Alcohol-related pathology, digestive system, cancer.

100. Husain, S. Drug problems among the elderly. The Spada Sage (Specialty Program in Alcohol and Drug Abuse), 1982, 3, 2-5.

Concentrated account of elderly alcoholics as a sociological influence upon ageism and reactions by the medical establishment. Clinical and administrative aspects of drug misuse, abuse, and potential misdiagnosis attributed to poor professional attitudes and faulty communication between physician and patient are expanded into projected problems for the future. Problems of iatrogenic and actual physical illness are identified as the need for abundant medication.

Descriptors: Medication, professional attitudes.

101. Hyman, M. M. Alcoholics 15 years later. Annals of the New York Academy of Sciences, 1976, 273, 613-623.

Follow-up results are reported of white male alcoholics in New Jersey discharged from a treatment center 15 years ago. Delineation of subjects appears in terms of demographics, social functioning, length of hospitalization, client-client interaction, and outcome results. Implied by the survey is that alcohol educational programs directed for outpatient care require more community support.

Descriptors: Demography, follow-up.

102. Irvine, R. E. Hypothermia. Modern Geriatrics, 1973, 3, 464-470.

Extensive review of hypothermic potential in elderly users of drugs such as phenothiazine, tranquilizers, alcohol, antidepressants, and barbiturates. When body temperature lowers from peripheral vasodilatation it may also cause decreased blood pressure and circulatory collapse in elderly. Reliable methods to protect hypothermic elderly during recovery are advised with strict admonishments against such common practices as gastric or tracheal intubation, bladder catheterization, and insulin administration. Moreover, symptoms of thermoregulatory failure in either deep body or hand temperature should receive modified treatments.

Descriptors: Hypothermia, alcohol-related pathology.

103. Jessen, P. Servicing Mental Health Needs of the Aged Through Volunteer Services. Rockville, MD: Alcohol, Drug Abuse, and Mental Health Administration, 1975.

Contents are primarily from a conference co-sponsored by the National Institutes of Health's Citizens Participation Branch and Section on Mental Health of the Aging. Topics concern the role of volunteers in local mental health operations described in language that is understandable by potential volunteers. Individuals involved in the provision of mental health services are classified into elderly and nonelderly volunteers and given techniques and strategies adaptable at different stages of the service relationship (recruiting, training, placing, retaining and accounting). Underlying these services is the role of elderly in effecting social change, personal attitudes, and why volunteerism is a social imperative.

Descriptors: Volunteerism, alcoholism and mental health.

104. Johnson, L. A. Use of Alcohol by Persons 65 Years and Over, Upper East Side of Manhattan. (Report no. NCAI-019198). Rockville, MD: National Institute on Alcohol Abuse and Alcoholism, 1974.

Questionnaire survey covers persons 65 years of age and older in New York City regarding their health, physical mobility, social activity, psychological adjustment, and attitudes about alcohol and medicinal drugs. Characteristics unique to this sample are high crime rates, minority group members and urbanization. Drinking elderly apparently indicate contentment, positive psychological health, and, despite periodical illness, sociability.

Descriptors: Questionnaire, drinking attitudes.

105. Johnson, L. C.; Burdick, J. A.; and Smith, J. Sleep during alcohol intake and withdrawal in the chronic alcoholic. Archives of General Psychiatry, 1970, 22, 406-418.

Sleep latency study involves "all-night" records on 14 chronic alcoholic patients during two days of alcohol intake and ten days without alcohol. Psychological measures taken in both conditions on anxiety, mood, and cognitive performance correlate with REM sleep patterns. Sleep during withdrawal is similar to that found in normal subjects aged 65 and over and especially in Stage 4, which is significantly diminished. Low REM sleep during alcohol intake improved to 20-25 percent after three days without alcohol. These and other results indicate sleep disturbances are considered symptomatic of the disease rather than clinically causative. Relationships of serotonin metabolism in sleep to schizophrenia induced by alcohol are explored for future research.

Descriptors: Sleep, withdrawal, cognitive abilities.

106. Jones, R. W. Alcoholism among relatives of alcoholic patients. Quarterly Journal of Studies on Alcohol, 1972, 33, 810.

Latitudinal investigation of alcoholism in relatives from 1,333 patients at an alcoholism treatment center. Alcoholic relatives make up 30 percent of female patients and 23 percent of male patients, with 16 percent of the total relatives sampled reported as 51 years and older. Indications of family inheritance and alcoholism are discussed.

Descriptors: Family and alcoholism, follow-up.

107. Keahey, S. P. Effects of Biofeedback Alpha Training with Alcoholics. (Report No. ZO-35532). Washington, DC: U. S. Veterans Administration, Department of Medicine and Surgery, 1974.

Reviews the hypothesis that the production of alpha rhythms for relaxation and "tranquility" can replace relaxation responses derived from drinking. Personality variables that change in response to alpha rhythm production are decreased anxiety and improved self-esteem. Fifty consenting subjects are randomly assigned either to experimental (biofeedback) or control (no biofeedback) groups and receive no supplemental psychotropic medication. Phase 1 demonstrates the subjects' physiological reactivity and in subsequent phases a tone (feedback) is used to train successive approximations to alpha stability.

Descriptors: Biofeedback, relaxation training.

108. Kirk, J. Alcoholism: Complications it causes and other conditions. Resident and Staff Physician, 1976, February, 31-33.

Personnel survey asks 2,200 physicians the types of problems they encounter in alcoholic patients. In most cases, family physicians (82 percent) and hospital physicians (83 percent) identify the problem of prescribing medication for withdrawal syndrome symptoms, liver abnormalities, gastrointestinal ailments, trauma, and malnutrition. Physicians note the masking effect of heavy drinking that obscures an accurate diagnosis and the same for complications from neuroses, anxiety and depression.

Descriptors: Alcohol-related pathology, professional attitudes

109. Kolb, D. , and Gunderson, E. K. Prognostic indicators for Navy alcoholics in rehabilitation centers and units. U. S. Naval Health Research Center Report, 1975, February, 75-16.

Comparisons are made of younger and older alcoholic groups treated at U. S. Navy Alcohol Rehabilitation Centers and Units. Predictive variables studied in relation to outcome success are highest for pay grade and staff treatment ratings. Biographical and clinical variables beyond these two are also relevant for assessment but not used in the prediction equation.

Descriptors: Rehabilitation, prognosis, U. S. Navy personnel.

110. Korboot, P. , and Naylor, G. F. Patterns of WAIS and MIA in alcoholic dementia. Australian Journal of Psychology, 1972, 24, 227-234.

Patients diagnosed with "alcoholic dementia" (mean age: 56 years) are given a psychological battery for assessing their maximum rate of information acceptance (MIA). WAIS subtest scores on two different occasions, separated by six months, reveal patterns that are comparable to scores obtained by Korsakoff patients and also by normal similar-aged subjects. MIA patterns are consistently low across different diagnoses. Possible relationships between dementia, the aging process, and nonfocal brain damage are explored.

Descriptors: WAIS, maximum rate of information, neuropsychology.

111. Koskenvuo, M.; Kaprio, J.; Langinvainio, H.; Romo, M.; and
     Sarna, S.   Coronary-prone behavior in adult same-sexed
     male twins: An epidemiological study.   Progress in Clin-
     ical Biology Research, 1981, 69, 139-148.
        Demographic analysis explores the suspected correlation
between coronary heart disease and alcohol as "inheritable" family
traits.   Monozygotic and dizygotic studies in psychology showing
different temperaments in the adult twin have traced smoking and
substance abuse problems to paternal and maternal influences.   Complications of these results in interpreting social trends are examined.
        Descriptors: Twins, alcohol-related pathology, epidemio-
        logy.

112. Kurzinger, R.   Der alkoholabbau bei alten bei menschen.
     Deutsche Gesundheitswesen, 1963, 18, 1224-1230.
        Alcohol effects in older people appear more pronounced in
an examination of metabolism rates.   During the rise of the blood
alcohol curve there is no manifest tolerance to alcohol.   Indications
are that alcohol susceptibility of older people must be due to the
greater sensitivity of nerve cells to extroceptive stimulation.
        Descriptors: Metabolism rate, alcohol-related pathology.

113. Lamy, P. P.   Misuse and abuse of drugs by elderly: Another
     view.   American Pharmacist, 1980, 20, 14-17.
        Recognizes the precedency of elderly substance abuse and
in particular alcoholism.   Drug utilization studies offer predictive
evidence of an upward spiral trend toward more elderly abuse cases
unless physicians are more sensitive to misprescribed medication and
situational stresses involved in drinking.
        Descriptors: Prescriptions, stress.

114. Lancaster, J.   Maximizing psychological adaptation in an aging
     population.   Topics for the Clinical Nurse, 1981, 3, 31-43.
        Issues regarding the disruption in psychologically adapting
to old age are discussed in contrast to social theories about stereotyping, discrimination, and psychological development.   Aging persons who are also alcoholic or overmedicated mislead the public's
perceptions of their polymorbidity.   Examined in this context are
difficult social adjustments expected of the elderly by both physicians
and society.
        Descriptors: Social adjustment, attitudes.

115. LaPorte, D. J.; McLellan, A. T.; Erdlen, F. R.; and Parente,
     R. J.   Treatment outcome as a function of follow-up diffi-
     culty in substance abusers.   Journal of Consulting and
     Clinical Psychology, 1981, 49, 112-119.
        Study regards the practical application of follow-up systems
to be problematic in most substance abuse rehabilitation (treatment)
centers.   Recidivism rates, though largely unchanged in residential
facilities, may inaccurately reflect annual follow-up success because
so many clients are unavailable for evaluation.   Follow-up research
is advised to adopt safeguard methods to assure that data are representative of treatment outcomes.
        Descriptors: Follow-up, elderly recidivism.

116. Larson, A. Intoxication as a defense in workmen's compensation. Cornell Law Review, 1974, 59, 398-417.
    Article reviews several court decisions regarding the award or denial of workmen's compensation in cases where "intoxication" is used as a defense against payment. State imposed criteria are different but will vary in terms of (a) definition of intoxication, (b) blood alcohol concentration level, (c) intoxication as "volitional" conduct, (d) causal relationships between intoxication and injury, and (e) employer participation or knowledge prior to the injury. Causal connections between intoxication and injury range from "intoxication while the injury occurs" to "proof beyond a reasonable doubt that intoxication caused the injury. " Courts are likely to minimize the prospect of employee fault and maximize interest in protecting the family and family of employee.
    Descriptors: Law and legislation, occupational safety, industry.

117. Lattanzio, S. , and Bruder, G. A. Analysis of Deficiencies in the Verbal Memory Processes of Amnesic Patients. (Report no. ZO-33574 1). Washington, DC: U. S. Veterans Administration, Department of Medicine and Surgery, 1974.
    Memory deficits of Korsakoff patients are examined using tasks and concepts applicable in normal memory test batteries. Two experiments comparing Korsakoff with alcohol control patients suggest that Korsakoff patients can use word meaning to overcome deficits. Information organized into a system (mnemonic, associative) would at least facilitate memory performance, since most of the deficit lies in long-term storage rather than retrieval difficulty.
    Descriptors: Memory, cognitive ability, amnesic.

118. Leber, W. R. , and Parsons, O. A. Premature aging and alcoholism. International Journal of the Addictions, 1982, 17, 61-88.
    Recent attention has been paid to organic neurological impairment (right hemisphere) involved in persistent alcoholism. Cognitive and other psychological deterioration resulting from chronic ethanol abuse is suspected to cause premature aging in the central nervous system. Conceptual issues related to this topic and the scientific utility of pursuing it are discussed in depth.
    Descriptors: Alcohol-related pathology, neuropsychology, premature aging.

119. Lerebouleet, J. L'espérance de vie des alcooliques. Revue de l'Alcoolisme, 1968, 14, 279-289.
    Correlative data regarding mortality and alcohol-related pathology are interpreted from British and American insurance companies. Findings that alcoholism greatly reduces life expectancy correspond to the French, American, and Swedish literature reviewed in the article.
    Descriptors: Alcohol-related pathology, mortality.

120. Lerner, J. Chronic alcoholism--after thirty years some second thoughts. Journal of the American Geriatrics Society, 1967, 15, 137-141.

Exploratory discussion on problems that arise from the commercialization of alcohol. Chronic elderly alcoholism is gradually transmuted into an accepted illness but the treatment of alcoholism is still rejected by societal standards. A retrospective glance over 30 years shows that little societal change has resulted; alcohol is still readily available and in large part encouraged. The author articulates that a constructive program to reduce or prevent youth and elderly susceptibility to alcoholism would include dismantling the misconceived glamour of drinking.

Descriptors: Drinking attitudes, commercialization.

121. Linde, T. F. Left-right Differences in Auditory Perception in Alcoholic Patients. (Report no. ZO-34281). Washington, DC: U. S. Veterans Administration, Department of Medicine and Surgery, 1977.

Study describes results of manual perceptual-motor performance in a group of aging right-handed, brain-damaged alcoholics. Verbal instructions are to move certain geometric shapes when a certain color appears and stipulate which hand to do it with. Responses typically show the following patterns: (a) responding correctly on all trials; (b) reversing the correct shape-color combination on each trial; (c) reversing the shape-color response midway through the set; and (d) randomly responding (generating) a private set of "contingencies". Implications are that performance by brain-damaged alcoholics depends on such variables as hearing loss, localization of damage, task complexity, type of reinforcement, and transference between tasks.

Descriptors: Memory, neuropsychology, perceptual-motor coordination.

122. Lucas, M. L'alcoolisme dans les hospices de vieillards de la région parisienne. Revue de l'Alcoolisme, 1969, 15, 268-284.

Cultural assessment of 304 elderly chronic alcoholic patients is provided. Seventy percent admit to drinking, whereas 60 percent drink one to two liters of red wine or its equivalent daily, 12 percent drink more than two liters, 19 percent are intoxicated daily, 47 percent drink every week, and 30 percent drink every month. Attempts to trace recurrent drinking patterns in each classified group are discussed.

Descriptors: Drinking patterns, cultural trends.

123. MacAndrew, C. What the MAC scale tells us about men alcoholics. An interpretive review. Quarterly Journal of Studies on Alcohol, 1981, 42, 604-625.

Subscales of MMPI are considered to have potential interpretive value for rating the psychiatric status of alcholic middle-aged adults. Case reviews are among the evidence for wider application of this psychological test during intake assessment.

Descriptors: MMPI, assessment.

124. McKnight, A. J. , and Green, M. A. Safe Driving Knowledge Dissemination and Testing Techniques. Volume II. Final

Report. (Report no. D2963A4). Washington, DC: National Highway Traffic Safety Administration, 1977.

A set of seven driver license manuals and tests are developed for the following groups: (1) new drivers; (2) youthful drivers; (3) renewal applicants; (4) older drivers; (5) traffic violators; (6) accident repeaters; and (7) drinking drivers. Manuals tested out on 30,000 drivers, primarily from Virginia, make it possible to determine their effectiveness for acquisition, retention, and application of safe driving information. Following this test, a one-hour audiovisual presentation covers contents of recently added material. Interestingly, older drivers show a slight gain in overall retention of the material over other groups tested.

Descriptors: Highway safety, educational materials.

125. MacLean, H.; Steward, A. W.; Riley, C. G.; and Beaven, D. W. Vitamin C status of elderly men in a residential home. New Zealand Medical Journal, 1977, 86, 379-382.

Results of a study reveal that plasma and leukocyte vitamin C levels in men over 70 years of age decrease with increased alcohol intake. Thirty-five subjects from a residential home, measured for grams per day of vitamins and alcohol intake, are shown to account for only 6.1 percent of their plasma vitamin C from alcohol. Suggested directions for improving daily allowances of vitamin C are in the discussion.

Descriptors: Vitamins, alcohol-related pathology.

126. Malikovic, B.; Divac, M. B.; Biagojevic, M.; and Kirkovic, M. Osobenosti grupne psihoterapije alkoholicara starijeg zivotnog doba. Socijalna Psihijatrija, 1976, 4, 67-76.

Traces evolutionary and contemporary development of group psychotherapy of elderly alcoholics in a homogenous age group held in a therapeutic community. Basic results reported include (a) hospitalized elderly alcoholics display less intense recovery, (b) poorest therapeutic success found in primary alcoholics with initial dementia, in paranoid persons and in persons with character deviations, and (c) best therapeutic results shown in adventitious (recently becoming) alcoholics, or those for whom drinking offered an escape from some traumatic event. It is concluded that group psychotherapy in conjunction with "other" modalities has more prognostic value.

Descriptors: Group therapy.

127. Marden, P. G. Alcohol Abuse and the Aged. (Report no. NCAI-026923). Rockville, MD: National Institute on Alcohol Abuse and Alcoholism, 1976.

Description of alcohol abuse among the aged against a backdrop of national demographic and sociological trends. Suggestions are given for appropriate services and programs akin to financial and housing problems faced by the elderly. Generally, author contends that although the proportion of elderly drinkers is significant, drinking declines with age. Modifications in existing services are proposed to NIAAA and directed toward stronger advocacy and community dissemination.

Descriptors: Demography, service programs.

128. Mayer, M. J. Alcohol and the elderly: A review. Health and Social Work, 1979, 4, 128-143.
Review article on anticipated growth of elderly alcohol abuse and why social workers should focus their future research on identification (case-finding) and diagnostic issues. Population figures indicating higher unemployment and hence early retirement are interpreted as being predictive of depression and other psychological distress symptomatic of substance abuse. Efforts toward an expansion of projects in methods of treatment are advised.
Descriptors: Demography, social casework.

129. Mayfield, D. G. Alcohol problems in the aging patient. In Drug Issues in Geropsychiatry. Baltimore, MD: Williams and Wilkins Company, 1974.
General overview presented on alcohol problems in aging client, noting that elderly alcoholics tend to be undetected, undiagnosed, and untreated. Author asserts that the aging alcoholic is a better candidate for rehabilitation than younger alcohol abusers. Details examining this prospect in view of the sociopolitical structure around which abusers live are analyzed with implications for treatment intervention.
Descriptors: Demography, rehabilitation.

130. Medhus, A. Alcohol problems among male disability pensioners. Scandinavian Journal of Social Medicine, 1976, 4, 145-149.
Swedish males (N = 235) who are granted a disability pension in 1964 and another group randomly chosen from pensioners in 1974 (N = 235) complete a survey on their alcohol problems. Few pensioners have criminal records, while one in ten in each group experience compulsory treatment for alcoholism. Disability compensation received for alcoholism is less common than for mental disorders, particularly by subjects who are in compulsory treatment. Both groups, however, show high frequencies of divorce and relatively low social status.
Descriptors: Disability compensation, industry.

131. Mellstrom, D.; Rundgren, A.; and Svanborg, A. Previous alcohol consumption and its consequences for aging, morbidity, and morality in men aged 70-75. Age and Ageing, 1981, 10, 277-286.
Longitudinal comparisons are made between 468 seventy-year-old men surveyed first in 1971-1972 and again in 1976-1977 and another group of 489 seventy-year-old men. The epidemiological measure is the number of registrations at the Temperance Board (index of recidivism). Results of the 1976-1977 evaluation indicate that recidivists have higher morbidity rates of diabetes and chronic bronchitis, consumption of drugs, and mortality rate. Functional ability on cognitive tests, muscle strength, and skeleton density among recidivists also parallel these results. Adjunctive analyses are provided on differences between blood and physiology.
Descriptors: Polymorbidity, alcohol-related pathologies, Sweden.

132. Merry, J. Alcoholism in the aged. British Journal of Alcohol and Alcoholism, 1980, 15, 56-57.

Case histories of nine women between ages 70 and 80 and hospitalized for problem drinking are examined. Marital and social complications contribute heavily to their inebriety. Because 80 percent of this sample is still hospitalized, author is skeptical about institutional and aftercare preparation for independent community living Supportive measures for bereaved and lonely elderly women are scarce and could benefit from service extensions that are reachable and usable by elderly after discharge.

Descriptors: Rehabilitation, alcoholic females, diagnosis.

133. Mishara, B. L. , and Kastenbaum, R. Wine in the treatment of long-term geriatric patients in mental institutions. Journal of the American Geriatrics Society, 1974, 22, 88-94.

Describes the improvements upon earlier research using wine in the form of therapy. Long-term geropsychiatric patients who drink controlled amounts of wine find it induces sleep and stimulates congenial socialization. Contraindications of wine in traditional psychotherapy are inconsistent with these data and are examined for questionable validity.

Descriptors: Wine, geropsychiatry.

134. Mishara, B. L. , and Kastenbaum, R. Alcohol and Old Age. New York: Grune and Stratton, 1980.

Current perspectives on cultural and pharmacological indications of elderly alcoholic potential are brought forth under a single cover. Positions presented are twofold. First, alcohol use is dangerous at any age and even more deleterious for elders. Second, alcohol use does provide medicinal benefits under proper therapeutic conditions and supervision. Topics cover a broad range of introductory and controversial issues including (a) historiographic use of alcohol by elderly, (b) physiological effects of ethanol and the congeners of alcoholic beverages, (c) criticism of current epidemiological data, (d) evaluation of problem drinking, and (e) review of studies identifying possible beneficial effects of moderate amounts of alcohol consumption.

Descriptors: Demography, alcohol-related pathology, pharmacology.

135. Mishara, B. L.; Kastenbaum, R. ; Baker, F. ; and Patterson, R. D. Alcohol effects in old age: An experimental investigation. Social Science and Medicine, 1975, 9, 535-547.

Assessment of psychological and physical effects of alcohol covers two different elderly populations (nursing home and residence). Randomly chosen subjects receive two servings of different beverages and then are interviewed about medical and psychological information or subjected to physical examinations (electrocardiograms, blood tests, etc.). Negative psychosocial and physical changes are not attributable to alcohol consumption, whereas increased morale, improved cognitive ability, and better sleeping habits did correlate. Implications for structured use of alcoholic beverages are discussed.

Descriptors: Alcohol benefits, psychosocial changes, therapy.

136. Municchi, L. Studio statîstico-clînico sulle psicòsi alcoòlica
asservate nel-l'ospedale psichiàtrico de alessandria nel
perîodo 1954-1965. Rassegna di Studi Psichiàtrichi, 1967,
56, 433-456.
   Alcoholic psychosis is observed at the psychiatric hospital
of Alessandria between 1954 and 1965. During this 12-year period
the admissions show a steadily rising incidence of alcoholism among
elderly patients unrelated to concurrent fluctuations in socioeconomic
patterns. Reasons for this increased incidence include longer life
expectancy and freer accessibility to alcohol and medication.
   Descriptors: Hospital admissions, cultural trends.

137. Murdock, H. R. Effect of table wines on blood glucose levels
in the geriatric subject. Geriatrics, 1972, 27, 93-96.
   Clinical study reports on whether table wines have adverse
effects on blood glucose levels in elderly people. Regular wine and
table wine (or dilute aqueous solutions of ethanol comparable to
ethanol content of wine) are given to 100 subjects. Regular wine
produces a definite decrease in blood glucose, but it remains the
same for diluted ethanol. Glucose stability is probably due to car-
bohydrates in the wine being too low to affect glucose levels. Effects
of relaxation and tranquility, also produced from regular wine, are
absent after ingesting diluted alcohol.
   Descriptors: Blood glucose level, alcohol-related pathology,
diluted alcohol.

138. Myers, A. R. Evidence for cohort or generational differences
in the drinking behavior of older adults. International
Journal of Aging and Human Development, 1981-82, 14,
31-44.
   Intensified cross-sectional study of Boston's elderly indicates generational (cohort) pattern of drinking behavior. Examined
are possible epidemiologic conditions endemic to Boston that foster
drinking tendencies within the mainstream of metropolitan and surrounding urban areas.
   Descriptors: Epidemiology, drinking patterns.

139. NIAAA Information and Feature Service, December 31, 1982.
   Special issue is devoted to an extensive coverage of current
debate and issues concerning elderly alcoholic problems. Research
and treatment conflicts compounded by both professionals and public
media are clarified in short articles written by guest columnists.
Directory assistance is provided to clinical agencies and clearinghouse materials for addicted elderly or direct service workers (para-
professionals, volunteers, etc.) involved in elderly programs.
   Descriptors: Clearinghouse, current issues.

140. Negrete, J. C. , and Macpherson, A. Comparative study of
matrimonial adaptation of "active" and "cured" alcoholics.
Acta Psiquiatrica y Psicológica de America Latina, 1966,

12, 251-256.

Study investigates three types of couples--with alcoholic husbands, with cured alcoholic husbands, and with nonalcoholic husbands. Demographic similarities are held constant (Anglo-Saxon, white, Protestant, well-educated, middle-aged Canadians). Significant differences for nonalcoholic husbands related to household administration and social functioning. Sexual adjustment and anxiety control, however, are more significant for husbands who are alcoholic. Marital satisfaction and relations with other family members are additionally split between alcoholic and nonalcoholic husbands.

Descriptors: Marital satisfaction, alcoholic men.

141. Neurobiological interactions between aging and alcohol abuse. Alcoholism: Clinical and Experimental Research, 1982, 6, 1-53.

Seven articles drawn from a symposium on neurobiological correlates examine aging and alcoholism. They describe experimental findings gathered on behavioral effects of ethanol, brain structure, premature aging, cognitive patterns, and advancements in evoked brain potential research. Theoretical articles appearing also include toxicity effects and the Continuum (evolutional) account of natural aging.

Descriptors: Alcohol-related pathology.

142. Nolan, A.J., and Peretz, D.I. Beer as an adjunct to the low sodium diet. British Columbia Medical Journal, 1973, 15, 300-302.

Describes use of beer for providing relief from the "monotony" of low sodium diets without adding significantly to the sodium input. Qualities of beer highly regarded include its "salty" taste, appetite-stimulant, and mild diuretic effect. Sodium potassium content in domestically brewed beers in British Columbia are explored in the management of geriatric patients.

Descriptors: Beer, sodium potassium.

143. Nussenfeld, S.R.; Davis, J.H.; and Nagel, E.L. Alcohol benefit for the geriatric patient. Journal of the American Medical Association, 1974, 227, 439-440.

Examined carefully are results of the "Miami Sudden Cardiac Death Study." After examining autopsies of 118 consecutive cases, harmful effects on heart tissue are not significant between heavy alcohol users and nonusers with respect to chronic coronary artery stenosis or acute heart vessel or muscle damage. These results contravene previous reports of a possible alcohol benefit to geriatric patients and protective effect of alcohol on a myocardial infarction.

Descriptors: Coronary disease, alcohol-related pathology.

144. Older problem drinkers. Alcohol Health and Research World, Spring 1975, 12-17.

Capsulating review of elderly alcoholism and the problems responsible for it. Advancing age engenders problems of boredom, poor health, inadequate support and increasing isolation from community and family. Elderly individuals who turn to alcohol for consolation are among the least visible alcoholics in society and have special needs inadequately being met by senior service agencies. Reported here are also confirmatory data from a New York study of 65- to 74-year-olds revealing that elderly widowers are the most highly susceptible candidates for drinking.

Descriptors: Aging, social service needs.

145. Opstelten, G. E. Island of Sobriety for the Frail Elderly. Paper presented at the San Francisco Conference on Aging and Alcoholism, San Francisco, August 1981.

Program alternatives for elderly inebriates are offered in this position paper that incorporates didactic and experimental data collected by North of Market Senior Alcohol Program. Comprehensive training is for (a) alcohol-related problems (b) illness of alcoholism, and (c) problems related to legal drug use or abuse. Called "Island of Sobriety for the Frail Elderly," it represents a continuum of care philosophy targeted for home and community counseling. Specific program components include (1) modified medical detoxification, (2) residential treatment program, (3) extended residential room and board, and (4) community follow-up.

Descriptors: Social casework, community programs.

146. Pace, C.; Riboni, E.; and Taffon, C. L'elettrocardiogramma nell'alcoolismo crònico: Studio dell'onda. Minerva Cardioangiol, 1972, 20, 231-233.

Electrocardiogram (EKG) readings taken of 80 alcoholics, aged 30 to 60 years, are reported regarding abnormalities. Abnormal and modified "U" and "T" waves indicate altered permeability of membranes, or disturbances due to abrupt or gradually diminishing changes in the intermediate mitochondrial metabolism. Utility of EKG in prediagnostic measures is considered.

Descriptors: Alcohol-related pathology, electrocardiogram.

147. Pader, E. Clinical heart disease and electrocardiographic abnormalities in alcoholics. Quarterly Journal of Studies on Alcohol, 1973, 34, 774-785.

Results of EKGs of 100 alcoholic men (ages 46 to 64) are randomly selected from employees in a medical department. Incidence of preliminary heart disease was questioned in subjects drinking beer and spirits, spirits alone, and beer alone. Among cardiac abnormalities are enlargement of hearts, resting tachycardia, sinus bardycardia, rhythm disturbances, first-degree A-V block and discontinuous T and P waves. Hypothesized is that abnormalities emerging in early stages of alcoholic cardiomyopathy may be potentially reversible with abstinence.

Descriptors: Cardiomyopathy, electrocardiogram, alcohol-related pathology.

148. Parker, B. M. The effects of ethyl alcohol on the heart. Journal of the American Medical Association, 1974, 228, 741-742.

Recognition that ethyl alcohol may be associated with heart disease and is a direct myocardial toxin is supported by clinical focus on its pathology and potential treatability. Author examines this morphologic abnormality in elderly alcoholics based on four observations:

First, patients with myocardial disease of unexplained cause are frequently alcoholics. Second, ingestion of alcohol creates dysfunctional release of phosphate, potassium, glutamic oxaloacetic transaminase, and isocitric and malic dehydrogenases. Third, alcoholics without apparent heart disease manifest decreased myocardial contractility. And fourth, cardiac failure in a nutritionally balanced alcoholic is common after ingesting 12 to 16 ounces of Scotch whiskey daily.

Descriptors: Cardiomyopathy, alcohol-related pathology.

149. Pascarelli, E. F. , and Fischer, W. Drug dependence in the elderly. International Journal of Aging and Human Development, 1974, 5, 347-356.

Contravening evidence is shown that alcoholism and drug dependence persist with old age. Elderly street addicts continue drug use while making certain economically motivated changes in drug selection, dosage, or purchasing strategies. Since considerable misuse of legal drugs is reported among elderly, authors consider the elderly prone to dependency on psychotropic compounds dispensed for treatment of loneliness and aging. Alternative approaches are proposed for public policy dealing with alcohol and drug abuse in the geriatric population.

Descriptors: Drug abuse, policy changes.

150. Patients drink beer in hospital pub. Journal of the American Medical Association, 1970, 212, 1801-1804.

Attempts to use beer therapy in a geropsychiatric ward are elaborated. Induced social activity and overall improvements in psychopathology are among the immediate changes observed. Support for beer therapy is weighed against conflicting reports regarding its impact on development of heart disease.

Descriptors: Beer, cardiac disease.

151. Patterson, R. D. ; Abrahams, R. ; and Baker, F. Preventing self-destructive behavior. Geriatrics, 1974, 29, 115-118.

Survey results of a representative sample of 445 persons over 65 in Boston who reportedly engage in self-injurious habits. Alcoholism accounts for only seven respondents, most of whom develop it in old age. Self-inflictions indirectly related to alcohol and drug abuse largely constitute the percentage of dermatologic and nutritional problems.

Descriptors: Self-injurious behavior.

152. Peck, D. G. Alcohol abuse and the elderly: Social control and conformity. Journal of Drug Issues, 1979, 9, 63-71.

Argued is that alcohol use and abuse by the aged has been improperly addressed by gerontological and alcohol literature. Demographics on elderly alcoholic abuse in the United States are compared to national aging trends. Author also explores aspects of sociological theories on deviance (conformity to social establishments, etc.) that apply to medical noncompliance and attitudinal change by society.

Descriptors: Epidemiology, review.

153. Pemberton, D. A. A comparison of the outcome of treatment in female and male alcoholics. British Journal of Psychiatry, 1967, 113, 367-373.
    Tabulated results are drawn from social, psychological, and psychiatric measures of 50 male and 50 female elderly alcoholics recently discharged from the hospital. Statistically significant findings include (a) fewer females remained abstinent, (b) "neurotics" were reasonably curable, and (c) intellectual impairment resulting from alcohol conformed to a poor prognosis. Relatively few score variables are different on psychological tests (e. g. , MMPI, 16PF, etc.).
    Descriptors: Treatment outcome, intelligence.

154. Peppers, L G. , and Stover, R. G. Elderly abuser: A challenge for the future. Journal of Drug Issues, 1979, 9, 73-83.
    South Carolina pilot program shows that 5, 279 of 5, 500 elderly persons (55 and over) indicate alcohol as a primary substance abuse problem. Characteristics of the sample relevant to results are that subjects are predominately white, unemployed, have low educational levels, median annual household incomes (estimated $12, 200), and are married living with spouses. Primary and secondary referrals made by social and medical agencies to both in- and out-of-state programs account for under half of the targeted subjects. Implied by these data is that elderly abuse is underestimated and underreported, resulting in inadequate treatment modalities.
    Descriptors: Drinking patterns, referral services.

155. Plutchik, R. , and Discipio, W. J. Personality patterns in chronic alcoholism (Korsakoff's syndrome), chronic schizophrenia, and geriatric patients with chronic brain syndrome. Journal of the American Geriatrics Society, 1974, 22, 514-516.
    Comparative study of chronic alcoholics (with Korsakoff's syndrome), chronic schizophrenics, and geriatric patients with chronic brain (organic) syndromes drawn from a long-term state hospital facility. Personality traits of being gregarious, obedient, timid, and having poor self-control appear for Korsakoffs, which is tantamount to patterns noted in geriatric patients. Typological similarity seriously questions the need for a "unique" alcoholic personality category.
    Descriptors: Personality patterns, Korsakoff's syndrome.

156. Plutchik, R.; McCarthy, M.; and Hall, B. H. Changes in elderly welfare hotel residents during a one-year period. Journal of American Geriatrics Society, 1975, 23, 265-270.
    Describes a survey study of 100 hotel occupants in Manhattan (17 elderly alcoholics) who participate in structured interviews one year after a new program for residents began. Alcoholic residents report positive changes in greater proportion than other residents, possibly because an alcoholic counselor is a full-time member on the project staff. Residential in-house training developments are advised for similar facilities and for programs involved in outreach services.

Descriptors: Training program, residential facility.

157. Porch, B. E. , and Rada, R. T. Alcohol and Language Function. (Report no. ZO-37820 1). Washington, DC: U. S. Veterans Administration, Department of Medicine and Surgery, 1977.
Effects of chronic alcoholism on language function are examined in 35 diagnosed alcoholics, none of whom have known histories of verbal deficits, central nervous sytem trauma, severe or chronic medical disease, liver or neurologic disease, or psychosis. Inpatient subjects undergo a psychometric battery (Index of Communicative Ability, Raven's Coloured Progressive Matrixes, Word Fluency Test, and Token Test) during the first and third week. Lower performance by subjects compared to control groups suggests that effective communicative skills lost while drinking are possibly reversible.
Descriptors: Language, psychometric tests.

158. Posey, E. , and Windham, G. D. Problem Drinking and the Aged DWI Offender. Conference paper at Mississippi State University, 1977.
Study attempts to locate problem elderly drinkers and determine if they differ significantly from the nonproblem drinker in driving reports (cf. Miss. Alcohol Safety Education Program). Apart from types of alcohol consumed, groups differ in that higher proportions of drinkers experience preadult socialization with alcohol. Advantages from the Gordon Parent Effectiveness Training for parent-adolescent problems are provided.
Descriptors: Alcoholic socialization, DWI.

159. Price, J. H. , and Andrews, P. Alcohol abuse in the elderly. Journal of Gerontological Nursing, 1982, 8, 16-19.
Reported statistics show that approximately 10 to 15 percent of general elderly populace suffers from alcoholism. Types of elderly susceptible to drinking and drug-drug interactions are described along with tables and charts. Refuted is the contention that infrequent referrals are due to health professionals' belief that elderly are too old for beneficial treatment. Advancing the nurse's role in appropriate therapy is a proposed solution to alleviate this and several concomitant problems that are enumerated.
Descriptors: Alcohol-related pathology, nurses, referral service.

160. Rathbone-McCuan, E. , and Bland, J. A treatment typology for the elderly alcohol abuser. Journal of the American Geriatrics Society, 1975, 23, 553-557.
Unrecognized aspects of elderly alcohol abuse are attributed to the clinician's frequent failure to understand alcoholism and to physical, mental, and social problems that complicate diagnosis. Presented is a diagnostic and treatment typology that facilitates the implementation of social support systems and affordable resources for prospective clients. Long-range benefits include an integrated and comprehensive treatment service.

Descriptors: Referral services, treatment programs, attitudes.

161. Rathbone-McCuan, E. , and Hashimi, J. Elder alcohol abuse and isolation. In Isolated Elders: Health and Social Intervention. Rockville, MD: Aspen Systems, 1982.
Treatment barriers preventing the resolution of depression and emotional isolation are interpreted as links to alcoholism. Elderly victims of this social stagnation go unnoticed. This chapter introduces alternative ways to treat aging alcoholics through intervention strategies in which eligibility for third-party payment is necessary. Full reimbursement of services would serve a motivational function in the casefinding process.
Descriptors: Third-party payment isolation, service delivery systems.

162. Rathbone-McCuan, E.; Lohn, H.; Levenson, J.; and Hsu, J. Community Survey of Aged Alcoholics and Problem Drinkers. (Report no. 1R18-AA01734-01). Rockville, MD: National Institute on Alcohol Abuse and Alcoholism, 1976.
Sociodemographic survey taken of 695 persons aged 55 and over in domiciliary settings in Baltimore. Interview data on health status, medication, alcohol consumption, social participation and service utilization show the rate of problem drinking to be highest in single, divorced or separated males who are unemployed. Highest prevalence by domiciliary residents also includes more alienation, poorer health status, and approximately 85 percent not receiving treatment for alcoholism. Several report taking medications that preclude alcohol use but without adequate education about repercussions. One option recommended concerns day care centers.
Descriptors: Demography, service delivery systems.

163. Rathbone-McCuan, E. , and Roberds, L. A. Treatment of the older female alcoholic. Focus on Women: Journal of Addictions and Health, 1980, 1, 104-129.
Program evaluation issues are raised in two sections devoted to older female alcoholics. First, planning and treatment provisions are outlined. Secondly, data from a pilot study in a Midwest treatment center contrast younger, middle-aged, and older women with respect to multiple drug abuse, areas of treatment relative to aging, and availability of inpatient hospital programs offering relief for the emotional aspects of abuse behavior.
Descriptors: Alcoholic females, treatment goals.

164. Rathbone-McCuan, E. , and Triegaardt, J. The older alcoholic and the family. Alcohol Health and Research World, 1979, 3, 7-12.
Describes a survey undertaken by a school of social work of alcoholics in inpatient treatment programs. Results challenge the belief that family involvement in treatment is unnecessary, since 34 cases (of 63) reveal some pattern of family involvement. Families realize their previous behavior is inadvertently supportive of drinking and would limit the older person's entry into treatment. Encouragement is given to expand existing family networks in alcohol

education.
Descriptors: Family, service delivery.

165. Regodon, V. G. Alcoholism in old age. Actas Luso-Españolas de Neurología, Psiquiatría y Ciencias Afines, 1974, 2, 3-14.
     The notion of "belated alcoholism" is defined as onset of alcoholism after 60 years of age. Precipitating characteristics explored include traumatic development, progressive decline in alcohol consumption (before 60), and generally good prognosis. Anecdotal events related to antisocial behavior, institutionalization and "skid row" typology offer further distinctions.
     Descriptors: Precipitation, prognosis, "belated alcoholism."

166. Reic, P.; Borcic, R.; Luksic, P.; Uglestic, B. Effect of alcoholism on the course and prognosis of cerebral vascular disease. Alcoholism, 1972, 8, 65-70.
     Investigates effects of alcoholism on atherosclerosis in patients with cerebrovascular disease over a span of four years. Alcoholism is shown to exert influence on increasing the incidence of cerebral hemorrhage and higher mortality rates. Similar distinctions are absent for cases of cerebral thrombosis. Conclusions are that alcoholism may aggravate or delay recovery of patients from cerebrovascular damage.
     Descriptors: Cerebrovascular disease, therapy.

167. Riccitelli, M. L. Alcoholism in the aged--modern concepts. Journal of the American Geriatrics Society, 1967, 15, 142-147.
     Overview of sociologic concepts in alcoholism literature arguing that alcoholism is a mental and physical disease that is progressive and produces irreversible pathology. Assumptive evidence is presented on the interplay between factors of heredity, environment, and personality. Diagnostic hazards in misprescribing alcohol for pain-relieving purposes are attributed to the difficulty physicians have with distinguishing social drinkers from alcoholics. Effective therapy is recommended that requires more definite delineation between etiology and treatment.
     Descriptors: Demography, alcoholism concepts, etiology.

168. Richardson, A. M. Androgyny: How it affects drinking practices: A comparison of female and male alcoholics. Focus on Women: Journal of Addictions and Health, 1981, 2, 116-131.
     Prediction analysis techniques guide the study of comparisons between men and women alcoholics selected from Washington, D. C. Measures of androgyny and drinking behaviors from the Michigan Alcohol Screening Test and the PRF ANDRO (for sex identification) lend support to the hypothesis that women who possess androgynous sex role identities drink less than nonandrogynous women. Theories of sexism inherent in mental health interventions complement these findings. Androgyny data also presumably offer a better standard for mental health than does the traditional masculine and

feminine stereotypes.
Descriptors: Androgyny, drinking patterns.

169. Riege, W. H.; Cherkin, A.; and Greenblatt, M. Development of a Modernized Set of Quantitative Tests of Memory Function in Patients. (Report no. ZO-35157 2). Washington, DC: U. S. Veterans Administration, Department of Medicine and Surgery, 1976.

Memory dysfunctions are typically too elusive for precise measurement. The addition of "content reference" in a memory test battery enables the assessment of 112 geriatric patients from psychiatric and rehabilitation services. Experimental and multidimensional evaluations of differently categorized patients reveal two major results: material-specific memory deficits and inconsistent retrieval. For chronic alcoholics, retention of verbal or visual-spatial information (not auditory) is impaired as much as for Korsakoff patients. Collaborative studies showing there are emotional correlates to memory loss are considered in reference to lateralized brain pathology.
Descriptors: Memory, neuropsychology, Korsakoff.

170. Riege, W. H.; Greenblatt, M.; Cherkin, A.; and Jarvik, L. F. Quantitative Tests of Memory Function in Patients. (Report no. ZO-39951). Washington, DC: U. S. Veterans Administration, Department of Medicine and Surgery, 1977.

Memory functions manipulated through a psychological battery suggest changes in cerebral pathology. Component memory and perceptual processes descriptive of cognitive ability are measured in elderly alcoholics using quantitative memory tests that are sensitive to discrepancies between impairment and focal brain pathology. After removing covariant influences, data suggest the retraining of memory failures may involve context-specific techniques and recognition of emotional trauma.
Descriptors: Memory, neuropsychology, cerebral pathology.

171. Rix, K. J. Elderly alcoholics in the Edinburgh psychiatric services. Journal of the Royal Society of Medicine, 1982, 75, 177-180.

Elderly alcoholics in the Edinburgh psychiatric services are interviewed during a five-month period and matched against 30 young alcoholics. Groups show similarity except in terms of chronic organic brain disease and in generational attitudes. Excluding organic-syndromed elderly, the older alcoholics should be treated in age-mixed groups in general psychiatry specialized alcoholism services. Departure from traditional age segregational systems is encouraged.
Descriptors: Age differences.

172. Rodstein, M. Ischemic and hypertensive heart disease in the aged: Prognostic and therapeutic factors. Journal of the American Geriatrics Society, 1980, 28, 388-397.

Review of critical heart disorders with special attention on ischemic and hypertensive heart pathology induced by moderate ingestion of whiskey, wine, or beer. These compounds are high risk factors because they elevate high-density lipoprotein cholesterol levels in about 10 percent of abstainers. Correlations are also noted between alcohol consumption and absence of occlusive coronary artery disease in persons over 60. Finally, angina and coronary heart disease are predicted from prescriptive amounts of exercise and alcohol.

Descriptors: Coronary heart disease, exercise.

173. Rosenberg, N.; Goldberg, I.; Irving, D.; and Williams, G. W. Alcoholism and drunken driving: Evidence from psychiatric and driver registers. Quarterly Journal of Studies on Alcohol, 1972, 33, 1129-1143.
Residents registered on the Md Psychiatric Case Register (those receiving services around District of Columbia) are matched against those on the National Driver Register, with licenses revoked, suspended or withdrawn. Registrants who are psychiatrically diagnosed as alcoholic correlate on sociopathic scales to nonalcoholic residents, but have more organic brain disorders reported. Estimated by this study is that 7 percent of convicted white male drunk drivers are alcoholics.

Descriptors: Drunk driving, organic brain syndrome.

174. Rosin, A. J. , and Glatt, M. M. Alcohol excess in the elderly. Quarterly Journal of Studies on Alcohol, 1971, 32, 53-59.
Details are presented on precipitating causes, demographic characteristics, beverage preferences, and excessive drinking habits of 103 elderly patients in England. Half of the geriatric patients are over 80, with their prominent personality factors being dementia, bereavement, and loneliness. Study concludes that environmental circumstances contribute more than personality factors to elderly alcoholism, although they easily can distort diagnostic impressions or contaminate physiologic correlates of alcoholism.

Descriptors: Personality factors, environment.

175. Ruben, D. H. , and Kaiser, W. W. Morality and alcoholism: Tracing the origin and dangers of a cultural myth. Spada Sage (Specialty Program in Alcohol and Drug Abuse), 1983, 3, 4-11.
Historiographic analysis of the morality-alcoholism myth from its origin in pre-Hellenic periods to the establishment of social constructs and attitudes in contemporary theory. Data tracing this evolutionary pattern and effects on special populations (elderly, disabled, etc.) are gathered from a number of book and journal publications. Moral adulterates in medical, legal and psychological institutions largely responsible for the misguided perspectives of alcoholism are explored and replaced by reformulated concepts.

Descriptors: Historiography, psychology, morality.

176. Ruben, D. H.; Perra, R. G.; and Baker, R. J. The validity and standardization of drug addict population norms for the Rathus Assertiveness Schedule. Spada Sage (Specialty Program in Alcohol and Drug Abuse), 1983, 3,1-4.
Study attempts to succeed prior research on social skills development by focusing the evaluation question on standardization and validity of the Rathus Assertiveness Schedule (RAS) norms for drug

addict and alcoholic populations. Participants included 23 male and female outpatients between 16 and 77 whose primary diagnosis is substance abuse. Two interview sessions (both recorded on audio-tape) and the completion of the RAS and another matched test (A-RAS) reveal distinctions on the RAS inconsistent with previous research. Findings further stress the practical application of analogue assessment methodology to supplement traditional face-to-face intake.
Descriptors: Rathus Assertiveness Schedule, social skills, outpatients.

177. Schenkenberg, T.; Dustman, R. E.; and Beck, E. C. Changes in the Excitability Cycle of the Visual Evoked Response During Aging. (Report no. ZO-31436 4). Washington, DC: U. S. Veterans Administration, Department of Medicine and Surgery, 1975.
Reviews year-long study of nervous system affecting the visual and somatosensory evoked responses of middle-aged alcoholics and normal elderly. Perceptual, intellectual, and sensory tests administered to these subjects show striking similarity. Evoked responses on the sensory-perceptual tests also proved similar, although manifested differences are explored for future research.
Descriptors: Sensory evoked responses, perceptual ability.

178. Schmitt, A. F. Study of personality characteristics as predictors of treatment outcome of young and old alcoholic patients. Dissertation Abstracts International, 1976, 76-19758.
Personality characteristics are examined as predictors of alcoholic recovery in young (17-25 years) and older (26 and over) patients. Psychological profiles consisting of MMPI, The Comprey Personality Scale, and State Trait Anxiety Inventory provide comparisons on success and failure rates. Younger patients leave facilities with more "mature" attitudes and their level of depression decreases below number of psychosomatic complaints. Older patients entering with more diverse characteristics stay longer in the treatment facility.
Descriptors: Personality characteristics, treatment outcome.

179. Schuckit, M. A. Phenomenology and treatment of alcoholism in the elderly. In W. E. Fann (ed.) Phenomenology and Treatment of Alcoholism. Jamaica, NY: Spectrum Publishers, 1980.
Rehabilitative process by which elderly undergo recovery from alcoholism is interpreted within an historical, epidemiologic and individual process. Chapter's focus on phenomenology explores the personal transition from resistance to acceptance by the client during clinical course of treatment. Suggestions for directive versus non-directive group psychotherapies appear in context.
Descriptors: Phenomenology, rehabilitation, group therapy.

180. Schuckit, M. A. Alcoholism and the Elderly. Paper presented at the San Francisco Conference on Aging and Alcoholism.

San Francisco, August 1981.

Scope of diagnostic problems in identifying sociocultural and natural history are sorted regarding elderly alcoholism. Review also covers alcohol-related pathologies and reasons that health care deliverers mistake neuropsychological (organic brain) syndromes for symptoms of the aging process.

Descriptors: Alcohol-related pathology, demography.

181. Schuckit, M. A. The history of psychotic symptoms in alcoholics. Journal of Clinical Psychiatry, 1982, 43, 53-57.

History of psychotic symptomatology is reviewed in 220 male admissions. Group comparisons revealed in the survey are that symptoms are associated with less early life stability, higher levels of adult antisocial behavior, and significant use of illegal drugs. Psychotic versus nonpsychotic groups show no correlation between symptoms and personal or familial history of schizophrenia. Transient hallucinations and delusions appear for 43 percent of the sampled psychotics.

Descriptors: Mental health, psychosis, history.

182. Schuckit, M. A.; Atkinson, J. H.; Miller, P. L.; and Berman, J. Three-year follow-up of elderly alcoholics. Journal of Clinical Psychiatry, 1980, 41, 412-416.

Mental health evaluation consists of 280 consecutive seniors after three years from discharge. Course of alcoholism is either active or in remission for 11 percent, whereas 20 percent of those surviving remain abstinent. Affective disorders and dementia are prominent psychiatric symptoms arising during follow-up interviews. Diagnosed symptoms also characterize a percentage of the sample with higher mortality rates over three years.

Descriptors: Mental health, program evaluation.

183. Schuckit, M. A., and Gunderson, E. K. Alcoholism in young men. U. S. Naval Health Research Center Report, 1975, January.

Two samples of young Naval alcoholics when compared to older alcoholics indicate higher number of hospitalizations for younger group. Authors argue that heavy drinking by young men is insufficiently predictive of alcoholism but rather suggests an underlying character disorder poorly diagnosed. Revised criteria for alcoholism admission standards are advised for reducing misdiagnosis caused by false assumptions and stereotypes.

Descriptors: Age differences, Navy personnel, demography.

184. Schuckit, M. A., and Miller, P. L. Alcoholism in Elderly Men: A Survey of a General Medical Ward. Presented at the 6th Annual Medical-Scientific Session of the National Alcoholism Forum, Milwaukee, April 1975.

Determined rates of alcoholism in geriatric patients admitted to different medical wards is reported using three instruments (besides an interview): Memory-for-designs test, the pfeiffer tests, the mental status questionnaire, and the face-hand test. Self-reported accounts of social and drinking behavior are verified after interviewing significant others. Inactive and active alcohol abusers typically are younger, married more often, more likely to divorce or be separated, or achieve higher educational and occupational levels. Examined in depth are demographic interrelationships between psychiatric and alcoholic patients.

Descriptors: Mental health, memory, drinking patterns.

185. Schuckit, M A.; Miller, P. L.; and Berman, J. Three year course of psychiatric problems in a geriatric population. Journal of Clinical Psychiatry, 1980, 41, 27-32.
    Psychiatric disorders are examined in 276 elderly men admitted for various surgical and medical problems three years ago. Identified disorders diagnosed during initial interview include affective disorders, atherosclerotic dementia, and senile dementia. Surviving patients (N = 7) who originally received no diagnosis are now chronic alcoholics. Interpreted for research are the weighted advantages in outcome follow-up of alcoholic patients.

Descriptors: Psychiatry, mental health.

186. Schuckit, M. A.; Morrissey, E. R.; and O'Leary, M. R. Alcohol problems in elderly men and women. Addictive Diseases, 1978, 3, 405-416.
    Traces developmental stages in alcoholic dependency of elderly. Male and female patients from two different treatment centers undergo interviews about the events precipitating their drinking. Women over 55 have two to three years of alcoholism before hospitalization, and middle-aged patients frequently lose their jobs, have car accidents, or are divorced and separated before hospitalization. Older men drink up to 15 years before hospitalization and show less prevalence of psychiatric illness.

Descriptors: Etiology, mental health, psychiatry.

187. Shropshire, R. Hidden faces of alcoholism. Geriatrics, 1975, 30, 99-102.
    Discusses problems physicians face in diagnosing alcoholism. Attitudes toward alcoholism and the drinker, symptomatic complications, substance abuse, and procedural barriers enter into the overall phases of decision. Physicians are encouraged to recognize alcohol as a drug compounded by both pharmacologic and disease considerations rather than to treat it as a moral issue. Subacute and chronic elderly alcoholics viewed in this perspective would enable positive attitudes toward younger alcoholics.

Descriptors: Attitudes, age.

188. Silverman, E. M., and Silverman, A. G. Granulocyte adherence in the elderly. American Journal Clinical Pathology, 1977, 67, 49-52.
    Granulocyte adherence is studied in 57 elderly as compared to 50 control patients. Those ingesting alcohol within 24 hours of the evaluation show lower mean adherence. Elderly persons in both beer-drinking and distilled-spirit groups have similar results and this persists after ingestion of aspirin, chlorothiazides, methyldopa, digitalis, antihistamines, and barbiturates. Major difference presented is the higher adherence in older over younger patients.

Descriptors: Granulocyte adherence, alcohol-related pathology.

189. Simmons, H. J.; Hainsworth, W. C.; and Ishler, G. H. The Psychobiological Assessment of Brain Damage. (Report no. ZO-31889-3). Washington, DC: U. S. Veterans Administration, Department of Medicine and Surgery, 1975.
   Chronic brain syndrome is put into perspective with respect to excessive alcoholism, sensory-motor deficits, and subcortical factors. Results show that subcortical functions playing a more significant role than cortical mechanisms (when nervous sytem deficits are present) may render standard neuropsychological tests of little use. Neurologic correlates are analyzed according to psychological and physiological factors, chronic brain syndrome diagnoses, and treatment factors of alcoholism.
   Descriptors: Chronic brain syndrome, alcohol-related pathology, neuropsychology.

190. Simpson, D. D. , and Lloyd, M. R. Alcohol use following treatment for drug addiction. A four-year follow-up. Quarterly Journal of Studies on Alcohol, 1981, 42, 323-325.
   Recidivist rate of elderly alcoholics following treatment for varying drug abuse is statistically significant in comparison studies. After-care programs for recovered elderly abusers are insufficiently protective against interest in alcoholism, unless support is provided from polydrug users. Therapeutic alternatives to anticipate titrational effects of polydrug use are described.
   Descriptors: Follow-up, polydrug.

191. Smart, R. G. , and Liban, C. B. Predictors of problem drinking among elderly, middle-aged and youthful drinkers. Journal of Psychoactive Drugs, 1981, 13, 153-163.
   Factor analysis performed on employment status, drinking frequency, and socioeconomic status of adults aged 18 and over are interpreted as predictors to potential alcohol abuse. Questionnaire surveys show four consistent patterns. First, younger (18-25 years) persons drink more than those in the elderly group (60 years and over), but elderly alcoholism is harder to predict. Second, profile of the elderly alcoholic is characterized as male, not retired, in lower income bracket, and frequently drinking in small quantities. Third, prevalence of dependency symptoms is high among all groups surveyed. And fourth, several background variables unexplained by diagnostic evaluation are attributed to dependency symptoms.
   Descriptors: Drinking patterns, age comparison.

192. Smith, P. Nonpenal rehabilitation for the chronic alcoholic offender. Federal Probation, 1968, 32, 46-50.
   Experimental program for alcoholic offenders with a history of multiple arrests is an alternative to routine penal detention. Voluntary treatment involves a 60-day modified sentence and participation in rehabilitative programs. Success or failure in the study is more significantly related to age than education or intelligence. Older offenders (40 and above) remain in the program longer despite their

chronicity and resistance to other forms of treatment. Implications are that disabled elderly rather than law-breakers may benefit more from current program.

Descriptors: Penal system, rehabilitation.

193. Snyder, P. K. , and Way, A. Alcoholism and the elderly. Aging, 1979, 291, 8-11.

Identification of the elderly problem drinker represents a shifting paradigm in medical diagnosis. Educational programs for medical personnel are recommended to increase recognition of alcohol symptoms. So, too, education for the elderly could alert them to dangers of mixing alcohol with medications. Outlook for alcoholism in existing social service network for senior citizens is explored and developments in gerontology reviewed.

Descriptors: Education, social services, treatment.

194. Snyder, V. Aging, alcoholism, and reactions to loss. Social Work, 1977, 22, 232-233.

Discusses the rejection of elderly and elderly alcoholics who channel emotional grief over loss in socially unacceptable ways. Imposed perceptions on old age are persistent obstacles to understanding the bereavement process. Social expectations of behavior tend to be "age-related" rather than focus on how the removal of meaningful situations invoke atypical reactions. Reformulated perspectives on viewing the elderly reaction in reference to situations are given.

Descriptors: Social behavior, attitudes.

195. Sober Days, Golden Years: Alcoholism and the Older Person. Minneapolis, MN: Johnson Institute, 1981.

Explanatory manual focuses on medical, social, and treatment issues pertinent to the etiology and rehabilitation of elderly alcoholism. Alcohol and polydrug abuse is a topic warranting increased attention by community programs in Minnesota. This manual thus provides a list of agencies and organizations in Minnesota appropriate for referral.

Descriptors: Johnson Institute, etiology, social services.

196. Special Population Issues: Alcohol and Health Monograph No. 4. Washington, DC: U. S. Government Printing Office, 1982.

Unrecognized special populations of alcohol and drug abuse have certain needs described in this collection of research papers. The most recent scientific contributions in areas of biological consequences, prevention, diagnosis and treatment, traffic accidents, and educational programs clearly remove the traditional myths and assumptions believed true for certain racial and ethnic groups. Alcoholic females, youth, elderly, and American Indians are among the representative populations covered.

Descriptors: Special populations, research.

197. Squires, S. Alcoholism and the elderly. Democrat & Chronicle, 1982, September 12.

Newspaper article explaining the rapid influx of national concern over elderly alcoholism. Cited statistics for age-related pathology show an unprecedented 70 percent of elderly alcoholics contract a disease after age 60. Prominent factors in the alcoholic's evolution consist of loneliness, stress, health problems, bereavement, self-doubts about death, and society's prevailing unsympathetic attitude toward the aged. Treatment statistics on the outcome success with elderly are contrasted to disadvantages in public costs absorbed by medicare services.

Descriptors: Medicare, alcohol-related pathology, attitudes.

198. Study of Alcohol Effects on Old Age. Boston, MA: Socio Technical Systems, Assoc. , 1973.

Physical and emotional characteristics of elderly people varying with alcohol consumption are examined within an agency with long-term residents. Questions about subjective feelings and physiological, endocrinologic, and psychological tests compare two groups for acute or chronic effects over a period of time. Prior drinking history is summarized for each subject.

Descriptors: Alcohol-related pathology, test batteries.

199. Teige, B. , and Fleischer, E. Fatal drug alcohol poisoning investigated at the Institute of Forensic Medicine, University of Oslo, during 1977-1979. Tidsskrift Nor Laegeforen, 1981, 101, 1563-1566.

Study traces annual cases admitted to the University of Oslo Forensic Medicine Center during a two-to-three year period of time. Poisoning from alcoholic intoxication, analgesics, barbiturates, and propoxyphene largely comprise the cases and account for several reported suicides. Increases in mortality rate due to adolescent and elderly poisoning are compared longitudinally across admissions of previous year.

Descriptors: Poisoning, mortality, forensic medicine.

200. Treatment of Alcoholics: An Ontario Perspective. (Report no. NCAI-040008). Rockville, MD: National Institute on Alcohol Abuse and Alcoholism, 1978.

Assessed is the magnitude of alcoholism in Ontario and present and future demographic trends expected. Alcoholism-specific resources for elderly (and other populations) are outlined, including hospital and community treatment centers. Basic types of existing treatment resources and projected service costs by alcoholics are contained in different chapters focused on youthful, elderly, female and various ethnic group alcoholics. Ontario's growth in expanding alcoholic recovery opportunities is apparently the underlying theme.

Descriptors: Social services, Ontario.

201. Turner, T. B. ; Bennett, V. L. ; and Hernandez, H. Beneficial side of moderate alcohol use. Johns Hopkins Medical Journal, 1981, 148, 53-63.

Case studies attesting to medicinal benefits from moderate alcohol consumption serve to contrast published evidence against alcohol use. That alcoholic beverages can reduce myocardial infarction

and improve the elderly's general quality of life is based on measured ethanol intake levels at which no adverse health effects are
observed. Authors indicate, however, that current documentation is
inadequate to exclude possible effects of mild consumption on driving
and prenatal health. Contradictory evidence to these studies is examined critically.

Descriptors: Alcohol-related pathology, alcohol benefits.

202. Twigg, W. C. Alcoholism in a home for the aged. Geriatrics,
1959, 14, 391-395.

Individual case history exemplifies that placement of the
elderly alcoholic in a communal facility increases treatment success.
Prognostic indicators in determining if the facility meets a practical
criterion are outlined with recommendations for social reform.

Descriptors: Communal facility, prognosis.

203. U. S. Department of Health, Education and Welfare. Alcohol
use in special population groups. In D. A. Ward (ed.) Alcoholism: Introduction to Theory and Treatment. Dubuque,
IA: Kendall/Hunt, 1980.

Alcohol use in special populations is examined in reference
to women, elderly, American Indians, Spanish-speaking persons, and
Blacks. Accultural aspects inherent in the sociocultural units
of their lives will largely determine which needs are important for
prevention and treatment. American Indians have the highest reported incident of drinking problems and the Black women are proportionally heavier drinkers than white women. Stress factors apparent
in the lifestyle of nearly every group covered are partly to blame for
development of drinking habits.

Descriptors: Special populations, drinking patterns.

204. Van De Vyvere, B. ; Hughes, M. ; and Fish, D. G. Elderly
chronic alcoholic: A practical approach. Canadian Welfare, 1976, 52, 9-13.

This study by a social services department focuses on
living accommodations of 64 elderly chronic alcoholic men. Factors
which facilitate or inhibit individual adjustment in the community are
associated with setting conditions, among which include middle-class
family care home, downtown family care home, downtown hotels, and
downtown boarding homes. Four facilitative variables are that (a)
residents accept elderly as alcoholic, (b) residents tolerate the alcohol consumption, (c) residents find mechanisms to control the drinking, and (d) residents apply sanctions when rules are broken. Boarding homes provide more of these variables than do personal care
homes in which conventional rehabilitation strategies are used.

Descriptors: Resident (environment) social services, rehabilitation.

205. Vannicelli, M. ; Pfau, B. ; and Ryback, R. S. Data attrition in
follow-up studies of alcoholics. Quarterly Journal of Studies on Alcohol, 1976, 37, 1325-1330.

Sixty alcoholic inpatients (ages 20 to 65) are in the original
follow-up sample. Of those responding, the post-treatment evaluation

shows a significant improvement rate. Nonresponders, however, may bias these data and revised procedures to account for missing replies are reviewed. To this extent, methodological changes may greatly challenge the validity of prior follow-up research done on alcoholics and particularly on populations (elderly) rarely accessible after hospital discharge.

Descriptors: Follow-up, methodology.

206. Vestal, R. E.; McGuire, E. A.; Tobin, J. D.; Andres, R.; Norris, A. H., and Mezey, E. Aging and ethanol metabolism. Clinical Pharmacology and Therapeutics, 1977, 21, 343-354.

Effects of aging on eliminative and distributive functions of ethanol in the body are studied in 50 healthy subjects (21 to 81 years old). Injections of ethanol are in a continuous, one-hour infusion at a calculated mean rate, with serial blood samples being taken to verify the concentration. Peak ethanol concentrations in blood water at the end of the infusion period are correlated differently with age. Results suggest that age-related changes in body composition are contributing factors to ethanol metabolism and conjunctive pharmacologic effects.

Descriptors: Ethanol metabolism, alcohol-related pathology, pharmacology.

207. Vojtechovsky, M.; Brezinova, V.; Simane, Z.; and Hort, V. An experimental approach to sleep and aging. Human Development, 1969, 12, 64-72.

Investigates the intimate relationship between sleep and aging in two sleep deprivation experiments. Deprivations of 66 hours for normal subjects and 127 hours for abstainers occur before subjects receive clinical tests. Middle-aged subjects have better mental tolerance to short-term sleep deprivation but more delayed biological reactions to stress. Somatic discomfort and improved mental capacity followed in treatment with centrophenoxine. Implications for use of this therapy in insomniacs and elderly alcoholics are explored.

Descriptors: Sleep, physiology, stress.

208. Voorhees, L.; Stern, B.; and Hilferty, J. Intervention Techniques for the Aging Alcoholic. Presented at the 1981 San Francisco Conference on Aging and Alcoholism, San Francisco, August 1981.

Dynamics of the family systems approach to treatment intervention are helpful in describing the stages of family growth during adjustment of an alcoholic member. Stages consist of denial, control of problem, disorganization, and disassociation. Family stability issues and the "survival roles" parents and siblings will assume in each stage are provided with techniques and described within the therapeutic framework.

Descriptors: Family therapy.

209. Walter, M. A. Drink and Be Merry for Tomorrow We Preach: Alcohol and the Male Menopause in Fiji. IASER Conference on Alcohol Use and Abuse in Papua New Guinea, Waigani, March 1981.

Beneficial accommodations of alcohol in the Lau Islands are contrasted to Western culture. Traditional secularity of distilled spirits in the culture's history accounts for its current acceptance. but only by citizens unconcerned with their figure of authority in the tribe or city-state. Young drinkers alter their preoccupancy with homebrew preparations as they grow older and acquire responsibilities in the community and church.

Descriptors: Cultural patterns, Lau Islands, cultural traditions.

210. Warshaw, A., and Lesser, P. B. Amylase clearance ratio is specific test for pancreatitis. Annals of Surgery, 1975, 181, 314-316.

Hyperamylasemia in older patients with peptic ulcer disease is usually not indicative of acute secondary pancreatitis and treatment may focus on the ulcer. The renal clearance of amylase is a useful approach to confirm or exclude acute pancreatitis from the diagnosis. Testing this hypothesis, 34 subjects hospitalized for abdominal pain, pancreatitis (associated with alcoholism), and significantly elevated serum amylase levels reveal varying clearance ratios of the pancreatitis. Those subjects with no peptic ulcer and those with an ulcer show clearance ratios three times higher than the normal range. Peptic ulcer patients with no pancreatitis had normal clearance ratios.

Descriptors: Pancreatitis, alcohol-related pathology.

211. Wattis, J. P. Alcohol problems in the elderly. Journal of the American Geriatrics Society, 1981, 29, 131-134.

Seven case reports of alcoholism in the elderly are presented to underlie fundamental differences in age-related drinking patterns. Socioeconomic indicators interact with the abrupt or gradual psychological and physiological changes elderly persons experience as their social support systems (family, friends, etc.) dissipate. Equivocations in the aging service network regarding policy and planning strategies that are impractical receive some attention.

Descriptors: Age-related drinking, social services.

212. Webb, J. D.; Ford, J. L.; and Sanjur, D. Food patterns among elderly hospitalized alcholics. Journal of Nutrition for the Elderly, 1980, 1, 101-112.

Food consumption patterns in the elderly's diet greatly reflect personal characteristics. Hospitalized alcoholic veterans with nutritional deficits are evaluated for types and amount of food consumed prior to and during admission. Extent of ethanol effects on deteriorative physical condition and interventions to prevent continual malnutrition are reviewed.

Descriptors: Nutrition, alcohol-related pathology.

213. Wells-Parker, E., and Spencer, B. G. Drinking Patterns, Problem Drinking, and Stress in a Sample of Aged Drinking Drivers: Final Report. (Report No. NCAI-059407). Rockville, MD: National Institute on Alcohol Abuse and Alcoholism, 1980.

Investigated are temporal relationships between onset of stress and drunk driving behavior for individuals over age 60. History surveys conducted on 92 drunk driving offenders and 68 nonoffenders reveal potentially stressful events over a five-year period. Types of stress follow three patterns. First, older offenders with no prior record vacillate between acute and chronic drinking. Second, first time offenders report more stressful events within 12 months from arrest. And third, overall incidence of stress in life space is consistent for first time and repeated offenders. Elaboration of results includes several models of drinking behavior and directions that treatment research should take.
Descriptors: Drunk driving, stress.

214. Wilkinson, P. Alcoholism in the aged. Journal of Geriatrics, 1971, November, 59-64.
Probing concerns in recent epidemiologic models of elderly alcohol and drug abuse are examined in this treatment of prevalence, prognosis, complications, and potential therapy. Alcoholism assumes responsibility for physical and mental discomfort in the aged and, in most cases, has evolved through long dependency histories. That excessive drinking is precipitated by severe emotional crises (such as bereavement or retirement) suggests that the prognosis is better than for younger drinkers. Psychopathology, except for chronic brain damage, is clearly less progressive in the elderly's reactional adjustment to problems.
Descriptors: Epidemiology, chronic brain damage.

215. Williams, E. P.; Carruth, B.; and Hyman, M. M. Alcoholism and Problem Drinking Among Older Persons. (Report No. C6474E3). Rockville, MD: National Institute on Alcohol Abuse and Alcoholism, 1973.
Findings are reported from a comprehensive reappraisal of community care providers, treatment centers, and private facilities targeted for relief to elderly alcoholics. Substantial numbers of alcoholic elderly suffering from medical disorders are oblivious to service agencies and, contrariwise, structured agencies for the elderly mistake alcoholic for nonalcoholic afflictions. Commitment to action by community task forces is necessary to establish effective prevention and detection programs. Research evaluation toward achievement of these and similar goals appears in detail.
Descriptors: Social services, medical services.

216. Wilson, J. Plight of the elderly alcoholic. Geriatric Nursing: American Journal of Care for the Aging, 1981, 2, 114-118.
Tulsa County Health Department's project to expand health delivery and supportive services to the growing needs of elderly uncovers the areas of weakest assistance. This article shows the project's resources at work for one particular client. Issues most relevant to the client include (a) familiarity with service systems, (b) planning factors carefully focused on developmental and coping mechanisms, (c) barriers encountered during admission to medical-surgical hospital units and misdiagnosis, (d) absence of appropriate treatment facility, and (e) discriminatory practices of health providers.

Case history identifies the current failure in diagnostic procedures to provide adequate methods for recording the extent of alcohol or drug misuse.
    Descriptors: Social services, psychological adjustment, health.

217. Winter, D. J Senior Adults Traffic Safety and Alcohol. Presented at the 1980 Annual NCA Forum, Alcohol and Traffic Safety Session, Seattle, May 1980.
    Driver and pedestrian programs geared to reduce accidents are part of the National Highway Traffic Safety's agenda on steps toward protection for senior citizens. Sensing, deciding, and acting skills essential for driving safety also determine proper coordination for nonvehicle interaction with traffic. Decreasing psychomotor skills compounded by alcohol consumption can manifest considerable vulnerability of seniors to traffic fatalities. An educational program on traffic safety that discourages drinking is briefly described.
    Descriptors: Drunk driving, education, perceptual-motor.

218. Wood, W. G. Aging and alcoholism: The need for an animal model. In K. Eriksson (ed.), Animal Models in Alcohol Research. New York: Academic Press, 1980.
    Alcohol consumption in animals at different ages and parameters of the drinking cycle provide a workable analogue model to elderly alcohol abuse. The need for an animal model stems from scarcely controllable conditions under which elderly can be assessed in terms of multiple effects. Since alcohol consumption is a "strain" and "stock" dependent, it may be influenced by varying concentrations. Preliminary research studying the functional performance of "older" mice (22-24 months) shows more severe and prolonged withdrawal symptoms than in younger mice (4-6 months). Controlled inducements of "premature aging" are another possibility being considered.
    Descriptors: Animal model, experimentation.

219. Yamane, H.; Katoh, N.; and Fujita, T. Characteristics of three groups of men alcoholics differentiated by age at first admission for alcoholism treatment in Japan. Quarterly Journal on Studies of Alcohol, 1980, 41, 100-104.
    Case records of 20 inebriates with affective psychiatric disorders admitted to a Japanese hospital are selected from among younger, middle-aged, and elderly groups. Incidence of multiple neuropathy and various psychoses is higher for younger than older groups, although the latter experience socioeconomic and familial adjustments. Recurrent factors also found in the elderly sample include hypertension, incontinence, hemiparesis, and carelessness with fire. Drinking-related profiles of the age groups are enumerated in further statistical comparisons.
    Descriptors: Alcohol-related pathology, neuropsychology, drinking patterns.

220. Zimberg, S. Alcoholism and drug addiction in the elderly: The geriatric alcoholic on a psychiatric couch. Geriatric Focus, 1972, 1, 6-7.

Article argues that the incidence of alcoholism peaks beyond the age of 50 and is therefore a serious geriatric problem. Hospital medical patients typically show 15 to 38 percent for men and 4 percent for women. Of 933 individuals aged 60 and over, arrested for different reasons by one city's police department, 82 percent receive charges of drunkenness. Articulated by these data is that older persons beset by depression, loneliness, and aging in general respond well to therapeutic regimes that combine depressant drugs with resocialization. However, increased attention to potential signs of abuse is warranted by both the public and medical profession.

Descriptors: Psychiatry, socialization, epidemiology.

221. Zimberg, S. The elderly alcoholic. The Gerontologist, 1974, 14, 221-224.

A critical review is presented of literature on alcohol and elderly stressing treatment orientation. Prevalence of elderly alcoholics is highest in widowers, but affective disorders and sensory-motor incapacitation can lower an older person's resistance to intoxicants. Weighed against the deleterious effects of alcohol are studies showing its therapeutic benefits, especially in nursing homes.

Descriptors: Prognosis, therapy, nursing homes.

222. Zimberg, S. Two types of problem drinkers: Both can be managed. Geriatrics, 1974, 29, 135-136.

Admissions to a Harlem hospital are categorically analyzed into two types of elderly drinkers: Those continuing a lifelong habit, and those reacting to stress. Patients between ages 50 to 69 in whose traceable history there appears cyclical drinking episodes fall into the first category. Elderly persons unable to recover from traumatic emotional loss, death, or isolation aptly belong to the second category.

Descriptors: Alcohol typologies, hospital, diagnosis.

223. Zimberg, S. Diagnosis and treatment of the elderly alcoholic. Alcoholism: Clinical and Experimental Research, 1978, 2, 27-29.

Based largely on data accumulated over the last 12 years, it is held that alcoholism among elderly is an ignored problem. Article discusses community-based studies in Manhattan and in the Baltimore metropolitan area shown to compute significant prevalence rates in the samples surveyed. Specific criteria for diagnosing alcoholism in elderly alcoholics are also presented, supplemented by the caveat against stereotypical symptoms.

Descriptors: Social survey, epidemiology.

224. Zimering, S. , and Domeischel, J. R. Is alcoholism a problem of the elderly? Journal of Drug Education, 1982, 12, 103-111.

The vulnerability of elderly persons unequipped to overcome social and financial burdens is considered one reason for drinking. Stress provokes the aversive circumstances to which elderly are responding by, at first, moderate levels of consumption. Solutions to this growing crisis require the adoption of educational training

programs in public institutions and within most private sector businesses in which the elderly are employed.
Descriptors: Education, cultural trends.

225. Zylman, R. Age is more important than alcohol in the collision-involvement of young and old drivers. Journal of Traffic Safety Education, 1972, 20, 7-8.
Repeated offenses in traffic collisions by very young and old alcoholics indicate that age is a more predictable variable than alcoholism. Findings from a Grand Rapids study show that (1) over-involvement of young drivers is substantially reduced after manipulations (exposure or nonexposure) to the official licensing records, (2) collision involvement is worse for nondrinkers, and (3) collision vulnerability is increased after two or three drinks. Alcohol thus mitigates important variables with larger contributory impact on driving performance (e. g. , experience, time of day, etc.).
Descriptors: Drunk driving, diagnosis, traffic accidents.

2. ILLEGAL AND LEGAL DRUGS:
USE AND ABUSE

226. Abelson, H. I. , and Atkinson, R. B. National Survey: Main
      Findings 1974: Public Experience with Psychoactive Sub-
      stances. Rockville, MD: Social Research Group, National
      Clearinghouse for Drug Abuse Information, 1977.
      Interpretive results are presented from a 1974 national sur-
vey on experiences and beliefs about psychoactive use and abuse, both
legal and illegal. Data presented on older adults reflect patterns of
addiction, frequency of use, types of drugs, and ways of coping with
stress related to use. Also included are questionnaires in the appendixes.
      Descriptors: Epidemiology, types of drugs.

227. Allgulander, C. Diagnosis of drug dependence in open health
      care. Lakartidningen, 1980, 77, 428-429.
      Presents results of diagnostic survey in medical facilities
involved with drug abuse. Hypnotics and sedatives account for the
primary substance dependence by middle-aged and elderly patients,
many of whom are not ambulatory. Non-hospital treatment centers
in Sweden also report higher prevalence among female elderly in
comparisons between sex and age characteristics.
      Descriptors: Sedative-hypnotics, treatment centers.

228. Alvarez, C. W. Analgesic drugs. Geriatrics, 1967, 22, 95-
      96.
      Discusses elusive problems caused by the structural formu-
las of codeine, heroin, "Bentley's compound" and morphine. Bentley's compound, in particular, because it produces marked respiratory depression and is dangerously addictive, is contraindicated for
relief of severe pain. Most analgesic compounds are nonaddictive
but there is no satisfactory theory to explain why certain molecules
are analgesic. Benzomorphans, morphinons, and synthetic drugs
(e. g. , nalorphine) may counteract many analgesics' physiologic effects
at the risk of side-effects (hallucinations, etc.). Ultimately the
prescriber should consider if the aged user of analgesics (especially
morphine) is dying in great pain and may not live long enough to become addicted.
      Descriptors: Opiates, pharmacology, side-effects, ethics.

229. Anstett, R. E. , and Poole, S. R. Depressive equivalents in
      adults. American Family Physician, 1982, 25, 151-156.
      Reviews unrecognized symptoms of depression and the
atypical syndromes manifested in older age. Common depressive

56

symptoms include depression without sadness, without an obvious source, somatic symptoms, chronic pain, intensification of personality styles, and intensification from substance abuse or other psychosocial disorders. That early signs of depression do not fit the classic syndrome indicate directions for etiology.

Descriptors: Etiology, depression, mental health.

230. Are barbiturates a bigger problem? Nursing Times, 1969, 65, 946.

Briefly identifies women between 35 to 50 years as being more addicted to barbiturates than teenagers to narcotics. Newly admitted hospital clients requesting sleeping medication are frequently the same persons who alternate between physicians collecting prescriptions. Middle-aged women, in particular, account for an increasing number of outpatient addicts psychologically helpless against miseries of old age.

Descriptors: Barbiturates, outpatient, prescriptions.

231. Barnes, G. E. Solvent abuse: A review. International Journal of the Addictions, 1979, 14, 1-26.

Literature summary on effects of solvent abuse. Over 110 sniffing deaths not attributable to suffocation indicate an increasing shift toward street drug use, although specific solvents are still not precisely delineated. Brain damage and blood abnormalities due to solvent inhalation undergo some evaluation, with emphasis greatly placed on environmental conditions that lead to psychological vulnerability of solvent users. Highest prevalence, for instance, seems to occur for native persons in some cultural transition. Methods of intervention proposed in the literature are compared to reformulated approaches.

Descriptors: Solvents, review, inhalants.

232. Barsky, A. J.; Stewart, R.; Burns, B. J.; Sweet, R.; Regier, D.; and Jacobson, A. M. Neighborhood health center patients who use minor tranquilizers. International Journal of the Addictions, 1979, 14, 337-354.

Predominantly elderly (single or widowed) medical patients who use tranquilizers for varying lengths are interviewed on questions regarding medical care. Hypotheses drawn from the survey include that, first, patients who repeatedly obtain prescriptions have more medical problems than infrequent prescription users. And second, patients obtaining tranquilizer prescriptions evidence more psychiatric symptomatology and anxiety. National trends for tranquilizer use and abuse help to evaluate its therapeutic efficacy.

Descriptors: Tranquilizers, follow-up, psychiatry.

233. Behmard, S.; Sadegi, A.; Mohareri, M. R.; and Kadivar, R. Positive association of opium addiction and cancer of the bladder. Results of urine cytology in 3,500 opium addicts. Acta Cytology, 1981, 25, 142-146.

Registered opium addicts in Fars province in southern Iran are part of this case-control study exploring associations between opium addiction and cancer of the bladder. Urine cytology in the sampling subjects reveal cases of transitional cell carcinoma, most notably in the population over 20 years. Results further indicate the need for routine urine cytology for opium addicts and long-term users of opiate alkaloid in early detection of carcinoma of the bladder. Preliminary data confirming these incidence rates and correlational demographics are reviewed.

Descriptors: Opium, urine cytology, drug-related pathology.

234. Bergman, H.; Borg, S.; and Holm, L. Neuropsychological impairment and exclusive abuse of sedative or hypnotics. American Journal of Psychiatry, 1980, 137, 215-217.

Study examines 55 consecutively admitted abusers of sedatives and hypnotics. Neuropsychological performance is significantly lower and intellectual impairment more frequently diagnosed over matched control groups drawn from the general population. Cerebral disorders related to sedative-hypnotic abuse are hypothesized in middle-aged and elderly groups subjected to later onset of emotional problems.

Descriptors: Sedatives, hypnotics, neuropsychology.

235. Biener, K. Health problems in prisoners. Sozial- und Präventivmedizin, 1980, 25, 228-230.

Prisoners in northern Switzerland are interviewed for determining preponderant abuse problems. Cannabis, heroin and lysergic acid diethylamide (LSD) accounted for 46 percent of the sample, and 32 percent smoked more than 20 tobacco cigarettes a day. Relationships of substance abuse to psychological disorders such as suicide and sexual dysfunctions are common in several middle-aged and older prisoners.

Descriptors: Cannabis, heroin, LSD, prisoners.

236. Biener, K. The drug problem in the opinion of working women--representative study. Offentliche Gesundheitswesen, 1981, 43, 578-582.

Sampling study conducted in West Germany on substance abuse and prevention programs indicates that the majority of the populace is middle-aged, and uses cannabis heavily. Occupational correlates in female users are significantly higher when considering the cost and toxicity of selected drugs. Adult and aged women keenly sensitive to legislative constraints on drug use may still prefer illegal access to their supplies.

Descriptors: Cannabis, occupation, women.

237. Bosse, R.; Garvey, A.J.; and Glynn, R.J. Age and addiction to smoking. Addictive Behaviors, 1980, 5, 341-351.

Study investigates the hypothesis that smoking fluctuates with age toward higher levels of psychological and pharmacological addiction to tar and nicotine consumption. Former smokers, male volunteers, and longitudinal surveys of aging at outpatient Veterans Administration clinics serve in the sample. Suggested is that two distinct kinds of addiction dominate older groups as measured by the Horn-Waingrow Smoker Survey in 1973 and 1976. First, older cohorts apparently generate more reasons or motives for smoking, although in comparative measures they consume less tar and nicotine than younger smokers.

Descriptors: Nicotine, veterans, psychopharmacology.

238. Boston Collaborative Drug Surveillance Program. Clinical depression of the central nervous system due to diazepam and chlordiazepoxide in relation to cigarette smoking and age. New England Journal of Medicine, 1973, 288, 277-280.

Frequency of clinical depression of the central nervous system is compared among light smokers, nonsmokers, and heavy smokers receiving diazepam, chlordiazepoxide, or phenobarbital for anxiety. After affected by two benzodiazepines, central nervous system depression is less intense in proportion to number of cigarettes smoked. Benzodiazepine effects are more evident with increasing age but unreplicated with phenobarbital. Increased benzodiazepine metabolism in cigarette smokers and decreased metabolism in older age may explain these results.

Descriptors: Nicotine, benzodiazepines, central nervous system (CNS).

239. Bourne, P. G. Drug abuse in the aging. Perspective on Aging, 1973, 2, 18-20.

Reasons outlined for drug abuse in elderly are compared across age populations, with suggestions for treatment and rehabilitation. The aging addict is of growing concern to institutional and local community agencies severely deficient in procedures for early detection. Alternative solutions on policy and legislative issues are discussed.

Descriptors: Age-related, rehabilitation.

240. Bueno, J. R. Drug dependency--physical dependency. Jornal Brasileiro de Psiquiatria, 1972, 21, 127-137.

Development of nicotine addiction in adolescent and elderly is discussed within the framework of drug and alcohol dependency. Physiological dependence persists in the adult smoker despite knowledge of its harmful effects. Under a specific treatment, the psychological pathology accompanying addiction involves resolution of the conflict between pleasure and struggle for will-power. Reports on similar reasons for nicotine indulgence in adulthood are reviewed.

Descriptors: Nicotine, physiological and psychological dependency.

241. Butler, R N., and Lewis, M. I. Drug and electroshock therapy. In R. Butler (ed.), Aging and Mental Health. St. Louis, MO: Mosby, 1973.

Chapter discusses the amelioration of recognized symptoms of mental disorder manifested by elderly substance abusers who suffer problems of aging. The variety of modalities reviewed include drugs, social activities, physical exercise, and psychotherapy. Depression and agitation, two frequent concomitants, are treatable with psychotropic medication (antidepressants, tranquilizers, hormones, etc.) as one component of the organized treatment plan. Safeguards and monitoring are necessary for sedative-hypnotic prescriptions and may be replaced by electroshock treatment. Another modality questioned for use (especially for chronic brain syndrome) is hyperbaric oxygenation. Lastly, much disputed claims regarding benefits of wine and alcohol for therapy are explored in terms of long-term safety and susceptibility to narcotic abuse.

Descriptors: Mental health, psychotropic medication, electro-convulsive therapy.

242. Cameron, P. , and Boehmer, J. And coffee too. International Journal of the Addictions, 1982, 17, 569-574.

Interviews are taken of 272 persons between ages 11 and 80 regarding their reasons for trying coffee, tobacco, liquor, and marijuana. Generated from these reasons is a guilt-shame index on which coffee and cannabis register lower than tobacco and liquor. Most tobacco users describe motives that are regrettable and reflect reactional adjustment and possibly defiance against the contentment they feel in regard to less "offensive" habits.

Descriptors: Guilt-shame, caffeine, cannabis, nicotine.

243. Capel, W. C. ; Goldsmith, B. M. ; Waddell, K. J. ; and Stewart, G. T. The aging narcotic addict: An increasing problem for the next decades. Journal of Gerontology, 1972, 27, 102-106.

Sociologic interpretation is provided on the growing epidemic of opiate abuse in elderly residents in New Orleans. White male addicts aged 48 to 73 are interviewed about their length of addiction, drug choices, marital status, work habits, arrests, imprisonments, and life-style. Opiate abuse is not only greater in proportion to younger abusers, but is apparently resistant to presently conceived treatment modalities. Moreover, increases in younger opiate addiction hold serious implications for future generations of elderly addicts.

Descriptors: Opiates, male addicts.

244. Carroll, J. F. Uncovering drug abuse by alcoholics and alcohol abuse by addicts. International Journal of the Addictions, 1980, 15, 591-595.

Substance abuse histories are explored of 1,544 addicts treated at federally funded centers. More than 80 percent who indicate sequential or concurrent abuse to other substances drink alcohol at some time during their lives, particularly after 40 years of age. Preponderant cases of polydrug abuse over single substance abuse is a noteworthy shift in diagnostic patterns, since admissions are routinely screened for only ostensible symptomatic categories. Lines of inquiry for improving diagnostic accuracy of alcohol abuse by addicts and drug abuse by alcoholics are provided.

Descriptors: Diagnosis, polydrug abuse.

245. Chandrasena, R. Management of opium dependence in a general hospital psychiatry unit. British Journal of Addiction, 1980, 75, 163-167.

Discusses follow-up evaluation of opiate addicted patients

released from a psychiatric hospital. Socioeconomic factors relevant to their current standing are correlational to both motivation and abstinence. Middle-aged patients undergoing severe withdrawal and showing minimal recovery while hospitalized eventually respond to treatment management.

Descriptors: Opiates, follow-up.

246. Cines, B. M. , and Rozin, P. Some aspects of the linking for hot coffee and coffee flavor. Appetite, 1982, 3, 23-34.

Food preferences are among items surveyed in adolescents, adults, and aged coffee drinkers. Temperature and flavoring agents apparently attract the strongest interest and may influence daily consumption rates over a period of years. Chemical properties besides these that contribute to physical caffeine dependency are elaborated upon using this survey.

Descriptors: Food preference, caffeine, physical dependency.

247. Cliche, S. T. , and Onge, G. Use of sleeping pills. A habit to be eliminated in the elderly. Infirmary of Canada, 1981, 23, 25-26.

Adverse effects of sedative-hypnotics taken by elderly females are briefly explained with encouragement to seek alternative forms of insomniac relief. Overuse of prescription sleeping pills can greatly disrupt a person's quality of life and depress central nervous system functioning to below safety margins at times. Nurses in hospitals and private clinics can exchange this information with clients during intake assessment.

Descriptors: Nurses, sedative-hypnotics, women.

248. Cohen, S. Drug abuse in the aging patient. Quarterly Journal of Studies on Alcoholism, 1976, 37, 1455.

Nervous system depressants shown to be increasingly preferred with advancing age are the result of community and hospital surveys. If extrapolated nationwide, these findings indicate about one million older alcoholics may comprise roughly two groups. One group has a lifelong history of excessive drinking. Another group, also managing to survive, starts to drink later in life in reaction to traumatic loss. Favorable use of antidepressants in both groups enables better adjustment. However, treatment directions are best toward resocialization programs.

Descriptors: Alcohol, depressants, national trends.

249. Coleman, J. H. , and Dorevitch, A. P. Rational use of psychoactive drugs in the geriatric patient. Drug Intelligence and Clinical Pharmacy, 1981, 15, 940-944.

Aspects of geriatric psychopharmacology included here are the pharmacists' unique position in mental health care systems and their role in drug surveillance in abuser patients. Rational therapeutic decisions about the safety and utilization of psychotropic medication is a major responsibility of pharmacists. Measures to maintain their competency and informed recognition of potential addicts are provided.

Descriptors: Psychopharmacology, psychotropic drugs, assessment.

250. Cooke, W. T. Laxative abuse. Acta Gastroenterol Belgium, 1981, 44, 448-458.
    Pharmacodynamics involved in the elderly's misuse of cathartics are brought to bear on related pathology and substance abuse. Colonic disease and hypokalemia diagnosed in adolescent and elderly groups relying on frequent use of laxatives illustrate the unforeseen repercussions in many of society's accepted over-the-counter medicines. Reversal of this reliance and implications for reliable diagnostics follow in the discussion.
    Descriptors: Laxatives, drug-related pathology, pharmacodynamics.

251. Cornacchia, H. J.; Bentel, D. J.; and Smith, D. E. Drugs in the Classroom. St. Louis, MO: Mosby, 1973.
    Various phases in the exploration of drug problems relative to American culture appear in different chapters of this book. Pill and drug takers in adolescence may defy authority, whereas the elderly abuser is alone and forgotten. Community relations, educational programs, and rehabilitation efforts to combat age-integrated solutions against an increasing incidence of nationwide cases are among the resource materials contained.
    Descriptors: Epidemiology, cultural patterns, age differences.

252. Cummings, J. H.; Sladen, G. E.; James, O. F.; Sarner, M.; and Misiewicz, J. J. Laxative-induced diarrhoea: A continuing clinical problem. British Medical Journal, 1974, 1, 537-541.
    This investigates complaints of middle-aged women who after 127 (average) days spent in the hospital for abdominal pain are given tests tracing the pain to excessive laxatives. All denied taking laxatives and no characteristic features of the effects of cathartics on the colon are detected after radiological examinations. Since hypokalaemia and other electrolyte abnormalities appear, reactions are due to a combination of severe diarrhoea and vomiting. Diagnosing this disorder ultimately requires either urinalysis or searching the patient's ward locker.
    Descriptors: Laxatives, drug-related pathology.

253. Drugs and the elderly. Focus on Alcohol and Drug Issues, 1980, 3.
    This special issue (vol. 3, no. 3) devotes itself to articles and assorted resource materials on medicine, drugs and the elderly. Featured articles delve into management issues in diagnosis, treatment, and program development around which many of the demographic data have revolved. Reviews of books and practical techniques to avoid misuse are clearly written in language understandable by elderly readers. The Focus is primarily for Miami residents but enjoys a fairly large national circulation.
    Descriptors: Reviews, education, self-help materials.

254. Eve, S. B. , and Friedsam, H. J.   Use of tranquilizers and
     sleeping pills among older Texans.   Journal of Psychoactive
     Drugs, 1981, 13, 165-173.
     Middle-aged male and female persons with diagnosed men-
tal disorders are shown to incline more regularly toward use of
tranquilizers and sedative-hypnotics.   Substance abuse from these
potentially addictive agents is common in Texans whose reclusive
life-style fosters loneliness and unhappiness.   Evidence of misused
tranquilizing agents indicates the need for rapid community involvement and re-entry into mainstream activities.
     Descriptors: Tranquilizers, mental health, sedative-hyp-
notics.

255. Fabrikant, B.   The use of hypnosis in the investigation and
     treatment of drug use and abuse.   Journal of the American
     Society of Psychosomatic Dentistry and Medicine, 1972, 19,
     88-97.
     Study conducted over a two-year period involves the use of
group and individual hypnosis for removal of personality structure
defects and treatment of drug abuse.   Young and middle-aged drug
users providing information on purity of drugs, frequency of use,
and quantity lead to four conclusions.   First LSD users and responsive to hypnosis.   Second, combinations of LSD and speed interfere with hypnotic concentration.   Third, the substitution of a hypnot-
ically induced "trip" can more effectively reduce drug dependency than
either aversion treatment or systematic desensitization.   And fourth,
opiate users are typically unresponsive to treatment.
     Descriptors: LSD, opiates, mental health, hypnosis.

256. Fidell, L. S. , and Prather, J. E.   Drug Use and Abuse in Wom-
     en.   Rockville, MD: U. S. Department of Health, Educa-
     tion and Welfare, 1976.
     Study discusses characteristics of middle-aged women who
take psychoactive drugs of various types (relaxants, stimulants, analgesics, antidepressants) and in varying degrees (regularly, infrequently, former use, nonuse).   Comparisons are made for mental and
physical health, attitudes, sources of satisfaction or dissatisfaction,
sources of stress, personality factors, and social and personal reinforcement derived from drug use.   The first phase of research is
entirely information-gathering, whereas in phase two prediction equations help to determine if certain women are at "risk. "
     Descriptors: Psychoactive drugs (general), drug-taking
patterns, women.

257. Gershon; S. . Sakalis, G. ; Oleshansky, M. ; and Aronson, M.
     Controlled Drug Evaluations.   Rockville, MD: U. S. De-
     partment of Health, Education, and Welfare, 1977.
     Clinical psychopharmacology research programs are co-
vered in regard to five central areas.   First is the exploration of the
dopamine hypothesis in relation to schizophrenia.   Second, a continuation of work as to possible links between blood levels of psychotropic drugs, their metabolites, and clinical responses.   Third, the
examination of aminergic theories underlying etiology and treatment

of affective disorders. Fourth, the relationship between psychopharm-acology and gerontology is studied. The fifth area concerns neuro-chemical agents. Preclinical evaluations of procedures in each area and their relevancy to differently aged groups are presented.

Descriptors: Psychotropic drugs, psychopharmacology, research.

258. Green, B. The politics of psychoactive drug use in old age. The Gerontologist, 1978, 18, 525-530.

Literature review stresses the abundance of psychothera-peutic drugs used by noninstitutionalized elderly. Precautions recog-nized by the patient are rarely exercised unless first explained by a physician or person in authority. Increased accessibility is another problem that health care workers encounter in long-term users. Diminished effectiveness at home, in occupations, and in mental and physical abilities all result from unaltered reliance upon medication. Pressured by family and friends, the chain of decision to seek treat-ment is described from different perspectives.

Descriptors: Psychotherapeutic drugs (general), drug patterns.

259. Guttman, D. A Survey of Drug-taking Behavior of the Elderly. Rockville, MD: National Institute on Drug Abuse, 1977.

Findings of 447 noninstitutionalized elderly around Washing-ton, D.C., surveyed about their drug-related characteristics, are reported here. Legal drug use, including alcohol, constitutes pre-dictably larger factions of the populace over demographic comparisons run ten years ago. Factor analysis further supports the conclusion that extensive proliferation of drugs in a metropolitan area greatly reduces longevity and is correlational to fatal accidents annually.

Descriptors: Cultural trends, demography.

260. Hale, W. E.; Marks, R. G.; and Steward, R. B. Drug use in a geriatric population. Journal of the American Geriatrics Society, 1979, 27, 374-377.

Questionnaires collected in a geriatric hypertension screen-ing program help to determine causal relations between drug use and behavioral disorders. Prevalent drug use is mostly of sedative-hypnotic origin and prescriptive medication. Elderly claiming to have long drug use histories are equally spread among those patients with inferior backgrounds but showing greater hypertension.

Descriptors: Hypertension, sedative-hypnotics, drug pat-terns.

261. Halmi, K. A.; Falk, J. R.; and Schwartz, E. Binge-eating and vomiting: A survey of a college population. Psychological Medicine, 1981, 11, 797-706.

Surveys college and middle-aged students about their eating habits in identifying prevalence of bulimia (binge-eating syndrome). Results indicate that although self-induced vomiting may accompany other symptoms, the vomiting is not a necessary symptom for diag-nosis. However, excessive vomiting interspersed with the taking of laxatives (termed "purging" behavior) occurs in 10 percent of the

sample. Bulimia students typically have histories of being over-
weight or in the upper portion of their normal weight range, thus
suggesting extensive unresolved substance abuse problems with "food."
Descriptors: Bulimia, food, laxatives.

262. Harrington, P., and Cox, T. J. A twenty-year follow-up of
     narcotic addicts in Tucson, Arizona. American Journal of
     Drug and Alcohol Abuse, 1979, 6, 25-37.
     Reports findings from a follow-up study of heroin addicts
in Tucson twenty years after their initial diagnosis. Focus is on
the maturation hypothesis that addicts will spontaneously cease narcotic use by age 40. Records from two agencies (law enforcement
corrections, treatment and welfare) provide the current status of
addicts' drug habits and in comparisons disprove the maturation
hypothesis. One possible explanation is that users grow up together
and live homogenously within the same subculture. In fact, 75 percent are still alive and presumed living within that subculture.
     Descriptors: Maturation hypothesis, heroin, follow-up.

263. Holm, L.; Bergman, H.; and Borg, S. Field dependence in
     patients with exclusive abuse of hypnotics or sedatives.
     Perceptual Motor Skills, 1980, 50, 987-992.
     Field dependence and independence are assessed in 47
middle-aged patients abusing sedative-hypnotics. Using the rod-and-
frame test, results of the pairwise, matched-control group and
abuser group show abusers are not more field dependent even though
prior research reveals them to have a higher incidence of intellectual
impairment. Suggests that discrepancies may be due to decreased
motor and perceptual coordination caused from prolonged depressive
effects on the central nervous system.
     Descriptors: Field dependence, drug-related pathology,
rod-and-frame test.

264. Jacobs, E. Hyperoxygenation Effect on Recent Memory in the
     Aged. State University of New York School of Medicine,
     1973.
     Study replicates pilot studies of the psychological effects
of increased oxygen intake on memory processes in elderly patients
with cerebral arteriosclerosis. Functional relationships also explored
include that between hyperoxygenation and psychological performance
in middle-aged, mentally defective, and normal young subjects. Experimental group first receives 100 percent oxygen breathing at 2.5
atmospheres for 90 minutes, twice daily for two weeks. Then, after
treatment, subjects undergo a standard psychological battery (e.g.,
Wechsler Memory Scale, the Bender-Gestalt, and Tien's Organic
Integrity Test). Ongoing studies with senile patients (as contrasted
with other groups) indicate that hyperoxygenation reduces vascular
insufficiency and improves test scores and general biomedical health,
except for memory deficits due to alcoholism and drug abuse.
     Descriptors: Hyperoxygenation, vascularity, psychological
battery.

265. Janicki, P., and Rewerski, W. Clinical pharmacology of ben-
     zodiazepine tranquilizers. Polski Tygodnik Lekarski, 1981,

36, 1313-1316.

Examines fundamental interactions of benzodiazepine toxicity with the metabolism (drug tolerance) effects upon female adults
and aged. The issues of pregnancy and related morphologic changes
disrupted by the biological availability of this drug (increased absorption rate, etc.) are raised as arguments against (and for) its therapeutic value.

Descriptors: Benzodiazepine, drug-related pathology, wom-
en.

266. Jarvik, L. F.; Matsuyama, S. S.; and Ku, T. Application of
cytogenetics to Management of Psychiatric Patients. (Report no. ZO-31478-6). Washington, DC: U. S. Veterans
Administration, Department of Medicine and Surgery, 1977.

Reports on yearly research projects in the psychogenetics
unit. Five ongoing projects include (1) drug effects on human chromosomes, including imipramine, morphine, amphetamine, and marijuana; (2) effects of morphine and amphetamine; (3) amphetamine-
like compounds on geriatric clients; (4) immunoglobulin levels and
intellectual functioning in the aged; and (5) chromosome changes with
age and the relationship to intellectual functioning. Chromosome
evaluations, in other words, attempt to elucidate genetic or biological
factors chiefly responsible for abusive habits.

Descriptors: Chromosomes, genetics, intellectual functioning.

266a. Johnson, R. P., and Connelly, J. C. Addicted physicians. A
closer look. Journal of the American Medical Association,
1981, 245, 253-257.

Physician impairment is attributable to several possible
reasons beyond the office itself. Addiction is one of them. Fifty
physicians undergo a psychiatrically oriented addiction program.
Physicians becoming addicted after age 40 are more apt to exhibit
psychopathology, from overt schizophrenia to subtle dementia. Physicians older than 40 years may further display organic brain impairment and depression. Discussed are predictors of treatment outcome
in relation to different addictive agents.

Descriptors: Physicians, psychiatry.

267. Kales, A.; Bixler, E.; Tijauw-Ling, T.; Scharf, M. B.; and
Kales, J. D. Chronic hypnotic-drug use: Ineffectiveness,
drug-withdrawal insomnia, and dependence. Journal of the
American Medical Association, 1974, 227, 513-517.

Middle-aged hypnotic users are monitored in a sleep laboratory while continuing to receive medication. Comparisons with insomniac control groups not receiving medication show less rapid eye
movement (REM) for users, although both groups experience difficulty
falling asleep. Abrupt withdrawal of ineffective drugs is seriously
questioned due to psychological and physiological changes that contribute to drug dependency action. Indications are that changes be
made for evaluating and advertising hypnotic drugs in public media.

Descriptors: REM, insomnia, hypnotics.

268. Khavari, K. A., and Douglass, F. M. The drug use profile (DUP): An instrument for clinical and research evaluation for drug use patterns. Drug and Alcohol Dependence, 1981, 8, 119-130.

Reports effective implementation of a profile form similar to that used by the Minnesota Multiphasic Personality Inventory. Overall drug patterns are based upon data collected from 4,984 (differently aged) respondents which have been transformed into standardized T scores. Pilot use of this profile suggests it is reliable and provides a quick diagnostic scan of person's drug practices, and is especially applicable for specific subgroups. Advancing utility of this instrument for routine examination is discussed.

Descriptors: Drug Use Profile, MMPI, diagnostics.

269. Krakowski, A. J., and Langlais, L. M. Acute psychiatric emergencies in a geriatric hospital. Psychosomatics, 1974, 15, 72-75.

Discusses the confusion when acute psychiatric emergencies resemble chronic degenerative mental illness, such as senile dementia, arteriosclerotic psychosis, or paranoid reaction of an organic type. Inadequate records, misinformation, or prejudgment by the family or paramedical personnel contribute to diagnostic errors. Commonly the organic factors precipitating psychiatric reactions include infections, operations, accidents, alcoholism, drug abuse, malnutrition (with deficiencies of vitamins A, B, or C), and emotional strain. Chemical agents affecting the central nervous system are even worse, among which are anesthetics, analgesics, psychotropic drugs, anticonvulsants, and antiparkinsonian agents. Return or reversal to premorbidity levels is gradually achieved through social interaction therapy and psychotherapy.

Descriptors: Psychiatry, mental health, CNS drugs.

270. Lancet Editors. Drug interactions. Lancet, 1975, 7912, 904-905.

Explains radically transitional changes in the concern for drug interactions. Potency and toxicity are substantially more relevant in the regular course of hospital treatment. Noted is that chronic ingestion of alcohol, cigarette smoking, or exposure to chlorinated insecticides, such as dicophane and lindane, will increase rate of metabolism in persons most susceptible to enzyme induction. Steps to improve communication about drug interactions are provided.

Descriptors: Drug interactions, metabolism, drug-related pathology.

271. Larsson, G.; Eriksson, M.; and Zetterstrom, R. Amphetamine addiction and pregnancy: Psycho-social and medical aspects. Acta Psychiatrica Scandinavica, 1979, 60, 334-346.

Middle-aged amphetamine addicted mothers are investigated by their psychosocial backgrounds. Predictive ratings then attempt to indicate subjects' chances of adaptation to motherhood. Only 17 of 69 subjects stopped taking drugs in the first months of gestation after they learned they were pregnant.

Descriptors: Amphetamine, motherhood, pregnancy.

272. Linn, L. S. , and Davis, M. S.   The use of psychotherapeutic
     drugs by middle-aged women.   Journal of Health and Social
     Behavior, 1971, 12, 331-340.
        Examines extent of psychotherapeutic drugs consumed by
middle-aged women based upon the concept called "illness behavior. "
Differently perceived symptoms are reacted to by seeking medication.
Measures of illness behavior (such as response to pain, recognition
of symptoms, attitude toward illness, utilization of health facilities,
and medicine compliance) apparently correlate to such sociocultural
factors as age, sex, and ethnic background.   Expanding upon this
concept, this study further defines the prevalence of psychotherapeutic drug use and, secondly, analyzes usage among demographic factors.   Drug-using women usually affiliated themselves with health-
oriented goals or defined their physical status as frequently chronic.
        Descriptors: Psychotherapeutic drugs, women, mental
        health.

273. Luban-Plozza, B.   The problem of tobacco cessation.   Schwei-
     zerische Zeitschrift für Hospitals, 1973, 6, 1-8.
        Covers various aspects of tobacco cessation, noting abso-
lute contraindications of smoking that include bronchitis, angina
pectoris, myocardial infarct, and thromboangitis obliterans.   Theoretical basis of smoking cessation programs should stress destruction of reinforcement for the habit and alternative reinforcement for
nonsmoking.   Genetics, personality factors, and experience also
complete the etiologic profile of resistant smoking behavior.   Organic
and subjective prognoses for smoking addiction in adolescents, adults,
and the elderly are outlined in methods such as hypnosis, smoking
substitute methods, and group therapy.   Nonmedication treatments include the use of filter and low-nicotine cigarettes, smoking only half
the cigarette, not carrying unsmoked cigarettes, and switching to a
pipe or cigar.
        Descriptors: Cigarettes, treatment, diagnosis, drug-
        related pathology.

274. Lushene, R. E. ; Coppinger, N. W. ; Eisdorfer, C. ; Wells, J. ;
     and Allee, J.   Study of SK & F 38462 in Geriatric Pa-
     tients.   (Report no. ZO-32498-3). Washington, DC: U. S.
     Veterans Administration, Department of Medicine and Sur-
     gery, 1975.
        Extensive data analysis on the drug SK&F 38462 shows that
it fails to discern significant effects on personality inventories.   Some
scattered marginal differences do not support previous findings and
methodological refinements may or may not guarantee the emergence
of altered symptomatology.
        Descriptors: SK&F 38462, personality.

275. McCarron, M. M. ; Schulze, B. W. ; Walberg, C. B. ; Thompson,
     G. A. ; and Ansari, A.   Short-acting barbiturate overdosage.
     Correlation of intoxication score with serum barbiturate
     concentration.   Journal of the American Medical Association,
     1982, 248, 55-61.
        Study reviews reactions to barbiturate overdose in male
and female adults, and aged upon the vascular system.   Hypotension

and hypothermia diagnosed during withdrawal from severe drug tolerance may quickly turn to coma, depending on the time factors involved. Accidental poisonings from barbiturate overdose typify these effects and each are classified in some detail.
Descriptors: Barbiturate, drug-related pathology.

276. McGlone, F. B. , and Kick, E. Health habits in relation to aging. Journal of the American Geriatrics Society, 1978, 26, 481-488.
Reports results from 52 patients over 80 years of age examined for alcohol, tobacco, coffee, or tea usage. Confirmed was the hypothesis that health habits have a positive effect on quality and quantity of life. Moderate alcohol use plus irregular smoking habits are apparently predictive of life expectancy according to results from other countries consistent with those reported here.
Descriptors: Drinking patterns, life expectancy.

277. Maletzky, B. M., and Klotter, J. Smoking and alcoholism. American Journal of Psychiatry, 131, 445-447.
Differential opinions are taken from hospitalized alcoholics and nonhospitalized control groups to clarify the relationship between alcoholism and cigarette smoking. Alcoholics apparently smoke more than nonalcoholics, particularly women alcoholics. Frequency of use and amount of alcohol also correlate with the number of cigarettes smoked daily. However, sudden decreases in smoking usually accompany abstinence. Also discussed are the implications of using cigarettes and alcohol for the oral drive and susceptibility models of addiction.
Descriptors: Alcoholism, cigarettes, models of addiction.

278. Maltbie, A. A.; Sullivan, J. L.; and Cavenar, J. O. Haloperidol treatment of a sixty-year narcotic addiction: Case report. Military Medicine, 1979, 144, 251-252.
Explores case of 82-year-old man shown to be addicted to opiates for 60 years. After withdrawn from methadone, subject is maintained on haloperidol alone. Haloperidol's pharmacologic advantages over methadone for drug treatment management in the elderly raise important considerations for cases of protracted addiction.
Descriptors: Haloperidol, opiates, treatment.

279. Mirimanoff, R. O. , and Glauser, M. P. Endocarditis during staphylococcus aureus septicemia in a population of nondrug addicts. Archives of Internal Medicine, 1982, 147, 1311-1313.
Microbiologic complications are frequently associated with infections from prolonged drug abuse. Staphylococcal infections in nondrug addicts may typically result from either hospital- or community-acquired diseases, but can vary at different age levels. Preschool through elderly patients suffering from staphylococcus aureus septicemia (from 1976 to 1979) undergo clinical examination to determine the degree of prevalence.
Descriptors: Infection, staphylococcal diseases, diagnosis.

280. Mollier, J. P. Migraines and the field of allergy. Journal de
     Medecine de Lyon, 1973, 1259, 1417-1418; 1421-1422; 1425-
     1426; 1429-1430; 1433-1442; 1445-1446; 1449-1450.
     Allergy testing of 126 migraine patients shows positive signs
of Allergy Y. Diagnosed groups are assigned either to migraine
treatment or allergy treatment, resulting in an 86 percent success
outcome from allergy treatment. Comparable factors, also treated
in the allergy group, are meteorological influences, alcohol consumption, changes in daily habits, and fatigue. Reduced migraine
in patients 40 years and over also required that they stop smoking
cigarettes.
     Descriptors: Migraine, cigarettes.

281. Neal, C. L.; Snow, J. B.; and Seda, H. J. An analysis of ther-
     apy for carcinoma of the tonsil. Transactions of the Amer-
     ican Academy of Ophthalmology and Otolaryngology, 1973
     (March-April), 97-104.
     Combined radiation therapy and surgical treatment for
squamous cell carcinoma of the tonsil is evaluated in 30 patients,
aged 41 to 76 years, who use tobacco and alcohol. Radiation treatment lasts about eight weeks with 8000 rads of mega voltage ir-
radiation given through bilateral, opposing ports of the primary tumor
area and 5000 rads to the same side of the neck. Radical resections
of the tonsillar fossa and other forms of surgery are discussed regarding potential complications from extensive cigarette smoking.
     Descriptors: Tonsil, radiation treatment, drug-related
     pathology.

282. Pankratz, L., and Levendusky, P. The Modification of Tal-
     win Addiction in an Elderly Male. (Report no. ZO-34969).
     Washington, DC: U. S. Veterans Administration, Depart-
     ment of Medicine and Surgery, 1974.
     Presents case of a 65-year-old retired army officer ad-
mitted to a psychiatric ward for chronic abdominal pain and social
withdrawal from prescriptions of Talwin. Self-control techniques,
such as relaxation training and visualizations, comprise one therapeutic component, while concurrently the subject is withdrawn by
diluting Talwin with normal saline. Following treatment, subject
resumed social activity and could relieve his pain without medication.
     Descriptors: Talwin, treatment.

283. Pascarelli, E. Alcoholism and drug addiction in the elderly:
     Old drug addicts do not die, nor do they just fade away.
     Geriatric Focus, 1972, 1, 4-5.
     Methadone maintenance programs serve higher percentage
of elderly patients than is socially known. Psychological and biological profile of elderly addict is presented with respect to resistance and participation within treatment programs. Diagnosed elderly addicts with 15- to 40-year histories resist methadone maintenance, but consider it their only option. Advancing age brings no
substantial diminution in their craving for narcotics and those addicts
economically unable to support their habit turn to legal drugs, short-
acting barbiturates, or alcohol, and persuade physicians to prescribe

them "geriatric medication. " Thus, polydrug abuse contributes to morbidity along with negligence in personal hygiene and nutrition. What elderly addicts apparently need most is personal attention from certain clinics.
Descriptors: Demography, drug patterns, barbiturates, medication.

284. Pascarelli, E. F.   Drug dependence in the elderly.   Gerontologist, 1973, 13, 56.
Explores recently reported characteristics of older drug addicts in view of pervasive trends toward new treatment and prevention strategies.   Methadone addicts, in particular, pass through stages of jail terms interspersed with experimentation with street and grey market drugs.   Aging addicts may maintain a low profile and avoid harassment, arrest or public attention, decreasing illegal and antisocial behavior.
Descriptors: Psychosocial drug patterns, aging.

285. Pascarelli, E. F.   Update on drug dependence in the elderly. Journal of Drug Issues, 1979, 9, 47-54.
In an overview of drug abuse the author estimates that older addicts clearly exceed demographic statistics and that concomitant use of alcohol and several depressants or tranquilizers is frequent.   Diagnostic problems inherent in determining primary from polydrug dependence is discussed.   Techniques to improve diagnosis and treatment are recommended for hospitals and medical schools.
Descriptors: Demography, diagnosis, treatment.

286. Pascarelli, E. F. , and Fischer, W.   Drug dependence in the elderly.   International Journal of Aging and Human Development, 1974, 5, 347-356.
Study of drug dependence in elderly refutes the common belief that long-term addicts die before they reach old age.   Contrariwise, dependency represents a serious problem in economically deficient elderly for whom methadone treatment is the only alternative. New approaches in public policy and advocacy recognize this growing epidemic, but are too distant for the changes needed within medical facilities and throughout educational training programs in gerontology.
Descriptors: Methadone, demography, education, treatment.

287. Paulus, I. , and Halliday, R.   Rehabilitation and the narcotic addict: Results of a comparative methadone withdrawal program.   Canadian Medical Association Journal, 1967, 96, 655-659.
Retrospective study compares relative effectiveness of regular methadone withdrawal treatment with prolonged treatment on adult and older patients.   Five years later, behavior improvement is detected in 43 percent of all cases and older addicts respond better to prolonged withdrawal.   Criteria for total rehabilitation include drug usage, work, criminal behavior, community associations, familial relationships, and friendship patterns.   Variations in the conventional methadone program are advised for enhanced efficacy.
Descriptors: Methadone treatment, rehabilitation.

72 / Drug Abuse and the Elderly

288. Peppers, L. G. , and Stover, R. G. The elderly abuser: A challenge for the future. Journal of Drug Issues, 1979, 9, 73-83.

Considers data on which conclusions to three questions are based: (a) who is the elderly abuser; (b) how does he become identified; and (c) how do treatment programs respond? Findings from a survey of 5,500 older individuals entering treatment during 1976 are primarily that abusers are white, male, and unemployed, mostly desire alcohol, and initiate treatment themselves or through encouragement from friends and family. Elderly abusers are also seldom treated in a holistic manner, suggesting an imperative for uniform interventions.

Descriptors: Demography, treatment, service programs.

289. Peterson, D. M. , and Thomas, C. W. Acute reactions among the elderly. Journal of Gerontology, 1975, 552-556.

Discusses how the national consumption rate of drugs places the elderly population at risk. Initial attraction to drugs for physical and psychiatric reasons soon yields to dependency and the problems of boredom, loneliness, and depression recover slightly. Most prescribed drugs for elderly include Valium, Librium, and the nonnarcotic analgesic Darvon. Documented dangers of medication misuse and acute drug reactions are reviewed against the backdrop of recommendations for protective services to aging addicts.

Descriptors: Demography, Valium, Librium, Darvon, medication, social services.

290. Peterson, D. M.; Whittington, F. J.; and Beer, E. T. Drug use and misuse among the elderly. Journal of Drug Issues, 1979, 9, 5-26.

Speculation about drug abuse among elders is replaced with factual information drawn from a review of relevant literature and summations of available research evidence. Particular emphasis is upon use of legal drugs, types and extent of misuse of legal drugs, and illegal drug abuse. Conclusions organize what is currently known regarding older drug abuse and directions feasibly foreseen for the next couple of decades.

Descriptors: Literature review, epidemiology.

291. Peterson, D. M ; Whittington, F. J.; and Payne, B. P. (eds.). Drugs and the Elderly: Social and Pharmacological Issues. Springfield, IL: Charles C. Thomas, 1979.

Major epidemiologic and pharmacologic issues surrounding elderly drug abuse and sociocultural conditions inherently involved are articulated in different chapters of this book. The clinical and community response to pronounced problems of elderly drug abuse expands upon earlier documented research and explores political as well as social constraints to effective management. Development of this theme continues in those chapters which present entrapments in the diagnostic system affecting both private and public sectors. Educational alternatives toward greater social alertness and attitudinal change are among several recommendations provided.

Descriptors: Epidemiology, pharmacology, social casework, attitudes.

292. Polichetti, E.   Smoking steatosis and hepatic cirrhosis.
   Epatologia, 1970, 67, 585-599.
   Indications of laboratory and anatomic-pathology research
for the causation of hepatic alterations are presented in relation to
cigarette smoking.   Alterations ranging from functional insufficiency
to degenerative processes, and from hepatic steatosis to cirrhosis
and cancerous cirrhosis suggest that the diseases are influenced by
increased consumption of cigarettes.   The effect of tobacco smoking
on the vascular system results in diseases whose synergistic effect
is critical to different types of lesions.   The nosology and symptomatology characteristic of these diseases are reviewed in ample detail.
   Descriptors: Drug-related pathology, cigarettes, hepatic
   cirrhosis.

293. Pontes, J. F.   The treatment, physiopathology, and etiopatho-
   genic aspects of duodenal ulcer.   Revista Paulista de Med-
   icina, 1972, 79, 165-174.
   Discusses the cause, nature, and treatment of duodenal
ulcers in search of correlative links between tobacco smoke, nicotine, and potential misuse of medications.   Older persons, in particular, are morphologically amenable to alteration of secretion or
gastric motility by tobacco smoke and nicotine but only a small
amount of demonstrable evidence is available.   In experiments with
dogs, the administration of nicotine producing some ulcerogenic pathology may hold useful implications for future research
   Descriptors: Duodenal ulcer, drug-related pathology, nicotine, tobacco smoke.

294. Poser, C. M.   The types of headaches that affect the elderly.
   Geriatrics, September, 1976.
   Examines many etiologies of headache potential.   Early
signs of vague neck discomfort that will later reach chronic states
are ineffectively curable with analgesics, local anesthetics, antidepressant drugs, and so forth.   Recommended for therapy is that
headache patients be understood, given compassion, and further examined for related biophysical disorders (e. g. , congestive heart
failure, cervical osteoarthritis) that may underlie or precipitate onset
of headaches.
   Descriptors: Headaches, treatment, physician-patient relationship.

295. Pottieger, A. E. , and Inciardi, J. A.   Aging on the street:
   Drug use and crime among older men.   Journal of Psychoactive Drugs, 1981, 13, 191-211.
   Heroin dependence wears thin on aging addicts whose long-
term habit is only sustainable, at times, by competing with street
politics.   Elderly drug addicts and skid row alcoholics average considerably higher in national statistics, as treatment agencies design
new wards or programs appropriate for prolonged users.   Presented
are typologic traits seen in street drug users and the inevitability of
criminal acts they commit to pay for or help obtain supplies.
   Descriptors: Street abusers, epidemiology, heroin.

296.　Preskorn, S. H.; Schwin, R. L.; and McKnelly, W. V.　Analge-
　　　sic abuse and the barbiturate abstinence syndrome.　Jour-
　　　nal of the American Medical Association, 1980, 244, 369-
　　　370.
　　　　　Discusses abstinence syndrome and sedative-hypnotic drugs
in clinical situations in which analgesic and barbiturates combined can
obscure diagnosis.　Differential diagnosis for most substance abuse
symptoms in adult and elderly addicts is less frequent than when
cryptic abuse of prescription drugs has occurred.　Potentiality of
side-effects and the pharmacodynamics underlying sedative-hypnotics
are two important features which geriatric physicians are obligated
to articulate better to their patients.
　　　　　Descriptors: Sedative-hypnotic, barbiturates, physician-
patient relationship.

297.　Probert, J. C.; Thompson, R. W.; and Bagshaw, M. A.　Pat-
　　　terns of spread of distant metastases in head and neck
　　　cancer.　Cancer, 1974, 33, 127-133.
　　　　　Adults with epithelial tumors are examined in most areas
of the head and neck for metastases attributable to cigarette smoking
or alcoholism.　Advanced primary tumors having metastases are in
patients who smoke one to two packages of cigarettes per day, al-
most 17 of whom might smoke beyond two packages.　Regarding alcohol consumption, predominantly more subjects drink heavily and
few drink socially or not at all.　Clinical autopsy reports spanning
1955 to 1967 account for the case studies reviewed.
　　　　　Descriptors: Cancer, cigarette smoking, alcoholism, tumors.

298.　Raffoul, P. R.; Cooper, J. K.; and Love, D. W.　Drug misuse
　　　in older people.　The Gerontologist, 1980, 21, 146-150.
　　　　　Study attests to misuse of prescription and over-the-counter
(OTC) drugs in 69 subjects over 60 years of age.　Misuse frequency
and its relationship to several psychosocial, medical, and pharmacological variables draw out the ostensible concern for immediate
community intervention, faced against shrinking financial and political resources within the senior services network.　Outlined briefly
are solutions generated from the literature for adducing both demographic and psychological evidence of the problem.
　　　　　Descriptors: OTC drugs, cultural practices, demography.

299.　Read, N. W.; Read, M. G.; Krejs, G. J.; Hendler, R. S.; Davis,
　　　G.; and Fordtran, J. S.　A report of five patients with
　　　large-volume secretory diarrhea but no evidence of endo-
　　　crine tumor or laxative abuse.　Digestive Diseases and
　　　Science, 1982, 27, 193-201.
　　　　　Examines five patients with chronic secretory diarrhea in
whom no evidence of an endocrine tumor or of surreptitious laxative
use could be found.　Diagnostic complications worsen when some patients had spontaneous and temporary remissions mistaken for symptoms of other chronic diseases.　Intestinal perfusion is the alternative that reveals secretion and abnormally low absorption of water
and electrolytes in the jejunum and low water absorption in colon.

Implied by these findings is that management of patients suspected of laxative abuse may benefit from closer attention to water absorption levels.
Descriptors: Laxatives, diarrhea, diagnosis, drug-related pathology.

300. Roberts, A. H.   A Normative Study of the Porteus Maze Test. (Report no. GWB-1420). Washington, DC: U. S. Department of Health, Education and Welfare and Social and Rehabilitation Services, 1974.
Describes the metric advantage in using the Porteus Maze Test (measures nonverbal intelligence) for clinical validity of brain injured and stroke patients undergoing drug rehabilitation. Samples of adults ranging in age from 20 to 85+, from whose scores evidence may be drawn about personality characteristics, are representative for the pilot study. Final results, although still underway, expect to prepare and revise this test for prognostic applications.
Descriptors: Porteus Maze Test, nonverbal behavior, treatment.

301. Robinson, G. M.; Sellers, E. M.; and Janecek, E. Barbiturate and hyposedative withdrawal by a multiple oral phenobarbital loading dose technique. Clinical Pharmacology and Therapy, 1981, 30, 71-76.
Substance withdrawal syndromes are explained regarding the intravenous phenobarbital loading technique. A more applicable method of oral ingestion is to achieve phenobarbital effects exhibited by the following: Nystagmus, drowsiness, ataxia, dysarthria, or emotional lability. Patients receiving varying phenobarbital doses did not develop seizures or similar forms of barbiturate withdrawal. Significant modifications in sedative-hypnotic treatment approaches using phenobarbital on adult aged are elaborated.
Descriptors: Phenobarbital, barbiturates, sedative-hypnotics, treatment.

302. Ross, B.; Greenwald, S. R.; and Linn, M. W. The elderly's perception of the drug scene. Gerontologist, 1973, 13, 368-371.
Older people are increasingly exposed to problems of drug abuse. Study focuses on attitudes of Miami senior citizens about current drug dimensions and its social impact on them. Correlations between the elderly's demographic data and scale responses are inconsistent, as senior citizens differ significantly from students and the police. Attitudes are largely stereotypic and agree with punitive statements concerning the treatment of users.
Descriptors: Demography attitudes, cultural practices.

303. Rumbaugh, C. L., and Fang, H. C. The effects of drug abuse on the brain. Medicine Times, 1980, 108, 37s-41s; 45s-46s; 48s-49s.
Exploratory review of the etiology primarily describing brain abscesses and injuries of animal and human (varying age) drug abuse. Case reports indicative of cerebral artery and cerebrovascular

disorders caused from chemically induced substances are examined through tomography and computed X-ray systems. Subjects shown to have neural diseases risk irreversible damage when the frequency of administration is high and this may complicate reliable detection of addiction.
Descriptors: Neurology, vascularity, drug-related pathology.

304.   Schachter, S.   Self-treatment of smoking and obesity.   Canada Journal of Public Health, 1981, 72, 401-406.
Study assesses effectiveness of therapeutic alternatives to obesity and smoking reduction. Adolescents, adults, and elderly participants of a program using self-help methods found they could significantly weaken habitual tendencies toward cigarettes smoked per day. Deceleration of eating habits, however, involves distinct adjustments to daily routine commonly overlooked by physicians and therapists.
Descriptors: Cigarettes, obesity, treatment.

305.   Schmidt, F.   Methods of smoking cessation.   Zeitschrift für Therapie, 1973, 11, 401-407.
Serous health hazards of nicotine addiction are explored and conclusions show that the responsibility for smoking cessation rests primarily on individual smokers. Methods from hypnosis to electro-shock produce less practical changes than group psychotherapy since group dynamics help motivate the individual. Autosuggestion and dietetic or drug therapy as concomitants are apparently more effective during illness when the flavor of smoking is aversive. General recommendations regarding benefits and risks of abrupt cessation versus stepwise reduction are indicated along with advice for people wishing to stop smoking.
Descriptors: Cigarettes, nicotine, treatment.

306.   Schuri, U. , and von Cramon, D.   Autonomic and behavioral responses in comas due to drug overdose.   Psychophysiology, 1980, 17, 253-258.
Physiopathologic indicators of toxicity during poisoning or drug overdose may surface in autonomic nervous system reactions. Middle-aged men and women entering into coma from a drug overdose experience respiratory and circulatory permutations that are diagnostically significant for expedient treatment. Possible complications due to unrecognized behavioral side-effects are reported with suggestions to overcome them.
Descriptors: Autonomic nervous system, drug overdose, coma.

307.   Singh, B. K. , and Knezek, L. D.   Characteristics and Treatment Outcomes of Older Patients in Drug Treatment Programs.   Paper presented at the 1978 Gerontological Society Meeting, Dallas, November 1978.
Examines characteristics and treatment outcomes of older patients (55 years and older) in federally funded drug treatment programs. Analysis of alcoholic patients, who later had opiate and psychotropic drug problems, indicates that older patients complete

treatment and substantially recover for extended periods of nonuse. Differences based on sex, primary drug problems at admission, and treatment milieu are also representative of outcome success. Policy and research implications draw from these data.

Descriptors: Demography, treatment, social casework.

308. Stash Capsules, September 1975.
Newsletter of the Student Association for the Study of Hallucinogens (Madison, Wisconsin) focusing on drug use among elderly. Review headings include prescription drugs, alcoholism, narcotic addiction, and drug use in nursing homes. Article clearly defines prevalence based on epidemiologic surveys around the nation and life expectancy trends over the next two generations. Problems in experimental methodology and measurability of drug history, frequency, and sociocultural pressures account for the many discrepancies in current research.

Descriptors: Epidemiology, literature review.

309. Stenback, A.; Kumpulainen, M.; and Vauhkonen, M. Illness and health behavior in septuagenarians. Journal of Gerontology, 1978, 33, 57-61.
Those alive out of 400 newborns in 1903 (called "septuagenarians") are studied for physical disease, illness behavior, and health behavior. Majority of respondents who consider themselves in good health maintain active interest in physical exercise and restrictive attitudes toward drinking and smoking. Implications for adopting ethical and moral attitudes during the aging process are discussed in contrast to the belief that elderly lose self-control after age 65.

Descriptors: Septuagenarians, drug-related pathology, morality.

310. Stephans, R. C.; Haney, C. A.; and Underwood, S. Psychoactive drug use and potential misuse among persons aged 55 years and older. Journal of Psychoactive Drugs, 1981, 13, 185-193.
Drug utilization among aging persons is examined in the context of ethnicity, socioeconomic income variants, and physiological and psychological dependency resulting from psychotropic medication. Males, more than females, predisposed to a medication regimen or under emotional stress from retirement, loss of companionship or physical malady, may actively increase their drug consumption in various ways. Reliance upon medical personnel is primarily the route taken by most addicted elderly inexperienced with street politics. Financial constraints which severely interfere with supply and demand issues are considered.

Descriptors: Demography, medication misuse, physicians.

311. Stojanovic, V. K.; Marcovic, A.; Arsov, V.; Bujanic, J.; and Lotina, T. Clinical course and therapy of Buerger's disease. Journal of Cardiovascular Surgery, 1973, 14, 5-8.
Examines treatment of 303 Yugoslav patients with thromboangitis obliterans who are heavy smokers. Patients showing sensitivity to nicotine react to minimal quantities of it with severe pain

in their limbs. Nicotine, excessive alcohol consumption, and commonly prescribed medicine may play an active etiologic role in the disease, although by comparison genetic traits exert the most predictive influence. Elderly persons in whose biological history there appear traces of vascular diseases are therefore at greater risk by smoking cigarettes.
Descriptors: Vascularity, nicotine, drug-related pathology.

312. Subby, P. Community Based Program for the Chemically Dependent Elderly. Paper presented at the 26th Annual Meeting of ADPA, Chicago, September 1975.
A community-based program in Hennepin County for chemically dependent elderly reports its current progress in assessment, intervention, and prevention. Program follows a systems approach with qualified volunteers assisting drug abuse specialists. Treatment methods and program commitments offer economically feasible directions for other communities concerned with elderly abuse. Organizational strategies are discussed at length.
Descriptors: Social casework, treatment.

313. Tamerin, J. S., and Neumann, C. P. Prognostic factors in the evaluation of addicted individuals. International Pharmacopsychiatry, 1971, 6, 69-76.
Generally accepted prognostic factors in addiction practice and research are tied together with confirmatory and supplementary evidence drawn from the Silver Hill Foundation. Additional prognostic indicators of value include age, drinking pattern, social stability, motivation, and diagnostic categories. For older patients the inclusion of sources of referral, acceptance of the problem, pain from the problem, willingness to change, sense of responsibility, capacity to relate to therapist, attitude toward treatment, and family or employment relationship are also significant. Clinical evaluations using these guidelines greatly reduce prognostic errors about addicted individuals.
Descriptors: Diagnosis, evaluation, prognosis.

314. Tulane University Medical Center. Drug abuse by the aged: An increasingly serious problem in the near future, Tulane study shows. Geriatric Focus, 1972, 11, 2-3.
Discusses extensive abuse of opiates by elderly who must adopt protective means of secrecy to avoid street harassment. Results from a Tulane University Medical Center study, which shows that obscurity and "helplessness" are two common patterns of elderly opiate addicts, confirm previous research regarding detachment theories. Investigative team also explores causation.
Descriptors: Opiates, helplessness.

315. Turner, J. A.; Calsyn, D. A.; Fordyce, W. E.; and Ready, L. B. Drug utilization patterns in chronic pain patients. Pain, 1982, 12, 357-363.
Chronic pain patients seen at multidisciplinary clinics typically are excessive or inappropriate users of medication. Study examines differences among pain patients who use all medications, those who use narcotics but no sedative medication, and those who use no

addictive medication. Medication-using patients accumulate more
pain-related hospitalizations and surgeries and score significantly
higher on MMPI hypochondriasis and hysteria than their cohorts.
Findings suggest that certain patients show more readiness to com-
plain or seek help for physical symptoms.
> Descriptors: Hypnotics, sedatives, MMPI, pain, med-
> ication.

316. Vestal, R. E. ; Norris, A. H. ; and Tobin, J. D. Antipyrine
metabolism in man: Influence of age, alcohol, caffeine,
and smoking. Clinical Pharmacology and Therapeutics,
1975, 18, 424-432.
Influences of age, alcohol consumption, caffeine consumption, and cigarette smoking on plasma half-life and metabolic clearance of antipyrine are examined in males aged 18 to 92. Older
subjects have plasma half-life to 16. 5 percent longer and antipyrine
clearance rate 18. 5 percent less than their younger cohorts. Antipyrine metabolism correlates with caffeine and cigarettes but insufficiently with alcohol, suggesting variations to theories on absorption rates. In large part smoking is responsible for more than 12
percent of metabolic clearance rate.
> Descriptors: Pharmacology, alcohol, caffeine, cigarettes,
> metabolism.

317. White, A. G. Medical disorders in drug addicts: 200 consecutive admissions. Journal of the American Medical
Association, 1973, 223, 1469-1471.
Cases of 200 patients consecutively admitted and analyzed
by their epidemiologic, demographic, and diagnostic characteristics
(13. 5 percent were 40 years or older) are presented in detail.
Whites, Blacks, Hispanics and Orientals have the following reasons
for admission: acute hepatitis, infections, detoxification, diabetes
mellitus, pulmonary disease, overdose, cardiovascular disease,
gastrointestinal disease, and venereal disease. Indications for
relatively simpler diagnostics within a large inpatient medical center
help to clarify potential problems that integrated symptoms may
impart on accurate judgment.
> Descriptors: Inpatient hospital, drug-related pathology,
> demography.

318. Worz, R. Abuse and paradoxical effects of analgesic drug
mixtures. British Journal of Clinical Pharmacology, 1980,
10, 391s-393s.
Discusses adverse effects of analgesic drug combinations
in middle-aged patients with chronic pain. Susceptibility to
barbiturate- and morphine-type dependency after prolonged administration of analgesics is observed to confirm that psychotropic
substances added to analgesics may hasten drug abuse. Chronic
pain patients dependent on analgesic drug mixtures, for instance,
had lowered experimental pain thresholds and tolerances. After
drug withdrawal, threshold and tolerance levels increase by gradual
amounts.
> Descriptors: Pain, drug interactions, analgesics.

319.   Wynne, R. D. , and Heller, F.   Drug overuse among the elder-
       ly: A growing problem.   Perspective on Aging, 1973, 2,
       15-18.
           Sharply increasing numbers of elderly drug abusers who
turn up in social agencies unkempt and financially disabled perpetuate
the stereotype of "Skid-Row" addicts.   Suggested is that elderly drug
abuse is symptomatic across all socioeconomic strata and particularly
noticeable among long-term medication recipients.   Prevalence of
abuse as interpreted by policy and planning networks provides further
background on this misinterpretation and social negligence.
           Descriptors: Stereotypes, demography, social casework.

3. MEDICATION: USE, ABUSE, AND COMPLIANCE

320. Aging and addiction in Arizona. (Report no. NCAI-040482), Rockville, MD: National Institute on Alcohol Abuse and Alcoholism, 1979.
   Reports problems of addiction among aging population in Arizona. Alcohol drinking is unsafe for nearly 70,000 persons over 55 years, many of whom abuse prescriptive medications. Physiological, psychological, and sociological conclusions drawn from county and regional assessments provide directions for improved strategies. A Phoenix-area mutual program and components for ideal treatment conditions are also discussed.
   Descriptors: Arizona, treatment, assessment.

321. Aikman, L. Nature's gifts to medicine. National Geographic, 1974, 146, 420-440.
   Provides a panoramic look at natural medicinal herbs in use since ancient Egyptian periods. From folk remedies to wonder drugs to enslaving narcotics, natural medicine meets modern pharmacology at the crossroads of human use and abuse. Elderly tribal leaders' relief from ailments typically would involve juices and applications extracted from highly addictive plants. Curative and dangerous reactions of these remedies and their implicit implications for adoption into society's code of approvable medication are pursued.
   Descriptors: Natural medicine, pharmacology, plants.

322. Albert, E. The task of the advisory psychiatrist in a home for the aged. ZFA (Stuttgart), 1980, 56, 327-340.
   Crucial diagnostic decisions are expected from psychiatric consultants. Nursing home psychiatrists facing mental disorders obscured by aging dementia, cerebral arteriosclerosis, and iatrogenic reactions may lose sight of abuse to tranquilizing agents. Substance dependence represents a major class of symptomatology easily confused for another nosological class. Psychiatric evaluations and methods of developing precautionary systems in diagnosis are explored.
   Descriptors: Nursing homes, psychiatry.

323. Analgesic abuse and the kidney. Kidney Internist, 1980, 17, 250-260.
   Case reports on aging patients with severe kidney pathology whose reaction to drug combinations is chemically, not psychologically, induced. Chronic kidney infection or failure caused by misuse of codeine or its analogs and derivatives is frequent among elders uninformed about potential deviation from the prescribed regimen.

Transplantation of homologous organs at that age raises serious risk factors that are avoidable with proper caution against misuse of analgesics (aspirin, caffeine, etc.).
Descriptors: Kidney, organ transplantation, analgesics, drug-related pathology.

324. Anandan, J. V. , and Matzke, G. R. Nephropathy as a hazard of analgesic abuse. American Journal of Hospital Pharmacy, 1981, 38, 1536-1539.
Analgesic nephropathy is discussed regarding patients with chronic renal failure and histories of excessive analgesic use. Analgesic abusers showing, in addition, psychoneurosis in terms of headaches, arthritis, or ulcers are possibly amenable to modified doses to decrease toxicity. Several mechanisms for this nephrotoxicity are, for example, that oxidative metabolites of phenacetin act in conjunction with aspirin to cause papillary necrosis. Clinical evidence of these symptoms is sufficiently detectable for pharmacists to avert progressive renal failure and unnecessary surgery.
Descriptors: Kidney, analgesics, drug-related pathology.

325. Ballin, J. C. Toxicity of tricyclic antidepressants. Journal of the American Medical Association, 1975, 231, 1369.
Introduction of imipramine hydrochloride in 1959 set forth the manufacturing and prescribing of tricyclic compounds for depressed patients. The predominant pharmacologic action of tricyclic compounds, cholinergic blockage, produces adverse side effects in aging persons, unlike the small dose for enuretic children. Frequent observation of pulse rate and EEG is advised for using these drugs in frequent administrations.
Descriptors: Tricyclics, depression, treatment.

326. Balter, M. B. ; Levine, J. ; and Manheimer, D. I. Crossnational study of the extent of anti-anxiety/sedative drug use. New England Journal of Medicine, 1974, 290, 769-774.
Results of international survey taken of patients in western European countries about their use of anti-anxiety and sedative drugs are discussed. Proportion of persons who use these drugs on one or more occasions varies from 17 percent to 10 percent, with female proportions being nearly always twice that of male cohorts. Persons aged 45 and over represent a high number among drug users, but only in terms of the reported census for different countries. United States appears in the middle position among the nine countries in question.
Descriptors: European survey, demography.

327. Baron, S. H. , and Fisher, S. Use of psychotropic drug prescriptions in a prepaid group practice plan. Public Health Reports, 1962, 77, 871-881.
Nonpsychiatric practice of psychotropic drugs carries great weight in determining health service considerations. A study is presented that explores variables which may influence number of prescriptions. Such factors as age, sex of client, and prescribing physician's specialty are among the potentials within a diagnostic and

therapeutic service (excluding psychiatry). On an a priori basis, factors identified include background variables on patients, on the physician, and the patient's symptomatology. Results indicate conformity with these factors and names alternative variables important for closer observation.

Descriptors: Patient characteristics, physician attitudes.

328. Basen, M. M. Elderly and Drugs: Problem Overview and Program Strategy. Rockville, MD: National Institute on Drug Abuse, Division of Resource Development, 1976.

Explored in this document is the prevalence of elderly substance abuse as a sociological problem. Elderly citizens make up 10 percent of the population, but use 25 percent of prescriptive drugs and hence spend approximately $877.5 million per year in proportion to receiving approximately 225 million prescriptions. Studies conducted between 1926 and 1975 are briefly reviewed for implications of today's pathological and social complications resulting from drug use and abuse. Lastly, functions of the National Institute on Drug Abuse are delineated with respect to elderly issues.

Descriptors: NIDA, epidemiology.

329. Beardon, W. O.; Mason, J. B.; and Smith, E. M. Perceived risk and elderly perceptions of generic drug prescribing. Gerontologist, 1979, 19, 191-195.

Perceived risks in taking drugs and dispensary facilities are compared between elderly drug users and nondrug consumers. Generic prescriptions readily accessible to users are nonthreatening, whereas obtaining medication from a physician may risk exposure of addict's dependency. Manipulative tactics users take to avoid this exposure differ greatly from the nonuser's form of avoidance.

Descriptors: Perceptions, attitudes.

330. Bender, A. D. Pharmacologic aspects of aging: A survey of the effect of increasing age on drug activity in adults. Journal of the American Geriatrics Society, 1964, 12, 114-134.

Pharmacologic activity of drugs is altered by aging physiology. A survey observes differences between man and animal regarding drug effects with increasing age, from young adult to elderly. Alterations in gastrointestinal tract, metabolism (absorption and elimination of drug), and motility cause declining reactivity to higher dosage levels. Stimulated by this research are efforts by physicians to improve communication with patients.

Descriptors: Aging, metabolism, drug effects.

331. Bender, A. D. Pharmacodynamic principles of drug therapy in the aged. Journal of the American Geriatrics Society, 1974, 22, 296-303.

Discusses certain precautions to be taken when prescribing a therapeutic regimen for the elderly. Increasing age in, especially, geriatric patients, brings about functional changes in many systems that control drug metabolism and evocative responses. Age delays or reduces absorption from gastrointestinal tract, impairs drug clearance and excretion by kidneys, and disrupts enzyme destruction.

Receptor interactions with various medication is another problem area. Decreased transmitter contact with affected tissues is accompanied by rigidity and overall declines in homeostasis.
Descriptors: Aging, drug-related pathology, receptors.

332. Bergman, S.; Forrest, J.; Betsill, W.; and Gillenwater, J.
Acquired upper ureteral stricture in a phenacetin abuser.
Journal of Urology, 1980, 124, 892-894.
Pathologies such as adenocarcinoma related to chronic kidney failure have traces of chemically induced, drug abuse symptoms. Kidney obstructions may result from side-effects of use or misuse of phenacetin compounds, directly routed from prescriptive medication. Casual use of phenacetin undetected by earlier diagnosis is only deleterious in unrestricted or unmonitored doses.
Descriptors: Kidney, phenacetin.

333. Bhasin, S.; Wallace, W.; Lawrence, J.B.; and Lesch, M.
Sudden death associated with thyroid hormone abuse.
American Journal of Medicine, 1981, 71, 887-890.
Drug-induced myocarditis has several possible causes. One cause consists of hyperthyroidism due to deliberate intake of excessive amounts of L-thyroxine. Effects of this drug on "instantaneous" death results, further, from ventricular fibrillation. Autopsies on three patients exhibiting hyperthroidism report that L-thyroxine abuse is still diagnosable in the absence of coronary artery disease.
Descriptors: Hyperthyroidism, myocarditis, drug-related pathology.

334. Bismuth, C.; Le Beelc, M.; Dally, S.; and Lagier, G. Benzodiazepine physical dependence. 6 cases. Nouvelle Presse Medicale, 1980, 28, 1941, 1945.
Substance withdrawal syndrome of benzodiazepine is discussed for middle-aged male and female clients. Symptoms include nightmares, insomnia, nausea, vomiting, muscular weakness or tremor, postural hypotension, hyperthermia, muscle twitching, convulsions, confusional state, and psychosis. Prominent features of withdrawal occur several days after treatment and are unknown to clients. Prevention issues discuss the gradual rather than abrupt removal of benzodiazepine treatment in patients receiving high dosages for more than one month.
Descriptors: Benzodiazepine, treatment, dependency.

335. Blum, R.H. Users of approved drugs. In R. Blum (ed.),
Students and Drugs: College and High School Observations.
San Francisco, CA: Jossey-Bass, 1970.
Explores characteristic differences of those who use medically and socially approved drugs with nondrug users. Student alcohol drinkers (at varying ages) are common, but only one-quarter of them also use sedatives. Intensive alcoholic and sedative usage begins at early age with tobacco and over-the-counter drugs. Comparisons between intensive and less intensive users also suggest directions for educationally-oriented programs which examine effects and long-term problems from uncontrolled addiction.
Descriptors: Drug patterns, students, sedatives.

336. Blum, R. H. , and Downing, J. J.   Staff response to innovation
    in a mental health service.   American Journal of Public
    Health, 1964, 54, 1230-1240.
        Study reports results of professional innovation survey.
Three innovation designs for improving patient care and staff efficiency are introduced in different clinics, after which a response measure
is taken of staff terminations and complaints from questionnaires.
Originally hostile and suspicious reactions dissipate after one year,
along with disruptions of staff prestige and informal relationships.
Noted is the significant success in the adult units partly due to outside expert consultants.   With exception to some uncooperative units,
resistance in most of the units is effectively overcome either during
or following desirable changes in patient behavior produced by innovations.
        Descriptors: Service delivery, training, drug unit.

337. Borgman, R. D.   Medication abuse by middle-aged women.   So-
    cial Casework, 1973, 54, 526-532.
        Descriptive study outlines results of psychosocial therapy
with 23 females treated for prescription medication abuse.   Employed
in a textile-furniture industry, clients earning a spendable salary
could manipulate physicians for wanted medication.   Their minimal
interest in vocational, educational, and marital goals and increasing
tendency toward illegal means of drug acquisition are identifiable signs
of deviance and infantile themes.   Psychosomatic symptoms in subjects who are demanding and enjoy uproars with their families may
have emerged through chronic subservience to their husbands and
children.   Activity therapy and restructuring the environment are conducive alternatives to developing the autonomy these subjects need.
        Descriptors: Age-integrated therapy, employment, treat-
    ment.

338. Burnett, K. R. ; Miller, J. B. ; and Greenbaum, E. I.   Transi-
    tional cell carcinoma: Rapid development in phenacetin
    abuse.   American Journal of Roentgenology, 1980, 134,
    1259-1261.
        Chemically induced cell pathology (transitional) in the kid-
ney is one adverse effect of phenacetin.   Article discusses time
factors in male elderly patients receiving drug therapy who in diagnosis show neoplasm staging.   Tomographic, X-ray, and radiographic
screens of potential kidney neoplasm in this case study tacitly imply
the need for precaution in extensive periods of phenacetin administration.
        Descriptors: Phenacetin, drug-related pathology, kidney.

339. Castleden, C. M. ; Houston, A. ; and George, C. F.   Are hyp-
    notics helpful or harmful to elderly patients?   Journal of
    Drug Issues, 1979, 9, 55-61.
        Hypnotics taken by elderly adults may be inappropriate since
insomnia (and other diagnostic symptoms) frequently results from depression, loneliness, and boredom.   The elderly's keen sensitivity to
adverse drug reactions, especially in drug-drug interactions, are
important considerations in medical assessment.   Few attempts are
known that reduce hypnotic doses in older patients.

Suggested are tactical additions to the intake process, such as length-
ier social histories and more intense examination of client. Medications should be selected on the basis of individual need rather than
taxonomous decisions.
Descriptors: Hypnotics, prescription practices.

340. Chappel, J. Physician attitudes and the treatment of alcohol
and drug dependent patients. Journal of Psychedelic Drugs,
1978, 10, 27-34.
Attitudinal interference in the diagnostic and treatment
stages of the physician-client relationship are presented for the alcohol and drug-abusing patient. Physicians unwilling or unqualified
to accept patients are still hesitant to make referrals. Treatment
that is undertaken can minimize the frustration by providing more
structure to patients with weak self-control. Currently the dominant
problem in resistant physicians is their infrequent exchange of feedback, as this can destroy the patient's confidence and hope for long-
term recovery.
Descriptors: Attitudes, physicians, treatment.

341. Chappel, J., and Krug, R. Substance Abuse Attitudes: Their
Role and Assessment in Medical Education and Treatment.
Presented at the National Conference on Alcohol and Drug
Abuse Education, November 1977.
Physicians' negative attitudes toward substance abusers and
the historical impetus for this bias are examined with respect to
various aspects of patient care. Description of efforts by career
teachers to develop educational programs conducive to more positive
professional attitudes provides the background and basis for discussion. Physicians seen as negligent in their selectivity of clients and
quality service delivery are encouraged to attend these programs.
Descriptors: Physician attitudes, education, medication.

342. Cohen, E. S., and Holman, R. C. An integrated approach to
iatrogenic drug abuse in a closed delivery system. Military Medicine, 1980, 145, 49-53.
Users of medication prescriptions of chlordiazepoxide,
diazepam, and doxepin run the risk of addiction under improperly
supervised organization and administration. Article discusses male
and female patients exhibiting iatrogenic effects of substance abuse
after being on these tranquilizing agents. Drug and narcotic control
within hospital care facilities is one alternative to iatrogeny and
increases the physician's awareness of drug toxicity. Military and
public hospitals rank high in incidence of iatrogenic illness and require regulatory standards for more intensive individual treatment
regimens.
Descriptors: Medication regimen, hospitals, iatrogenic
effect.

343. Cohen, S. A clinical appraisal of diazepam. Psychosomatics,
1981, 22, 761-769.
Oral administration of diazepam in children and older persons is therapeutically inadvisable for certain symptoms, the most

common being alcoholism. Discussed are the current diazepam treatment for various mental disorders (in drug therapy) and why dosage and adverse effects can impede control over substance abuse. Withdrawal potential varies by the drug administration schedule and degree of diagnosable anxiety. In the elderly, slower metabolism function is among the susceptible traits for severe drug interactions with diazepam, especially when duration of dose exceeds several years. Prevention strategies are suggested for the drug therapy. process with concomitant treatment for alcoholism.

Descriptors: Diazepam, drug interactions, mental disorders.

344. Conrad, K. A. , and Bressler, R. (eds.). Drug Therapy for the Elderly. St. Louis, MO: The C. V. Mosby Company, 1982.

Elderly afflicted with one or more chronic diseases, including drug abuse, constitute an increasing population. Chapters in this book address how chronic illness interfaces with pharmacodynamics of medication regimens and the changing physiology of aging. It elucidates topics on drug absorption, distribution, elimination, and effects, applying recent information to the prevalent concerns of mismedication, reactive (iatrogenic) diseases, and practical diagnostic errors in assessing drug clearance and homeostatic mechanisms. Emphasis is clearly upon the physician's educational needs.

Descriptors: Medication practices, pharmacology, drug-related pathology.

345. Daniel, R. Psychiatric drug use and abuse in the aged. Geriatrics, 1970, 25, 144-145; 148-151; 154-155; 158.

Mental symptoms of confusion in the elderly are also the result of underlying organic pathology and illness possibly brought on by barbiturate dosages. Frequently tranquilizers interrupt the cardiac and respiratory process and the symptoms caused by them are identified as the disease. More important is to treat the disease or underlying pathology as a whole. Measurement instruments able to detect this pathology are scarce and thus differentiating an acute confusional state from, say, chronic brain syndrome is difficult and raises practical problems for potential over- or under-estimations of dosage level.

Descriptors: Barbiturates, tranquilizers, holism.

346. David, J. Do-it-yourself medicine. Nursing Times, 1981, 77, 371-372.

Briefly describes the imminent dangers in self-prescriptive or nonprescriptive practices by economically disadvantaged elderly who pass through the "grey market. " Legal or illegal access to nonprescribed medication is a common alternative by virtue of the cost-free rewards in maintaining supplies. Because the supply is replete, grey market access will frequently result in medication errors or uncontrolled substance abuse which intensifies physical discomfort and the already strong alienation in the elderly's social life.

Descriptors: Self-medication, grey market, poverty.

347. Davis, R. H. Drugs and the Elderly. Los Angeles: Ethel
     Percey Andrus Gerontology Center, University of Southern
     California.
         Nine distinguished authors of different topics on elderly
     substance abuse present papers in this edited volume, originally part
     of a series at a career development institute sponsored by the Ethel
     Percey Andrus Gerontology Center. Drug effects, medication, at-
     titudes, clinical pharmacy, and geropsychological implications for
     drug abuse potential are among the issues covered. Primarily this
     text is for physicians acutely aware of undetectable manifestations
     of both developmental and iatrogenic illness associated with the dis-
     pensing of irregular doses and pitfalls in medication administration.
         Descriptors: Epidemiology, medication regimen.

348. De la Fuente, R. , and Weisman, M. N. (eds.). Proceedings
     of the 5th World Congress of Psychiatry, Mexico, November,
     December, 1971. New York: American Elsevier, 1973.
         Symposia papers are presented from the 5th World Congress
     of Psychiatry, held in Mexico in 1971 on correlative findings between
     psychiatric disorder and psychoactive drugs. Geriatric psychiatry
     relative to mental health includes topics concerning agression, drug
     dependence, alcoholism, metabolic aspects of psychosis, malnutrition,
     and psychosomatic medicine. Psychopathy and mental health service
     planning in general reflects the current Zeitgeist toward establishing
     a means of physician-patient channel of communication, more equipped
     in ways to educate the public.
         Descriptors: Drug-related pathology, mental health, geri-
     atric psychiatry.

349. Dirks, J. F. , and Kingsman, R. A. Bayesian prediction of non-
     compliance: As-needed (PRN) medication usage patterns
     and the battery of asthma illness behavior. Journal of
     Asthma, 1982, 19, 25-31.
         Discusses Bayes' therorem of patient noncompliance in
     asthmatic adolescent and adult patients undergoing drug therapy.
     Psychometric testing of eventual substance abuse reactions indicate
     there is a personalization of illness, where patients assume a "sick
     role. " As this role progresses, medication noncompliance is great-
     ly in jeopardy of producing substance abuse problems that might
     otherwise be misinterpreted as symptoms of aggravated respiratory
     illness.
         Descriptors: Asthma, iatrogenic illness, psychometry.

350. Do elderly patients take their drugs? World Medicine, 1968,
     3, 66-67.
         Survey reports that majority of geriatric patients (both
     living alone and with others) alter their drug treatment. Patients
     on fewer than four drugs per day and under good supervision are
     less deviant than those receiving barbiturates, diuretics, bendro-
     fluazide, ampicillin, and tuinal with little or no supervision. Grad-
     ual deterioration in their medication routine leads to incidences of
     suicide, increasing dementia, lethargy, and toxic confusion. Sug-
     gested is that by preventing unmonitored drug usage, incidences of

chronic drug abuse and psychiatric disorder can be reduced by half the national amount.
Descriptors: Medication regimen, psychiatric supervision, mental health.

351. Edwards, J. G.   Adverse effects of antianxiety drugs.   Drugs, 1981, 22, 495-514.
Antianxiety drug interactions on central and autonomic nervous systems are particularly important in vulnerable elderly.   Examined carefully are the adverse reactions (physiopathology) when antianxiety drugs are first introduced, increased, or are taken in combination with alcohol and other drugs.   Systems they affect (particularly from benzodiazepines) when tissue sensitivity is exaggerated are primarily cardiovascular and endocrine glands.   Authors make clear, however, that in some instances a causal connection with drugs is unclear and psychological disturbance is alternatively due to social conditions.   Precautionary measures for benzodiazepine prescription for elderly are an essential step against overprescription and general availability of effectively toxic, sometimes self-poisoning, antianxiety medication.
Descriptors: Antianxiety drugs, benzodiazepines, medicinal use.

352. Ellor, J R. , and Kurz, D. J.   Misuse and abuse of prescription and nonprescription drugs by the elderly.   Nursing Clinics of North America, 1982, 17, 319-330.
Attitudes toward health decline in the elderly among physicians and the public assume the bias that aging is a crippling and helpless syndrome.   Middle-aged and elderly persons in physical pain or on tranquilizers find they can avoid confrontations with the physician (and his or her attitudes) by self-administering medication.   Prescriptions typically desired (diuretics, barbiturates, etc.) are shown to be obtainable at the expense of dependency and exploitive mechanisms, both being learned during the adjustment period when physicians resist prescription renewal.
Descriptors: Medication errors, physician attitudes.

353. Finkle, B. S.; Caplan, Y. H.; Garriott, J. C.; Monforte, J. R.; Shaw, R. F.; and Sonsalla, P. K.   Propoxyphene in postmortem toxicology 1976-1978.   Journal of Forensic Science, 1981, 4, 739-757.
Propoxyphene analogs and derivatives are shown in toxicological analyses of 1,859 autopsies of suicidal deaths.   Period of investigation lasts from 1975 to 1978, in which a significantly high number of cases describe clearly defined psychiatric problems (e. g. , hypochondria, chronic depression, etc.) and multiple-drug toxicities.   Involvement of propoxyphene in many of these (suicidal) fatalities may be less revealing than incidences of what authors call "polypharmacy" and self-medication without appropriate medical surveillance.   These postmortem examinations seriously question whether propoxyphene is responsible for street-drug fatalities.   Implications for its use with alcohol and other central nervous system depressant drugs are suggested.

Descriptors: Propoxyphene, psychiatric disorder, drug-related pathology.

354.   Flexner, J. M. , and Abram, H. S.   A hostile patient: Fighting ire with ire. Hastings Center Report, 1978, 8, 18-20.
Describes encounters between physician and hostile patient who is both hemophiliac and drug addicted. Verbal exchanges involve derogatory and threatening behaviors which seriously question the physician's ethical role as service counselor. Noted is the ambivalence regarding therapeutic and beneficial value of the caregiver's treatment obligations under aversive circumstances, especially from patient resistance. Psychiatric consultation is seen as a threat to induce patient compliance and restore homeostasis in the physician-patient relationship. Psychological and sociological factors contributing to patient behavior are also discussed.
Descriptors: Ethical obligation, medication regimen, physician-patient relations.

355.   Ford, C. V. , and Sbordone, R. J.   Attitudes of psychiatrists toward elderly paitents. American Journal of Psychiatry, 1980, 137, 571-575.
Attitudes toward elderly inebriates and the stigma attached to aging in general are revealed in responses by 179 psychiatrists. Four clinical vignettes of younger and older patients with identical symptoms (ranging from neuroses to substance abuse) are rated based on desirability for treatment. Alcoholics rate lowest among the patients shown. Indications are that underlying clinical diagnosis are personal attitudes that greatly distort and impede accurate decisions.
Descriptors: Physician attitudes.

356.   Freeman, J. T.   Some principles of medication in geriatrics. Journal of the American Geriatrics Society, 1974, 22, 289-295.
Inappropriate and incorrect use of drugs is reflected in higher percentages of untoward effects. Discussed is that improper dosage, injudicious methods of administration and lack of awareness of drug interactions are common and associated with failure to quantitate reactive capacities of the aging body. The roster of confirmed pharmacologic data is infrequently translated in didactics between physician and patient and this adds to problems in following the medical regimen. Medication schedules which avoid the chances of primary or sequencing mishaps must involve observance of physical side effects and be responsive to reparative measures. Highlighted are predictable exogenous and endogenous changes in the body during drug interactions.
Descriptors: Medication regimen, physician attitude, education.

357.   Gaeta, M. J. , and Gaetano, R. J.   The Elderly: Their Health and the Drugs in Their Lives. Dubuque, IA: Kendall-Hunt Publishing Co. , 1977.
Book carefully and easily guides a general reading audience through chapters on basic problems encountered with physical reactions to drugs. Increasing age produces a measurable reduction

in efficiency of respiratory and other functional systems which professionals and patients may overlook in the course of drug therapy. Age differences in physical and mental capacity are stressed along with practical ways to avert medication errors and drug dependency. Both for professionals and lay public, this book dispels several myths about substance abuse and clarifies the potentiality of addiction.

Descriptors: Medication regimen, drug-related pathology, education.

358. Gehrhardt, B. A case of excessive drug collection. Zeitschrift für Ärztliche Fortbildung, 1981, 75, 1178-1179.

Case report describes coronary heart disease in an aged male suffering from iatrogenic substance abuse. Psychological disturbances in males on drug therapy regimens may account for high dropout rates or the increasing number of addicts but the cardiac damage from drugs is usually less reversible. Analysis is provided regarding preventive measures during initial stages of treatment to better assess coronary heart disease and contraindications for certain prescriptions.

Descriptors: Coronary heart disease, medication regimen.

359. Geiger, W. Bromine psychosis. Nervenarzt, 1955, 26, 99-106.

Discusses bromine psychosis based on seven observed cases of abnormal personality in patients prone to addiction. Elderly patients with cerebral arteriosclerosis or on salt-free diets are also apparently susceptible to bromine poisoning. Symptoms commonly associated with this condition include severe headache, slurred speech, tongue tremor, difficulty in swallowing, rigidness of gesture, and blank facial expression. Apathy, disorientation and hallucinatory reactions may accompany initial withdrawal episodes, rendering a differential diagnosis more difficult.

Descriptors: Bromine, psychosis, drug-related pathology.

360. Gillieron, C. M. A catamnestic study of the aging of toxicomanic patients: Catamnesis of 37 patients over the age of 65 years. Schweizer Archiv für Neurologie, Neurochirurgie und Psychiatrie, 1968, 102, 457-480.

A catamnestic study in elderly over 65 years of age with a history of psychiatric illness is described. Patients who are toxicomanic (except for alcoholism) are less nervous, more mature, and show improved social adjustment. Concluded was that toxicomania diminishes or is displaced by minor toxicomania (such as tobacco addiction). Further implications for correlations with psychiatric disease are reviewed.

Descriptors: Toxicomania, aging process, psychiatric illness.

361. Godber, G. E. Preventing the misuse of alcohol. British Journal of Alcohol and Alcoholism, 1977, 12, 2-4.

Recommendations to the health education council include a program against alcohol abuse rather than rejection of its use. Outlined is the idea that early, preventive health education is necessary before compulsive or continuous drinking develops, especially in elders accustomed to a routine drinking pattern. Health education would hopefully implant a belief in moderation over the tradition of abstention and alter most practitioners' conception of drinking as being morality-based. Strategies to encourage patients and families in seeking medical or psychological care are highly stressed.

Descriptors: Prevention, drinking moderation, physician attitudes.

362. Goldstein, S. E., and Birnbom, F. Hypochondriasis and the elderly. Journal of the American Geriatrics Society, 1976, 150-154.

Hypochondriasis is a poorly understood concept in its symptoms of primary and secondary (Pilowsky's categories) groups. Twenty consecutive cases of elderly patients analyzed for primary and secondary features are presented. Results show that primary hypochondriacs need neither intense therapy nor hospitalization whereas hospitalization, psychotropic drugs, therapeutic milieu and often electroshock therapy improve secondary hypochondriasis. Successful treatment differences in these two group types provide the basis for exploratory discussion on addiction.

Descriptors: Hypochondriasis, psychotropic medication, drug interactions.

363. González, D. H., and Page, J. B. Cuban women, sex role conflicts and the use of prescription drugs. Journal of Psychoactive Drugs, 1981, 13, 47-51.

Ethnologic survey of Cuban women using hypnotics and sedatives reveals they have several life complications, including stress and substance abuse. Tranquilizing agents are needed chiefly as the result of inadequate coping mechanisms against sex role identification conflicts in their culture. Male-dominated traditions transcend socioeconomic levels through successive generations within individual family histories. Women drug addicts are more amenable to prescriptive regimens and consequently comprise the largest percentage of medication misusers and accidental deaths. Etiological concerns are noted with respect to the culturalization of Cuban women.

Descriptors: Sex role identification, Cuba, medication regimen.

364. Greenblatt, D. J., and Koch-Wesler, J. Adverse reactions to intravenous diazepam. A report from the Boston Collaborative Drug Surveillance Program. American Journal of Medical Science, 1973, 266; 261-266.

Serious adverse reactions to intravenous diazepam in patients with hepatic decompensation or serious cardiac and pulmonary disease are discussed. Premedication use of diazepam before endoscopy, cardioversion or electroconvulsive therapy are the exception. Hospitalized patients with diagnosed agitation, drug use, alcoholism, and seizures are put on varying diazepam administration schedules. Implicated as possibly contributing to two deaths, diazepam is also hazardous in other patients because of hypoxia, hepatic decompensation, congestive heart failure, and central nervous system toxicity.

Descriptors: Diazepam (intravenous), drug-related pathology.

365. Greenblatt, S. <u>Social Aspects of the Use of Medication by the</u> <u>Elderly.</u> Paper presented at the Conference on Medication Use Among Older Adults, Chicago, April 1976.

  Overviews the meaning underlying much of the elderly's attraction for medication relief. The reliance on prescriptive medicine is the result of crippling physical condition and awareness of social collapse against which the elderly feel helpless. By creating a need for drugs, elderly disabled and those with low and unspendable incomes can both escape misery and surmount the ephemeral amount of pleasure in their lives. Overreliance also stems from misinformation about the purpose of substances and how chemical interactions can be simultaneously pleasurable and hazardous.

  Descriptors: Epidemiology, prescription medication.

366. Greer, M. Tracking down the cause of dizziness. <u>Geriatrics,</u> 1975, 30, 133-136.

  Presenting complaints of patients with dizziness may be vague and detail rotatory sensations that imply a disturbance beyond neurologic pathology. How to proceed in examining subjective reports of dizzy episodes is a critical consideration for accurate diagnosis. Careful questioning of the patient and his or her family about past history reveals involvement in drug abuse or other organic and learnable characteristics which clarify the direction of symptoms and render a physician's interpretation less difficult.

  Descriptors: Dizziness, drug-related pathology, neurology.

367. Griffin, N.; Draper, R. J.; and Webb, M. G. Addiction to tranylcypromine. <u>British Medical Journal,</u> 1981, 283, 346.

  Withdrawal syndrome is reported in a male elderly patient dependent on tranylcypromine. Evidence suggests that after prolonged administration the drug's therapeutic potential is highly suspect and may require a larger dose, contravening the safety margin before addiction occurs. Increasing tolerance to tranylcypromine is acutely possible in elderly because the drug is a frequent prescription.

  Descriptors: Tranylcypromine, case study.

368. Hajek, F., and Vojtechovsky, M. Drug treatment in the first 30 days of hospitalization in the Psychiatric Hospital in Horni Berkovice. <u>Activitas Nervosa Superior,</u> 1975, 17, 299-300.

  Surveys psychotherapeutic drugs administered to 139 admissions to a psychiatric hospital. Majority of patients show diagnostic signs either of schizophrenia or alcoholism, manic-depressive psychoses and organic psychosyndromes (of old age). Most frequently prescribed neuroleptic is chlorpromazine, the frequent depressant is dothiepin, and the common tranquilizer is diazepam. Interestingly, tranquilizers and antidepressants are rarely part of the medical regimen for alcoholism.

  Descriptors: Drug therapy, hospital, psychosyndromes of old age.

369. Hall, M. R. P. Drug therapy in the elderly. <u>British Medical</u> <u>Journal,</u> 1973, 4, 582-584.

  Drugs acting on organs and the body greatly affect sensory

reception in elderly patients. Pharmacokinetics of treating the elderly are closely reviewed with respect to commonly prescribed medications (e. g. : diuretics, etc.) and titrational effects. Guidelines for observing closer the possible physical or psychological impediments to positive drug responses are prepared in addition to recognition of basic pharmacologic principles.

Descriptors: Prescriptive medication, titration.

370. Health Care in the elderly: Report of the Technical group on use of medicaments by the elderly. World Health Organization. Drugs, 1981, 22, 279-294.

Patient compliance and noncompliance are among key issues raised in this report on prescriptive medicine, drug therapy, and elderly reactive effects. Self-care replaces the embarrassment of patients as they confront moral and attitudinal judgments by physicians. Emerging from this new trend are unsupervised drug manipulations, whereby dosage and frequency of administration undergo inappropriate changes and this develops into mental and physical disorders. When morphologic functions decline and require continuous monitoring the result is prevention of self-induced addiction.

Descriptors: Service delivery, iatrogenic disease, self-medication.

371. Helber, A.; Wambach, G.; B'ottcher, W.; Frinke, K.; and Hahn, R. Increased cardiovascular arteriosclerosis risk in patients with analgesic nephropathy. Deutsche Medizinische Wochenschrift, 1981, 106, 1369-1373.

Retrospective investigation covers 54 patients with analgesic nephropathy shown to have coronary sclerosis and an increased frequency of arteriosclerotic renal artery stenosis. Risk factors leading to the arteriosclerosis include hypercholesterolaemia and hypertriglyceridaemia, and arterial hypertension. The pathogenesis for arterial hypertension is still greatly unknown although complications may arise from excessive and improper use of dependency-developing chemicals. Adverse effects of analgesics in middle-aged and elderly patients causing kidney and blood diseases are elaborated.

Descriptors: Analgesics, drug-related pathology.

372. Hollister, L. Adverse reactions to phenothiazines. Journal of the American Medical Association, 1964, 189, 311-313.

Phenothiazine derivatives have multiple effects of clinical value. Treatment of many emotional disorders is, however, accompanied by antihistaminic, adrenergic blocking, anticholinergic, and metabolic-endocrine actions. Described are the classic central nervous reactions expected under phenothiazine medications and tactics for effective drug management. Allergic or toxic reactions to phenothiazines are not particularly different from those attributable to other agents, but, like other agents, their sedative effects are especially likely to have repercussions for the elderly.

Descriptors: Phenothiazine, drug-related pathology, drug-therapy.

373. Hollister, L. E. ; Conley, F. K. ; Britt, R. H. ; and Shuer, L. Long-term use of diazepam. Journal of American Medical

Association, 1981, 246, 1568-1570.

Administration of diazepam in middle-aged male and female patients is commonly for relief of pain or muscle spasm or anxiety and insomnia. Plasma concentrations of diazepam and its major active metabolite nordiazepam are measured in 108 neurosurgical patients taking the drug in doses of 5 to 40 mg/day for periods from one month to 16 years. Long-term use of diazepam seems to retain its efficiency, with minimal evidence shown of potential abuse. These data challenge the common recommendation for limited prescription of diazepam unless taken under controlled supervision. Kinetics related to drug consumption and treatment of physical pain are discussed.

Descriptors: Diazepam, adverse effects.

374. Horn, D. Public attitudes and beliefs relative to cancer prevention, cancer health care services and access thereto. Health Publication Monographs, 1973, 36, 11-17.

Actions considered to be related to cancer, such as tobacco and alcohol use, are examined regarding the need for periodic and early diagnosis. Acceptance by the patient to continue preventive actions and to substitute these hazardous behaviors is an attitude greatly lacking in most smokers. Most smokers recognize smoking as dangerous to their health but misevaluate smoking against other aspects of their lives. Carcinogens relative to alcohol and substance abuse both derived from prescription and illicit use are discussed.

Descriptors: Cancer, prevention, cigarette smoking.

375. Horn, J. Age and attitudes. Psychology Today, 1975, 12, 83; 87.

Reports results from a survey of 1,500 people that ascertains the relationship between age and attitudes on five major problems: Health, environment, drugs, national defense, and education. Respondents judge whether the government's financial budget is too steep or appropriately spent on domestic products. Older groups tend to agree that more funds are warranted for drug addiction research and issues rather than on national defense. Older respondents are also generally more conservative on most spending issues, considering their economic disadvantages and discouragement with appropriations to medical services.

Descriptors: Epidemiology, drug attitudes, economy.

376. Horstmann, P. Chronic ephedrine poisoning. Ugeskrift for Laeger, 1980, 142, 1502-1504.

Case report describes a substance-induced dependency on ephedrine. Poisoning resulting from nonadherence to the medication schedule by both adolescents and adults can ultimately produce a reaction that resembles psychosis. Etiologic foundations of ephedrine use and abuse are discussed.

Descriptors: Ephedrine, medication regimen.

377. Hubay, C. A.; Weckesser, E. C.; and Levy, R. P. Adrenal insufficiency may explain lack of response after surgery. Annals of Surgery, 1975, 181, 325-332.

Adrenal insufficiency is a consideration in patients unresponsive to usual therapeutic measures. Among different types, iatrogenic adrenal insufficiency results from taking more steroids than prescribed. A number of mechanisms involving surgical and medical intervention to determine level of adrenal function (especially in patients with Addison's disease) may greatly hasten the diagnosis and clarify confusion over which tissue destruction is caused by medication misuse or by premedication illness.

    Descriptors: Adrenal function, steroids, drug-related pathology.

378. Hubbell, J. G. Danger! Prescription-drug abuse. The Reader's Digest, April 1980, 100-104.

    Traces the growing prevalence of dependency on prescribed medication in America and the treatment monopoly by the medical establishment. Highly addictive drugs that are readily available from pharmacies or through physicians include the sedatives (e. g. , Chloral Hydrate and Valium), and opioid synthetics (codeine, etc.). Case reports of professionals and nonprofessionals experiencing the agony and resentment toward withdrawal and drug recovery help to provide coverage of current trends in the drug scene as perceived by experts in the field.

    Descriptors: Epidemiology, medical regimen, OTC.

379. James, M. Pharmacists and seniors: A gray area? Michigan Pharmacist, 1980, April, 4-8.

    Feature article comprehensively introduces and reviews the (Michigan) Governor's Task Force on Seniors and Substance Abuse Project. The Force is primarily creating a liaison committee to the governor's advisory group for the purpose of improving proper monitoring and use of medicines through increased consumer awareness and expanded availability of information. Illustrated cases depicting the oversight by physicians of social and physical debilitating conditions of senior citizens defines the vulnerable role of elderly persons placed on rather vague or routine medication schedules. Recommended by this Task Force is the inclusion of more articles relevant to prescription problems in the Michigan Pharmacist.

    Descriptors: Planning and development, medication prescriptions.

380. Jarvik, L. F. ; Greenblatt, D. J. ; and Harman, D. (eds.). Clinical Pharmacology and the Aged Patient. New York: Raven Press, 1981.

    This book attempts to resolve a myriad of complex considerations regarding use of drugs in patients of all ages. Biological, psychological, and socioeconomic factors interactive with the safe and dangerous sides of drug therapy are clearly explored, noting coexisting problems in the homeostatic capacity of the aged in general. Because drug reactions can mimic systemic illness or present nonspecifically organic disorders, information stresses certain age-related factors that typically complicate diagnosis and drug therapy.

    Descriptors: Etiology, medication prescriptions, drug therapy.

381. Johnson, J. C. An approach to the unresponsive patient. Journal of Indiana State Medical Association, 1980, 12, 802-804.

Case report describes a hypoglycemic and spinal injury emergency (including pregnancy) when the conscious patient resists medical services. Substance abuse complications are noteworthy in emergencies where the type of overdose is involuntary and due to medication nonadherence rather than suicidal ideations. Patients who are unconscious on arrival may later object to the medical intervention proceeding without consent. Practical strategies on the management of stubborn or unresponsive patients are included.

Descriptors: Medical emergency, physician-patient relations.

382. Judge, T. G. , and Caird, F. I. Drug Treatment of the Elderly Patient. Tunbridge Wells, Eng. : Pitman Medical Co. , 1978.
Approximately one in six old people takes three or more drugs a day, and perhaps one in sixteen, five or more a day. This incidence of a drug-taking problem among older persons is attributable to causes of morbidity commonly overlooked in geriatric medicine. This book attempts to remedy this deficiency by providing clinical guidance on relevant matters such as diagnosis and treatment precautions. Detailed factual information in the literature on elderly abusers includes topics on etiology but excludes those topics where the prescriber would be best advised to seek specialist advice before drug therapy is embarked upon (e. g. , ophthalmology and otology).

Descriptors: Etiology, drug therapy.

383. Junod, J. P. The anal incontinence in the geriatric treatment. Praxis, 1981, 70, 662-665.
Aged individuals with fecal incontinence (encopresis) are described during the duration of therapy involving cathartics, and sedative-hypnotics. Potential adverse effects from the impact of therapy on sphincter control indicates that cathartics may complicate patterns of diagnosed improvement. Tactical strategies allowing for maximal protection against drug dependency are discussed.

Descriptors: Encopresis, drug dependency, drug-related pathology.

384. Kayne, R. C. (ed.). Drugs and the Elderly. Los Angeles: University of Southern California Gerontology Center, 1978.
Compilation of papers providing information to assist practitioners and aged clients in drug management. Prevention issues within the aging network are explored along with detailed accounts of projected (or current) treatment programs offering specialized care for elderly abusers. Drug-related problems are viewed from different perspectives.

Descriptors: Medication prescription, physician-patient relationship, prevention.

385. Khan, A. ; Hornblow, A. R. ; and Walshe, J. W. Benzodiazepine dependence: A general practice survey. New Zealand Medical Journal, 1981, 93, 19-21.
Study evaluates dependence potential of benzodiazepines in 1,079 patients seen by general practitioners. Most users are middle-aged to elderly females with known chronic physical illness and drug histories ranging from one month to five years. Varying severity of

withdrawal symptoms are apparently not significant across socioeconomic levels.   Moreover, general trends in the prescriptive
practice are to replace barbiturates with benzodiazepines in preschool
(pediatric) and adult therapies.   Additional information drawn from
the questionnaire survey concerns substance dependence as an
adaptive-adjustment problem in society.

    Descriptors: Medication prescription, benzodiazepines,
general practitioner.

386.   Kleh, J., and Fazekas, J. F.   Effects of hypotensive agents on
      subjects with cerebral vascular insufficiency.   Journal of
      the American Geriatrics Society, 1956, 4, 18-23.

    Use of hypotensive drugs (hexamethonium, hydralazine, and
reserpine) in elderly subjects with hypertension and cerebral vascular
insufficiency has been both advocated and discouraged.   Discussed are
the objections that reduction of pressure may impair proper body
functioning, causing this insufficiency.   Sensitivity of the brain to the
ischemia attendant upon reduction of pressure is critical to evaluation
of hypotensive medication and would indicate directives for anticipating side-effects (habit-formation, withdrawal, etc.).   Investigated are
the actions of hypotensive drugs on selected patients.

    Descriptors: Drug-related pathology, hypotensive agents.

387.   Koch-Wesler, J.   Serum drug concentrations as therapeutic
      guides.   The New England Journal of Medicine, 1972, 287,
      227-231.

    Briefly surveys the efficacy of standard dosage schedules
that will or will not exert pharmacologic changes.   Drug toxicity is
noted as resulting from failure to reduce dosage levels as appropriate
to patient variables such as age and increased tolerance.   Optimal
dose requirements with respect to these variables are only easy when
the drug can be accurately quantified during its clinical use.   Otherwise, dosage adjustments may pose serious liability to stable treatment effects and possibly even engender new pathology.

    Descriptors: Dosage schedules, drug therapy, drug tox-
icity.

388.   Koch-Wesler, J.   Fatal reactions to drug therapy.   The New
      England Journal of Medicine, 1974, 291, 302-303.

    Almost all patients admitted because of adverse drug ef-
fects find themselves on acute medical services and a large share
of them with life-threatening drug reactions go to teaching hospitals.
Explored is the increasing prevalence of iatrogenic drug reactions
among different age populations in these services.   Issues of concern,
for instance, are that 7 percent of all deaths in this country are the
result of pharmacologic mishaps.   Intensive investigations of each
suspected drug-induced death would clearly involve a revitalization
of monitoring systems whereby the toxic potential of drugs would be
better indicated by the Food and Drug Administration.   Watchdog approaches to reactivity might prevent public consumption of those
drugs presently marketed in this country whose benefits do not out-
weigh their risks, especially where the benefit-to-risk ratio is quite
high.   Many lethal and adverse drug reactions vis-à-vis their clinical
facility are probed for debate.

Descriptors: Drug side-effects, prescription medication.

389. Koal, L. A.; Kosberg, J. I.; and Wegner-Burch, K. Perceptions of the treatment responsibilites for the alcoholic elderly client. Social Work in Health Care, 1981, 6, 69-76.
Sociopsychological factors affecting the elderly alcoholic both regarding adjustment and the attitudes of physicians are discussed. This questionnaire study looks at service providers' perceptions of sobriety in elderly. Majority of respondents indicate that few, if any, trained staff had specialty in elderly alcoholism or expected to receive in-service training on treatment methods. Interest in having this educational training is discouraged by the affordability of these programs.
Descriptors: Physician attitudes, prescription medication.

390. Kornetsky, C., and Mirsky, A. F. On certain psychopharmacological and physiological differences between schizophrenic and normal persons. Psychopharmacologia, 1966, 8, 309-318.
Evidence is presented to indicate control of schizophrenic behavior using all centrally acting drugs. Responsiveness is more intense than in normal persons, judging this reaction from a neuropsychological theory, namely, that schizophrenic patients are in a state of chronic hyperarousal. Neural dysfunction in those areas of the brain concerned with maintenance of arousal and attention (reticular activating system) is modifiable in cases of antisocial and addictive performance. Implications for addictive potential of drugs in elderly are offered.
Descriptors: Schizophrenia, drug-drug interactions, hyperarousal.

391. Kretschmar, J. H. The use of psychopharmacological drugs in the treatment of the aged. Therapiewoche, 1977, 27, 1345-1352.
Increasing importance of drug treatment in geropsychiatric disorders is indicated when any of the following signs are present: endogenous and organically based psychoses, neuroses, psychopathic disorders, epilepsies, vegetative symptoms, alcoholism and drug addiction. Explored are the psychosocial aspects germane to the patient's disease history and amenability for treatment. Prerequisites suggested for drug usage are that (a) drugs be selected carefully based on observation, (b) disorders be classified, (c) drugs dosage be introduced gradually, and (d) physician be familiar with side-effects unique to elderly. Noted problems are when side-effects of medication limit progress.
Descriptors: Psychiatry, drug-drug interaction, psychosocial.

392. Lader, M. H. Alcohol reactions after single and multiple doses of calcium cyanamide. Quarterly Journal of Studies on Alcohol, 1967, 28, 468-475.
Studies reactivity to alcohol after single doses (100 mg) of citrated calcium cyanamide. Comparisons made between alcohol and

and nonalcohol reactions on the drug are largely in cardiovascular symptoms. Facial suffusion and conjunctival reddening also appeared. Symptoms of headache, anginal pain (felt in older patients) and palpitations are also common. Since group differences are not significant, conclusions are that cyanamide is a feasible adjunct to outpatient therapy of alcoholics in regulating an abstinence schedule.

Descriptors: Calcium cyanamide, cardiovascular disorders, drug-related pathology.

393. Lader, M. Benzodiazepines--panacea or poison? Australian and New Zealand Journal of Psychiatry, 1981, 15, 1-9.

Adolescent, adult, and aging clients seen for anxiety disorders are frequent recipients of benzodiazepine drug therapy. Tranquilizing agents prescribed for diagnosed adjustment problems are also potentially addictive and will disrupt the therapeutic schedule once dependency intensifies. Examined are underlying etiologic concerns that physicians should raise about the risk-benefit ratio, and whether dose-response relationships require further investigation. Common mistakes in medication dosage level and consequently the development of accidental drug side effects are reviewed.

Descriptors: Anxiety disorders, benzodiazepines, prescription medication.

394. Lamy, P. P. Misuse and abuse of drugs by the elderly-- another view. American Pharmacist, 1980, 5, 14-17.

Discusses prescription drug problems among the elderly that are important for geriatric medicine practitioners and health care providers. Pervasive areas include (a) lack of appreciation for effects of primary and secondary aging, (b) inaccurate diagnosis, (c) use of unnecessary medications, and (d) deliberate overmedication. Physicians' attitudes also have much to do with rational drug decisions, knowledge of proper pharmacology, pharmacokinetics and toxicology of drugs. Treatment of elderly alcoholism and iatrogenic addiction (from benzodiazepines) should also recognize the sensitivity of interpersonal and emotional patterns accompanying somatic disease.

Descriptors: Physician attitudes, prescription medication.

395. Lamy, P. P. , Kitler, M. E. Drugs and the geriatric patients. Journal of the American Geriatrics Society, 1970, 19, 23-33.

Discusses reasons for caution in administering drugs to older persons. Medical record survey indicates that prescription practices vary between hospitalized patients and community patients. Emphasized needs in both settings are that drug dosage levels be monitored frequently and that complete instructions be given to older patients so they can anticipate realistic side-effects. Differences in attitudinal bias toward hospitalized geriatric patients are also explored.

Descriptors: Prescription practices, physician attitudes.

396. Larry, P. P.; Reichel, W. and Weg, R. Make age a factor in the drug equation. Patient Care, August, 1975.

Summarizes basic physiological processes of aging important in determining the dose of prescriptive medication. Routine practices are inadvisable and potential hazards to mis- and over-medication. Physicians learn of resultant implications of pharmacology for a safer administration of drugs.

Descriptors: Prescription medication, physician education.

397. Lee, P. V. Drug therapy in the elderly: The clinical pharmacology of aging. Alcoholism: Clinical and Experimental Research, 1978, 2, 39-42.

Reviews the principal cardiovascular disorders for which elderly receive medication. Orthostatic hypotension and syncope, when induced by several drugs (e. g. , alcohol) that act on the circulation, may worsen from use of diuretics or other drugs that affect central and autonomic nervous systems. Complications in drug therapy noted for older patients are in the diagnostic process and prevail during dosage reduction stages (withdrawal syndrome).

Descriptors: Cardiovascular disorders, drug-related pathology, alcohol.

398. Lemos, A. V. , and Moran, J. Veterans administration hospital staff attitudes toward alcoholism. Drug and Alcohol Dependence, 1978, 3, 77-83.

Surveys attitudes toward alcoholism and drug abuse in relation to (a) emotional problems that contribute to alcoholism, (b) loss-of-control, (c) possibility of recovery, (d) alcoholic as steady drinker, (e) character defects, (f) social status, (g) illness, and (h) harmless indulgence. Demographic variables such as sex and age correlate with results of the survey, showing more attitudinal change in certain staff members (depending on hospital role or function). Special alcohol and drug abuse training on attitudes is an alternative solution to the current strategies in practice.

Descriptors: Staff attitudes, demography, veterans hospital.

399. Levenson, A. J. (ed.). Neuropsychiatric Side-effects of Drugs in the Elderly. New York: Raven Press, 1979.

Volume 9 in the impressive Raven Press series on Aging explores the prevalence of iatrogenic neuropsychiatric side-effects in the elderly. Over-the-counter and prescribed medications are highest percentage of drugs that are routinely consumable. Chapters thus detail the pharmacoactive agents utilized by geriatrics and also the scientific rationale for understanding iatrogenic side-effects--how and why they are produced. The basic contention holds that iatrogenic side-effects of medications are preventable or potentially reversible if recognized and diagnosed early.

Descriptors: Iatrogenic illness, neuropsychiatric disorders.

400. Lewis, W. H. Medicine and the aging population. Journal of the American Medical Association, 1958, 166, 1412-1419.

Reports the abnormal processes and diseases in different age categories against the backdrop of physician responsibility. Scientific technology allows for greater inspection of longevity factors and age-linked diseases brought on by multiple (polymorbid) physical disorders. The physician's responsibility in medical management is to promote good health, duration, and quality of individual lives toward a long-term benefit of community welfare.

Descriptors: Technology, polymorbidity, physician responsibility.

401. Libow, L. S., and Mehl, B. Self-administration of medications by patients in hospitals or extended care facilities. Journal of the American Geriatrics Society, 1970, 18, 81-85.
Routine dispensing of medication on hospital wards is done by nurses. Then, after discharge, patients are expected to adhere to medication regimens which may include taking several different drug preparations of confusing sizes, shapes, and colors. Alternatively, this experimental study let patients self-administer medications during a two-week trial period and found surprising accuracy. Low number of medication errors would suggest that, in properly selected cases, self-administration is an advantageous opportunity to teach patients the skills needed in aftercare. Medication schedules and typical errors that complicate acquisition of the self-administered skills are examined with useful solutions.
Descriptors: Self-administered medication, hospitalization, drug therapy.

402. Lifshitz, K., and Kline, N. S. Use of an estrogen in the treatment of psychosis with cerebral atherosclerosis. Journal of the American Medical Association, 1961, 176, 501-504.
Reports the effects of treatment with a long-acting parenterally administered estrogenic substance in 90 men between 55 and 75 years of age. Estrogen-produced gynecomastia is apparent in patients suffering from atherosclerosis or senile psychosis. No significant differences are suggested between treatment and control (placebo) groups regarding mental functioning, except that psychological (demand) characteristics in placebo patients are stronger. Evidence that estrogens normalize the blood-lipid picture in patients and that they are of therapeutic value in physical and psychologic functioning of elderly women is brought into question.
Descriptors: Estrogens, drug-related pathology, prescribed medication.

403. Linn, L. S. Physician characteristics and attitudes toward legitimate use of psychotherapeutic drugs. Journal of Health and Social Behavior, 1971, 12, 132-140.
Study finds that physicians hold a range of attitudes toward two popular prescribed psychotherapeutic drugs, dexedrine and librium. Decisions to prescribe either drug tend to reflect their values, social position, and social background, and are less reflective of medical or scientific background. Prescribing habits of physicians in the context of both age-related prejudice and disregard for physical ailments resulting from socially unacceptable disorders (e. g., alcoholism and drug addiction) strongly suggest there is a need to investigate further the role of social factors in medical prescription.
Descriptors: Physician attitudes, prescribing habits, malpractice.

404. Linn, L. S., and Davis, M. S. The use of psychotherapeutic drugs by middle-aged women. Journal of Health and Social Behavior, 1971, 12, 331-340.

The well-documented concept called "illness behavior" says that symptoms of illness are differentially perceived, evaluated, and acted upon by different kinds of people in different social situations. This concept undergoes further clarity by measuring different types of illness behavior (pain, recognition of symptoms, attitudes toward illness, utilization of health facilities, etc.) in relation to social and cultural factors. To this extent, the study defines the prevalence of psychotherapeutic drug use (within their sample population), and analyzes these data as indicators of social, cultural, medical, and environmental influences. Noteworthy is their discussion of statistical reports that production and marketing of mood-altering drugs are evidence of an increased amount of public consumption.
Descriptors: Illness behavior, psychotherapeutic drugs, women.

405. Lipton, H. L. The graying of America: Implications for the pharmacist. American Journal of Hospital Pharmacy, 1982, 39, 131-135.
Current interest in substance abuse among older persons has clearly evolved from increased longevity of the U.S. population. For this reason, pharmacists aware of the demands by elderly for medication are in a better position to anticipate or identify cases of abuse. In addition, the ratio of men to women in the elderly population is decreasing and consequently more women, who already constitute a large medication group, will place greater demands upon pharmacies. This need for prescription medication imposes a financial burden on economically disabled elderly. Medication errors and noncompliance that result from having to obtain drugs elsewhere will contribute to overall physical and psychological problems and likely complicate any therapy. Prevention strategies recommended for the pharmacist are discussed.
Descriptors: Epidemiology, prescription medication, pharmacy.

406. Lundin, D. V. Must taking medications be a dilemma for the independent elderly? Journal of Gerontological Nursing, 1978, 4, 25-27.
Nursing advice is offered on strategies to instruct elderly persons on medication regimens to comply with the schedule. Frequent communication problems in the physician's instructions end up costing the patient both more money and the discomfort of physical side-effects, such as drug dependency. Patients unlikely to maintain continuous adherence are those persons on complex schedules or taking pills along with alcohol. The nurse's responsibility to intercede on the elderly's behalf is a first step toward taking the drug regimen seriously, but it must follow with the recruitment of public and community support.
Descriptors: Nurses, prescription medication, physician-patient relations.

407. Lundin, D. V. Medication taking behavior of the elderly; A pilot study. The Pharm-Chem Newsletter, 1979, 8 (#6).
Briefly describes a simple survey test to determine what drugs older persons are taking and to what extent their knowledge of

medications is lacking for effective drug therapy. Development of survey instruments is less important than finding the vulnerable elderly in community areas.

Descriptors: Medication prescription, self-administration.

408. Melmon, K. L. Preventable drug reactions--causes and cures. New England Journal of Medicine, 1971, 284, 1361-1367.

Modern therapeutic agents can contribute favorably to the physician's ability to interpret and treat diseases under most circumstances. Drug toxicity problems, however, largely account for the nation's high percentage of hospital admissions due to drug reactions, with approximately 30 percent of these patients suffering a second reaction during their hospital stay. Explored are the causes and long-term modifications of uncontrolled drug reactions. Age factors play a central role in measuring correct dosage levels. But especially in elderly groups, major causes of preventable drug reactions are that (a) too many pills are prescribed and (b) physicians may fail to set a therapeutic end-point for the drugs used.

Descriptors: Drug therapy, toxicity reactions, physicians' prescribing practices.

409. Mihatsch, M. J.; Hofer, H. O.; Gutzwiler, F.; Brunner, F. P.; and Zollinger, H. U. Phenacetin abuse I: Occurrence, per capita consumption and costs of treatment. Schweizerische Medizinische Wochenschrift, 1980, 110, 108-115.

Phenacetin abuse and its chemically induced pathology are reviewed. Legislative lobbying to establish sanctions against certain medication dispensaries are of relevant concern, since the number of aging persons in Switzerland is increasing rapidly. Treatment of kidney, bladder and ureteral neoplasms developed from prolonged abuse are also discussed.

Descriptors: Phenacetin, epidemiology.

410. Mihatsch, M. J ; Schmidlin, P.; Brunner, F. P.; Hofer, H. O.; Six, P.; and Zollinger, H. U. Phenacetin abuse II. Chronic renal insufficiency in Basel autopsies. Schweizerische Medizinische Wochenschrift, 1980, 110, 116-124.

Chronic terminal renal failure produced by unarrested use of phenacetin or paracetamol containing analgesics is examined in autopsies. Autopsied patients treated by hemodialysis and renal transplantation show such nephropathies as glomerulonephritis, diabetic nodular glomerulosclerosis, systic kidney disease, and vascular nephropathies. General results suggest the replacement of phenacetin by other, less toxic, analgesic compounds.

Descriptors: Phenacetin, analgesics, renal obstruction, drug-related pathology.

411. Miller, M. B. Iatrogenic and nursigenic effects of prolonged immobilization of the ill aged. Journal of the American Geriatrics Society, 1975, 23, 360-369.

Factors related to the kinesic, psychopathologic, and psychosocial effects of prolonged immobilization on the ill aged are examined over a period of 12 weeks. Iatrogenic and nursigenic

(induced by nurses) changes resulting in functional disabilities illustrate the ease with which immobilization can render aged patients
helpless. Prolonged inactivity causes severe physical and psychological harm to patients on rigid medication regimens who over a
short period of time develop social withdrawal, increasing apathy,
stupor and confusion. Reversibility of this immobilization syndrome
depends on the nursing staff realizing that their overassistance is
contraindicative.

    Descriptors: Iatrogenic and nursigenic illness, prescrip-
tion medication.

412.   Mirsky, A. F. , and Kornetsky, C. The effect of centrally-
      acting drugs on attention. In D. Efron (ed.), Psychopharm-
      acology: A Review of Progress 1957-1967. Washington, DC:
      USPHS, 1968.

    Reviews the recent literature and exploratory theories on
the effects of centrally acting drugs on attention responses. Dynamics of attention include symptoms of psychopathology and underlying
changes in humoral and physiological mechanisms. Viewing attention
as a behavioral reaction, devices to measure the nature and quality
of attention are corticalized tests and continuous performance tests.
Attentive errors made on these tests stem from lapses or from confusion, usually the result of biochemical interactions. Important in
this research are several reinterpretations of concentration and attentive potential under the influence of central nervous system drugs.

    Descriptors: Attention responses, drug-related behavior,
test battery.

413.   Munson, M. L. ; O'Leary, J. S. ; and Locke, B. Z. Use and non-
      use of medication by sufferers of selected symptoms of de-
      pression. Journal of Human Stress, 1980, 6, 20-27.

    Stress-related illnesses are major antecedents to overmedi-
cation and drug dependency. Explored is the expedient means of
alleviating stress in persons severely reluctant to seek nondrug forms
of therapy. Of the higher proportions of people reporting symptoms
of stress and psychological disturbance (in their survey), few resort
to medications on a continuous basis. Multiple standardization is
used to assess correlations of medication users to varying ranges of
socioeconomic status, education, race, sex, and marital status. Authors conclude that the popular belief that U. S. is a "pill-popping"
society is a misrepresentation of actual data.

    Descriptors: Stress, prescription medication.

414.   National Institute on Drug Abuse. The aging process and
      psychoactive drug use. National Institute on Drug Abuse:
      Service Research Monographs. Rockville, MD: National
      Institute on Drug Abuse, 1979.

    Monograph consists of three reports that correspond to each
part of the study. Part 1 examines the physiological and psychological aspects of aging and their relationship to drug use. Effects of
absorption, transport, tissue localization, metabolism, and excretion
of drugs vary widely among elderly by the number and chronicity of
pathologic diseases. Part 2 discusses patterns of psychoactive drug

use by the elderly. Highly disputed is the question of whether drug misuse and abuse really exists in older Americans. In the third part appears a review of operating programs established to prevent or treat drug problems of elderly. Few programs are exclusively for this purpose but may contain experts on staff or provide components of training specialty.

Descriptors: Epidemiology, service delivery systems.

415. Parkin, D. M.; Henney, C. R.; Quirk, J.; and Crocks, J. Deviation from prescribed drug treatment after discharge from hospital. British Medical Journal, 1976, 2, 686-688.

Study shows that out of 130 patients medically discharged on medication schedules, 66 deviate from the drug regimen. Faulty communication and medication error are primarily to blame for nonadherence, but the complexity of medication regimen is further explored. Medicines prescribed before admission to the hospital would compound the confusion, since often these are nonrenewable prescriptions. Implications for adaptive strategies within the ward to develop more compliant practices are offered.

Descriptors: Medication compliance, prescription medication, hospital discharge.

416. Parry, H. J. Use of psychotropic drugs by U. S. adults. Public Health Reports, 1968, 83, 799-810.

Mood-changing drugs continue to be in popular demand by middle-aged and elderly adults hoping to satisfy various needs. Three broad categories examined with respect to their national circulation include "hard drugs" (opium derivatives and cocaine), "psychedelic drugs" (e. g., LSD), and "psychotropic drugs" (e. g., sedatives, tranquilizers, and stimulants). Typological aspects of personality and sociocultural factors also define the use of each drug category. Urban slums and depressed minorities, for instance, will be typically associated with users of hard drugs, as will campus drop-outs be associated with users of psychedelic drugs. Psychotropic users apparently loom largely across many different socioeconomic strata.

Descriptors: Demography, drug-patterns.

417. Pattison, J. H, and Allen, R. P. Comparison of the hypnotic effectiveness of secobarbital, pentobarbital, methyprylon and ethchlorvynol. Journal of the American Geriatrics Society, 1972, 20, 398-401.

Summarizes the results of a placebo-controlled study on hypnotic effects of secobarbital, pentobarbital, methyprylon, and ethchlorvynol in 50 elderly with chronic diseases. Insomniac levels of improvement are rated by time of sleep onset and sleep duration (in half-hour units). Generally, pentobarbital is consistently more therapeutic over both placebo and other barbiturates, although each sedative is superior over placebo. Known risks in using barbiturates in elderly who are chronically ill may be prevented with methyprylon, considering its lower toxicity and faster hypnotic effects.

Descriptors: Barbiturates, insomnia, sedative-hypnotics.

418. Pavkov, J., and Stephens, B. The older adult and drug therapy: Part one. Special considerations for the community-based elderly. Geriatric Nursing, 1981, 6, 422-428; 441.
Community health nursing takes the service provider into home-based locations, quite different from the antiseptic hospital confines. Natural limitations in maintaining chronically ill elderly on drug regimens include no supervision, and noncompliance while on a self-administered schedule. Self-medication practices certainly permit greater autonomy to the aftercare patient, but may also hinder medical recovery if dosage and frequency of administration are inconsistent. Alternatives to mismedication involve health educational programs run by nurses on home-bound assignment.
Descriptors: Self-medication, nurses.

419. Pavlovsky, P.; Urban, E.; Hav'akov'a, B.; Petr'a'nov'a, V. Toxicomania in doctors hospitalized in a Prague psychiatric clinic. Ceskoslovenska Psychiatrie, 1980, 76, 331-335.
Physicians hospitalized for substance abuse undergo the care of the psychiatric treatment facility in Prague. Discussed are some etiologies and whether occupational involvement with drug therapy (especially in elderly physicians) is psychologically responsible for later addictive formation. Cultural aspects that impact on hospitalized physicians are noteworthy.
Descriptors: Physicians, Prague.

420. Pelle, R., and Von Loetzen, I. Phenothiazine deaths: A critical review. American Journal of Psychiatry, 1973, 130. 306-309.
Article questions whether "phenothiazine death" is a valid entity or is due to unrecognized lethal catatonia. Review of case studies attesting to this cause of death indicates less than affirmative answers about the chemical propensity for respiratory depression. Authors raise doubts regarding the currently held diagnosis and explore possible options involving cardiovascular effects.
Descriptors: Phenothiazines, drug-related pathology.

421. Pegel, L. A. Iron therapy for aged patients. Journal of the American Geriatrics Society, 1958, 6, 621-622.
Side-effects of iron therapy are common among aged patients, possibly because aging causes atropic changes in the mucous membranes and secretory cells of the gastrointestinal tract. Elderly patients suffering from even mild abdominal cramps will then resist or refuse further medication. Reported is the evaluation of a new iron preparation in the treatment of anemia which attends to side-effect issues.
Descriptors: Iron, drug therapy.

422. Peterson, D. M., and Thomas, C. W. Acute drug reactions among the elderly. Journal of Gerontology, 1975, 30, 552-556.
Analyzes records of patients treated for acute drug reactions. Examined characteristics show that (1) acute drug reactions are more likely to occur among whites and females, (2) a substantial

number of the reactions follow the ingestion of two or more substances, (3) one-third of admissions are related directly to suicide
attempts, and (4) the majority of acute drug reactions involve ingestion of legally manufactured drugs. Implications offer direction
for restricted availability of over-the-counter drugs.

Descriptors: Prescription medication, hospital admissions.

423. Pinsky, J. J.; Griffin, S. E.; Agnew, D. C.; Kamdar, M. D.;
Crue, B. L.; and Pinsky, L. H. Aspects of long-term evaluation of pain unit treatment program for patients with
chronic intractable benign pain syndrome: treatment outcome. Bulletin of Los Angeles Neurological Society, 1979,
44, 53-69.

Outcome assessment is part of this follow-up analysis of
former substance abuse patients experiencing intractable pain. Antidepressive agents, morphine derivatives, and various tricyclics are
analgesic relief during therapy that may have developed dependency.
Differences compared between younger and older patients in terms
of attitudes and aftercare adjustment reveal that more elderly are
on tranquilizing prescriptions. Indications for long-term evaluation
are that reactivity effects and possible withdrawal syndromes exacerbate pain.

Descriptors: Evaluation, pain, barbiturates.

424. Prien, R. F.; Haber, P. A.; and Caffey, E. M. The use of
psychoactive drugs in elderly patients with psychiatric disorders: Survey conducted in twelve veterans administration
hospitals. Journal of the American Geriatrics Society,
1975, 23, 104-112.

Survey results of detailed information collected on the use
of psychoactive drug use in 1,276 elderly psychiatric patients. Prescription practices relate to (a) choice of drugs, (b) prevalence of
drug use, (c) dosage, (d) combination of drug preparations, and (e)
antiparkinson agents. These factors largely vary with respect to
patient's age and initial or long-term diagnosis. Discusses vulnerability of hospitalized elderly who are on unregulated schedules of
psychoactive medicine and adverse effects they react to. Implications
for general hospital management and medical care delivery are offered.

Descriptors: Psychoactive drugs, veterans, demography.

425. Psychopharmacology in the aged. Journal of Geriatric Psychiatry, 1974, 7, 145-207.

A group of papers presented at the 13th Annual Science
Meeting of the Boston Society for Gerontologic Psychiatry include
topics on psychotropic medication, geriatric psychopharmacology,
and general commentary reflecting key issues pervasive to diagnostic
and treatment process.

Descriptors: Psychotropic medication, side-effects, pharmacology.

426. Raven, M. Pharmacists who save senior citizens from themselves. Drug Topics, November 1979, 60-61.

Retired pharmacists retrospectively appraise their reactions toward elderly substance users. Addressing health care professionals is the major thrust by this group, which recognizes apparent gaps in physician-patient communication. Pharmacists owe elderly the commitment to assure prescriptions are understood and followed with maximum adherence. Presumptions pharmacists make about physiology also should be dispelled, especially concerning the elderly's memory lapses being due to senility. Explicit guidelines to assist pharmacists and physicians in enhanced service delivery are organized with examples.

Descriptors: Prescription medication, pharmacy, physiology.

427. Rich, N.; Hobson, R. W.; and Fedde, W. Recognizing rare but dangerous iatrogenic vascular injuries. American Journal of Surgery, 1974, 128, 715-721.

Discusses vascular injuries associated with diagnostic and therapeutic procedures. Inasmuch as they are rare, those that occur require prompt restoration of arterial continuity and methods are given. Injuries are commonly from cardiac catheterization or general vascular angiography, surgical procedures, and remaining types are due to drug therapy. Vascular repairs made in the subjects observed include thrombectomy (surgical), vascular suture, autogenous vein by-pass, and repairs of arteriovenous fistula and false aneurysms. Discussed are protective and preventive mechanisms important to implement during treatment

Descriptors: Iatrogenic illness, drug-related pathology, vascularity.

428. Rickels, K. Psychopharmacologic agents: A clinical psychiatrist's individualistic point of view: Patient and doctor variables. Journal of Nervous and Mental Diseases, 1963, 136, 540-548.

Reviews typical physician perceptions in the clinical evaluation of psychiatric pharmacologic agents. Discussion first traces development of drug trial experiments as predictors of the physician's knowledge of presenting patient variables. These variables, either separately or by interaction, may overcome pharmacologic effects and depend quite heavily on personality characteristics, attitudes, and expectations of patient and physician. Studies claiming demonstrations of drug efficacy may or may not be sensitive to these variables.

Descriptors: Drug experiments, physician attitudes, physician-patient relationship.

429. Ritschel, W. A. Pharmacokinetic approach to drug dosing in the aged. Journal of the American Geriatrics Society, 1976, 24, 344-354.

Explores physiologic changes in elderly system that account for fluid and total cell mass effects on sensitivity to drug reactions. Equations are derived for calculating the loading dose and maintenance dosage of single and multiple drugs following different patterns (inhibitory, etc.) of dose-response relations. Noted is that the Minimal Inhibitory Concentration (MIC) pattern for, in particular, bacteriostatic drugs, provides a better therapeutic steady-state. Interest in developing this alternative pharmacokinetic approach derives from the fact that during multiple-dose therapy, elderly receive dose sizes that are too large for proper absorption, metabolism, and excretion if no corrections are made.

Descriptors: Drug therapy, pharmacokinetics.

430. Roberts, J.; Adelman, R. C.; and Cristofalo, V. J. (eds.).
Pharmacological Intervention in the Aging Process. New York: Plenum Press, 1977.

Pharmacologic information, of sorts, is taken from the Philadelphia Symposium on Aging in 1974. Chapters in this book reflect progress since that time regarding biomedical and psychological interface with drug reactions. Underlying this interface is an attempt to add greater insight into the nature of the aging process using interventions workable for several disciplines concerned with elderly drug users.

Descriptors: Pharmacology, aging process.

431. Rodriguez, G.; Bruzzone, M.; Gasparetto, B.; Montano, V.; and Rosadini, G. Statistical studies of the consumption of psychotropic drugs in an urban community. Archivio e Maragliano di Patologia Clinica, 1978, 34, 165-169.

Substance abuse occurrence in urban populations is greatest among adolescent and aged persons who take daily prescriptive medication. Psychotropic drug use observed in Italy is examined by factors of sex, occupation, and frequency of drug utilization, as compared to drug consumption trends over the last decade or so. Increasing usage in urban areas is speculatively due to drug accessibility and perceived benefits by consumers.

Descriptors: Prescription medication, demography, Italy.

432. Rosenbaum, J. Widows and widowers and their medication use: Nursing implications. Journal of Psychiatric Nursing, 1981, 19, 17-19.

Speaks to the pressing emotional aspects of grief and its devastation on medication compliance. Death of a family member fosters a state of bereavement frequently causing disruption in routine behavioral patterns as well as personal responsibility to health care. Bereaved subjects interviewed regarding their current use of psychotropic medication and alcohol report less drinking when depressed. Implications for nursing care for dying clients and the enhanced vulnerability of medication abuse are discussed.

Descriptors: Bereavement, psychotropic medication, nurses.

433. Ruben, D. H.; Shouse, D. W.; Page-Robin, E.; Simpson, C. D.; and Blevins, G. A. Drugs and the Elderly: A Manual on Substance Abuse (under review).

Chapters of this book carefully address the needs of service providers to the aging who have minimal background in pharmacology and its relevance to elderly populations. The sociology of aging the context of drug use, abuse, and misuse potential is followed by simplified descriptions of drug-drug interactions and common

communication barriers encountered in physicians' prescribing practices. Casefinding methods and models of therapy complete the full
circle around the ability of practitioners to better identify, prevent,
and treat potential drug abuse among older persons. National programs with established elderly treatment centers are briefly discussed.

Descriptors: Pharmacology, sociology of aging, educational manual.

434. Ruznisky, S. A.; Thauberger, P. C.; and Cleland, J. F. Rejection and the use of chemical agents. Social Science and
Medicine, 1981, 15, 205-210.

Drug-taking persons identified in Canada undergo a psychometric examination to determine whether the drug is desirable or un-
desirable. Rejection of alcohol and drug therapy is more pronounced
than attitudes toward cigarette smoking, although there are noticeable
fluctuations across different age groups. Investigated are the need
for efficient determinants of the patient's drug preference and understanding of chemical interactive effects.

Descriptors: Psychological battery, patient-drug attitudes.

435. Salzman, C.; Kochansky, G. E.; Shader, R. I.; and Cronin, D. M.
Rating scales for psychotropic drug research with geriatric
patients. II. Mood ratings. Journal of the American
Geriatrics Society, 1972, 20, 215-221.

Psychotropic drug research clearly relies on subjective
evaluations of preference or attitude by patients either currently on
or expected to begin prescriptions. Mood surveys that involve rating
scales require some degree of predisposing behaviors in order that
the ratings be measured as accurate depictions of patient opinion.
This study identifies as predisposing the following criteria: (1) that
the subject must be responsive and cooperative, (2) that the scale be
brief, with clear response choices, and (3) that the questions be
clear and relevant to the current situation of the patient. Noted by
the use of these criteria is that mood scales offer little advantage
over multidimensional rating scales.

Descriptors: Mood states, rating scales (tests), psychotropic medication.

436. Schwartz, D. The elderly patient and his medications. Geriatrics, 1965, 20, 517-520.

Discusses medication errors that frequently occur among
chronically ill and elderly patients. In a randomly sampled group
of patients, 60 percent are taking medication not prescribed, not
taking medicine prescribed, or taking incorrect dosages and at the
wrong time. Medication errors apparently begin when two or more
prescriptions are given at the same time without separate instructions.
Omission of specific instructions greatly contributes to the failure
to comply to medication regimens. Techniques for remedying or
avoiding these problems are reviewed.

Descriptors: Medication errors, prescription medication.

437. Schwartz, D.; Wang, M.; Zeitz, L.; and Gross, M. E. W.
        Medication errors made by elderly, chronically ill patients.
        American Journal of Public Health, 1962, 52, 2018-2029.
        Self-administration of medication in elderly with severe
ambulatory or health care problems poses risks that are explored in
this study. Factual data collected on "life-situation" and "nursing"
needs of hospital patients show that prescription of medicaments are
in frequent demand, but are proportionally greater than the number
of prescriptions given. Aftercare responsibilities of taking medication belong to the uninformed patient who is prone to the following
three mistakes: (a) take medication that is not ordered by physician,
(b) not take medication ordered by physician, and (c) take properly
ordered medication, but in wrong dose or at incorrect time intervals.
Evidence is shown to suggest how simple medication abuse can occur
shortly after discharge.
        Descriptors: Medication errors, prescription medication,
        self-administration.

438. Seixas, F. A. Drug and alcohol interactions: Avert potential
        dangers. Geriatrics, 1979, 34, 89-102.
        Annotated analysis of alcohol interactions with various types
of commonly prescribed medications for elderly patients. To illustrate them, a table offers a matrix comparison of specific drugs, the
type of known reaction, and possible adverse results. Guidelines for
alleviation of these potential interactions are suggested.
        Descriptors: Drug-drug interactions, alcohol, prescription
        medication.

439. Shapiro, S. , and Baron, S. H. Prescriptions for psychotropic
        drugs in a noninstitutional population. Public Health Re-
        ports, 1961, 76, 481-488.
        Information about the prescribing of psychotropic drugs out-
side the hospitals is fairly scarce. Data in this study reflect the
patterns of prescribing practices by family physicians and specialists,
written for different ranges of age groups. Increasing needs for
psychotropic drugs as indicated by the sample number of written prescriptions confirm the hypothesis that nonhospitalized drug users are
equally as prone to dependency problems or problems derived from
inaccurate medication regimens.
        Descriptors: Psychotropic medication, prescription med-
        ication.

440. Shoemaker, D. M. Use and abuse of OTC medications by the
        elderly. Journal of Gerontology and Nursing, 1980, 6, 21-
        24.
        Commentary identifies major dangerous over-the-counter
(OTC) preparations commonly sought by elderly consumers. Cathartics rank high on the list of nonprescription medicaments and are
extremely habit-forming unless taken under some semblance of supervision. The role of nursing care workers to inform and educate elderly about addictive potentials of OTCs and to be available for monitoring drug schedules is one of the concerns discussed.
        Descriptors: Nurses, OTC.

441. Shouse, D. Medication misuse by the elderly. Spada Sage (Specialty Program in Alcohol and Drug Abuse), 1983, 3, 5-8.
Summarizes crucial findings on the plethora of medication errors made by hospitalized and nonhospitalized elderly. Social, physical, and psychological aspects in the aging process involved with purchase and utilization of drugs help provide a basis for research. Also, conclusions by the National Institute on Drug Abuse on prescription misuse are clarified.
Descriptors: Prescription medication, sociology of aging.

442. Smith, D.; Chappel, J.; Griffin, J.; and Russell, K. Practicing physicians' view of the alcohol and drug abuse patient: A training and consultation model for analysis and change. In D. Smith (ed.), Multicultural View of Drug Abuse. Cambridge, MA: Schenkman Publishing, 1978.
Details the polydrug research project's availability of workshops for physicians who devote only a small percentage of time to substance abuse. Major findings are that attitudinal barriers exist against treating addicted patients or that absent sessions, unpaid bills, and lack of appreciation seem common among elderly. Objectives of the workshop training focus on clinical and pharmacologic changes of aging and why patient "negligence" is actually due to nonintentional behavior problems. Established at these workshops is a telephone consultation service for more expedient attainment of information.
Descriptors: Physician education, substance abuse.

443. Smith, M. C. Portrayal of the elderly in prescription drug advertising. The Gerontologist, 1976, 16, 329-334.
Discusses elderly and nonelderly models in advertisement for prescription drugs in two medical journals. Negative portrayals tend to strengthen false stereotypes of elderly abusers and communicate misrepresentative patterns leading to prescription needs. Chosen for examination are the journals Medical Economics and Geriatrics. Written opinions polled on the negative-positive depiction of elderly indicate this problem is more prevalent than believed.
Descriptors: Elderly in advertisement, prescription medication.

444. Solomon, J. R. The chemical time bomb: Drug misuse by the elderly. Contemporary Drug Problems, 1977, 6, 231-243.
Summarizes the general problems causing misuse of drugs by the elderly. Misinformation on the part of physician, pharmacist and patient contribute to initial medication errors, which are aggravated by noncorrective interventions. Specific problems for physicians to be aware of include overmedication, which can lead to acute organic brain syndrome, and sociocultural aspects that impact on adherence to the medical regimen. Directions are for elderly to encourage an open positive channel of understanding with the physician or pharmacist before commencing self-medication.
Descriptors: Self-medication, physician-patient relationship.

445. Solursh, L. P.   Use of diazepam in hallucinogenic drug crises.
     Journal of the American Medical Association, 1968, 208,
     98-99.
         Dangers of using phenothiazines in treatment of hallucino-
     genic (atropine-like) action are brought into question.   Since doctors
     should assume that ingestion of phenothiazines may be combined with
     a chemical having atropine-like action, chemotherapy with diazepam
     seems possible.   Testing of diazepam treatment on 69 hallucinogenic-
     drug crises patients shows it can supplement routine interventions.
     Discussion follows on using only restricted doses during the crisis
     and with different age groups.
         Descriptors: Phenothiazines, hallucinogens, drug-drug
     interactions.

446. Streltzer, J.   Treatment of iatrogenic drug dependence in the
     general hospital.   General Hospital Psychiatry, 1980, 2,
     262-266.
         Medically prescribed drugs for organic pathology are as
     addictive as over-the-counter or psychoactive medication.   Reviewed
     are patients under psychiatric consultation who are middle-aged and
     have no known drug history.   Associated with their medical condition
     is a narcotic dependence, possibly developing from medication to
     relieve headaches, insomnia, anxiety, and pain.   Although addictive
     potential goes unnoticed, there is a progressive constriction of social
     and occupational functioning which stymies medical recovery.   The
     primary physician's detection of this progressive deterioration should
     follow with the admission to detoxification units.   The authority of
     physicians makes it easier for them to encourage elderly abusers to-
     ward inpatient treatment.
         Descriptors: Iatrogenic illness, hospital care, physician-
     patient relation.

447. Studer, H. , and Straub, W.   Steroid withdrawal syndrome.
     A current problem of outpatient medicine.   Schweizerische
     Medizinische Wochenschrift, 1981, 111, 1462-1467.
         Iatrogenic adrenal insufficiency for patients on steroids is
     common enough to develop early detection or screening methods.
     Guidelines for outpatient detection include routine use of early morn-
     ing cortisol measurements, as well as knowledge of the multifaceted
     steroid-withdrawal syndromes (SWS) due to classical adrenal insuf-
     ficiency.   Symptoms occurring when the disease initially calls for
     steroid treatment is discussed with respect to psychological causes.
     Dose-response relationships in middle-aged males prone to adrenal
     pathology are explored.
         Descriptors: Iatrogenic illness, adrenal insufficiency, drug-
     related pathology.

448. Study of Legal Drug Use by Older Americans.   National Insti-
     tute on Drug Abuse, Services Research Report.   Washing-
     ton, DC: U. S. Department of Health, Education and Wel-
     fare, 1977.
         Official investigation into statistical use of prescription and
     over-the-counter drugs among the elderly.   Patterns of alcohol use

in combination with legal and psychotropic drugs suggest that heavy users are elderly women who live alone or are not married. Findings stress the ethnocultural and demographic diversity in elderly drug habits, although in general self-esteem and perceptions of physicians are fairly universal. The data are also in complete agreement with national predictive statistics reporting that omission of information on drug-drug interaction poses a dangerous threat to the elderly drinker.

Descriptors: Demography, epidemiology, drug patterns.

449. Substance Abuse Among Michigan's Senior Citizens: Current Issues and Future Directions Seniors and Substance Abuse Task Force. Lansing, MI: Michigan Office of Services to the Aging, August 1978.

The Governor's appointed task force to investigate senior drug abuse in the state of Michigan presents the result of their field survey. Implementation strategies in the initial field evaluation are briefly reviewed, followed by the Task Force's recommendations and proposed interventions. Among the seniors interviewed, a large majority regard medications as routine and necessary to relieve illness. Knowledge of side-effects and drug-drug interactions is problematic, as is the increasing attraction for legally sold preparations. Mechanisms proposed by the force to dispense drug information and reduce iatrogenic reactions appear in the discussion on the social network of service delivery.

Descriptors: Demography, education and prevention.

450. Tajiri, J.; Nakayama, M.; Sato, T.; Isozaki, S.; and Uchino, K. Pseudo-Batter's syndrome due to furosemide abuse: Report of a case and an analytical review of Japanese literature. Japanese Journal of Medicine, 1981, 20, 216-221.

Chemically induced symptoms of Batter's syndrome (e.g., vomiting, diarrhea, etc.) that are attributable to laxative and diuretic abuses may only be a metabolic mimic of the real disease. A middle-aged woman showing alleged signs of this syndrome as the result of self-administration of furosemide (for six years) also shows calcification of the bilateral renal medulla. Neural adverse reactions such as this are not reported for Batter's syndrome, unless symptoms constitute a pseudo-form of Batter's syndrome. Fourteen case reports in Japanese literature explore the characteristic symptomatology and etiology of Batter's disease and its link to drug abuse.

Descriptors: Batter's syndrome, drug-related pathology, iatrogenic illness.

451. Tandberg, D. How to treat and prevent drug toxicity. Geriatrics, 1981, 36, 64-73.

Elderly persons taking a collection of prescribed medication are physiologically predisposed to risk of toxic effects. Multiple medication increases medication error, the chance of poisoning, and usually has a correlation with attempted suicide. For seniors to self-administer dosage at reduced risks there must be developed new prevention and control programs (or therapy), designed to improve physician-patient communication.   Several possible options are mentioned.

Descriptors: Prescription medication, physician-patient relationship, drug toxicity.

452.   Taylor, C. B. ; Zlutnick, S. I. ; Corley, M. J. ; and Flora, J.
The effects of detoxification, relaxation, and brief supportive therapy on chronic pain.   Pain, 1980, 8, 319-329.
Describes study of seven chronic pain patients detoxified from analgesic medication.   Effects of relaxation training and supportive therapy lasting approximately six months are that reductions occurred in pain, mood and medication usage.   Mood ratings (self-reported) improve when pain and tension are removed concomitant with increased activity levels.   This form of rehabilitation appears to produce significant relief in middle-aged patients as long as motor activity is proportionally more frequent than intractable pain.

Descriptors: Analgesics, pain, relaxation training.

453.   Tyler, V. E.   Are generics a drug on the market?   Journal of Indiana State Medical Association, 1980, 73, 452-457.
Questioned is the therapeutic equivalency of generic drugs sold in readily accessible markets.   A cost analysis profile indicates the affordable benefits of generics are in sharp contrast with the cost-prohibitive nature of prescriptive medication.   Legislative trends in the United States toward regulation of generic medicines are discussed, as are the potential age groups most likely affected if regulatory constraints pass in congress.

Descriptors: Generic medication, prescription medication, economics,

454.   Viewig, W. V. R. ; Piscatelli, R. L. ; Houser, J. J. ; and Prouix, R. A.   Complications of intravenous administration of heparin in elderly women.   Journal of the American Medical Association, 1970, 213, 1303-1306.
Discusses heparin therapy administered intravenously to coronary care patients.   Elderly women in particular are susceptible to bleeding and congestive heart failure, but this is possibly due to parenteral administration into the buttocks of medications other than heparin.   Bleeding and other adverse side-effects of prolonged heparin use are observed in a controlled experimental study.

Descriptors: Heparin, drug-related pathology, side-effects.

455.   Wandless, I. , and Davie, J. W.   Can drug compliance in the elderly be improved?   British Medical Journal, 1977, 1, 359-361.
Tests three instructional schemes in older patients designed to improve compliance to medication regimen.   Each group is instructed verbally on the nature and amount of their medications using different cues and devices (either a tear-off calendar or an identification card).   After 14 days of self-medication, patients with calendars made fewer errors and those with either a card or calendar made fewer errors than those patients given standard instructions. Indications are that verbal and written prompts accompanying the

physician's instructions should be in a usable form (like calendars).
Descriptors: Self-medication, training program, prompts.

456. Wetli, C. V. , and Bednaczyk, L. R.   Deaths related to pro-
     poxyphene overdose: A ten-year assessment. Southern
     Medical Journal, 1980, 73, 1205-1209.
     Accidental overdose and suicidal overdose of the drug
propoxyphene is frequently due to its combination with alcohol.   Propoxyphene preparations alone are by no means harmless, but they
have a low rate of dependency and a low potential for recreational
abuse.   Deaths resulting from propoxyphene are in persons who already had chronic illness, polydrug addictions, and emotional distress.   Stressed is that dosage abuse warrants that this drug not be
reclassified to a Schedule II drug.
     Descriptors: Propoxyphene, overdose, polydrug addiction.

457. Widmer, E.   Nursing supervisor's workshop. Praktische
     Psychiatrie, 1970, 49, 229-239.
     Papers presented on the agenda of a 1970 workshop re-
garding Swiss psychiatric nursing supervisors are summarized.   New
developments in psychopharmacology give the field of institutional
psychiatry a different orientation, especially toward aging.   Elderly
persons should remain with their family; if hospitalization is unavoidable, the family can provide social outlets.   Information about
Geneva's growth of service programs and social network also stressed
the professional future of nurses in terms of their salaries and
utilization of time.
     Descriptors: Nurses, psychopharmacology.

458. Winstead, D. K.   Psychotropic drug use in the elderly.   Jour-
     nal of the Louisiana State Medical Society, 1982, 134, 88-
     93.
     Confronts the problems senior citizens have with taking
medication.   Nondrug interventions are advisable alternatives when
organic disorders are in remission.   Harmful effects in using or
overusing drugs, specifically psychotropic medicines, are observed
more in elderly alcoholics, in whom manifestations of self-neglect
and confusion are more salient.   Implications for treating elderly
alcoholics both on and off of psychotropic medication are discussed,
with suggestions to reduce prescription errors.
     Descriptors: Diagnosis, prescription medication, self-
medication, side-effects.

459. Wolf, F. W. ; Parmley, W. W. ; White, K. ; and Okun, R.   Drug-
     induced diabetes: Diabetogenic activity of long-term ad-
     ministration of benzothiadiazines. Journal of the American
     Medical Association, 1963, 185, 568-574.
     Observations during the treatment of hypertensive patients
suggest there is a diabetogenic activity of benzothiadiazine derivatives.
Examined are nonobese patients without a family history of diabetes
compared with patients who are obese and have this history.   Adverse
reactions resembling diabetic seizures are more likely to occur in
young or middle-aged hypertensives in whom there is a lengthy life

expectancy. Alternatives to hypotensive therapy are among the recommendations.

>Descriptors: Hypertension, benzothiadiazines, obesity,
>diabetes, drug-related pathology.

460. Zurrow, H. B. , and Sergay, H.   Lipoid pneumonia in a geri-
      atric patient.   Journal of the American Geriatrics Society,
      1966, 14, 240-243.

The dangers inherent in mineral oil preparations include
the incidence of lipoid pneumonia.   Symptoms of this pneumonia are
particularly contractable in elderly patients prone to self-medication
for constipation.   Over a period of time, self-medication errors
which exacerbate the pneumonia will usually be undetected in diagnosis
because patients rarely mention their use of mineral oil or its role
in the family history.   Examined are the postmortem findings of a
65-year-old woman whose sudden death from coronary heart disease
was suspected to have pneumoniac involvement.

>Descriptors: Lipoid pneumonia, self-medication, mineral
>oil.

4. EPIDEMIOLOGY: PSYCHOSOCIAL AND ECONOMIC FACTORS

461. Alcohol and other drug problems among senior citizens. Bottom Line on Alcohol in Society, 1978, 2, 21-24.
Details incidence rates of polydrug abuse in elderly populations in which nutrition and diet problems prevail. Prevention issues stress the need for efficient casefinding methods coupled with the early participation of Alcoholics Anonymous. Seniors suffering greatly from economic deficits are vulnerable to enhanced polymorbidity and medication misuse. Alternatives in community-sponsored relief programs are discussed.
Descriptors: Drug-taking patterns and culture.

462. Allen, R. C. Legal Rights of the Disabled and Disadvantaged. (Report no. 20402). Washington, DC: Social and Rehabilitation Service, 1969.
Laws defining and applicable to disabled and elderly individuals are explored with respect to mental and physical treatment rights. Alcoholics and drug addicts entitled to civil rights are frequent victims of social and economic abuse. Legal deprivations resulting from this abuse include denial of proper channels of rehabilitation and social services. Also described are legal entitlements for prisoners, offenders, and disadvantaged elderly.
Descriptors: Legal rights, drug abusers.

463. Anderson, O. J. Registration of the needs among lodgers and alcoholics without place of residence in Oslo. Tidsskrift om Edruskaps Sporsmal, 1978, 30, 30-32.
Study seeks to investigate necessary relief funding for 2,463 homeless alcoholics living in Oslo, Norway. Men 60 years and over (593) require greatest assistance and men between ages of 50 to 59 have been without residence for an average of 15.6 years. Economically disadvantaged men taking to alcoholism attribute this transition to several social factors including depression and isolation, but not to divorce. Exploratory options in providing temporary shelter to homeless elderly are discussed.
Descriptors: Homeless, economically disadvantaged.

464. Aron, W. S. Family background and personal trauma among drug addicts in the United States: Implications for treatment. British Journal of Addiction, 1975, 70, 295-305.
Evaluates composition of patients in three California state

hospital drug programs. Programs operate on a therapeutic community model, involving relatives and family whenever treatment permits. Results show that (1) most patients are middle-class, (2) nearly half come from homes in which one of the biological parents is absent, (3) several come from homes with broken religious ties, (4) families have evidence of parental drug or alcohol abuse, and (5) several personal traumas occurred in family life. Considering this background, authors hypothesize that addicts lack identity with a legitimate community and through drugs can discover a sense of belonging. Therapeutic communities offer an alternative route to personal realization and possibly restore growing interest in religious associations.

Descriptors: Therapeutic community, familial relations.

465. Ashley, M. J.; Olin, J. S.; le Riche, W. H.; Kornaczewski, A.; Schmidt, W.; and Rankin, J. G. Morbidity patterns in hazardous drinkers: Relevance of demographic, sociologic, drinking and drug use characteristics. International Journal of the Addictions, 1981, 16, 593-625.

Profile is given of socioeconomic factors affecting drug use and drinking patterns of selected inpatient alcoholics (several being elderly). Factors especially recognized include sex, skid-row status, social class, abnormal drug use and dependency, duration of drinking, and types of beverage. Clinical significance of this social and physical disease profile is to predict hazardous potentials when patients enter hostile and enriched environmental conditions. Implications for treatment planning and preventive programs using the profile are considered.

Descriptors: Socioeconomic factors, demography, predictive diagnosis.

466. Asogwa, S. E. Some characteristics of drivers and riders involved in road traffic accidents in Nigeria. East Africa Medical Journal, 1980, 57, 399-404.

The rising number of traffic accidents in Nigeria are associated with age- and substance-related etiologies. Middle-aged and elderly motorists under the influence of drugs or alcohol comprise a fairly sizable majority of fatal accident victims reported during the last decade. Adolescent victims and comparisons between male and female victims account for commonly unexplained trends in accident characteristics.

Descriptors: Driving accidents, drug abuse.

467. Atkinson, D.; Fenster, C. A.; and Blumberg, A. S. Employer attitudes toward work-release programs and the hiring of offenders. Criminal Justice and Behavior, 1976, 3, 335-344.

Work-release programs offering rehabilitative service to employed offenders and drug users tend to create bias in employer attitudes. Questionnaires administered to a group of potential employers surveys the general attitude representative of city and county workers. A majority are sympathetic toward hiring ex-offenders, unmatched by the hesitancy felt by employers who previously hired them.

Murderers, rapists and muggers are the least desirable persons for hire, while those most employable are car thieves, burglars, drug addicts, and embezzlers. Criticism and commentary analyze the value of work-relief programs being either on the prison grounds or in the community.
Descriptors: Work-relief programs, ex-offenders.

468. Baer, P.; Merin, K.; and Gaitz, C. M. Familial resources of elderly psychiatric patients: Attitude, capability and service components. Archives of General Psychiatry, 1970, 22, 343-350.
Discusses four groups of elderly patients diagnosed as having organic brain syndrome. Organic syndromes with alcoholism, without alcoholism, and forms of functional psychosis are traced to sociocultural factors inherently manifested in familial relations. Family capability is similar within the groups, but family attitude is more positive with organic brain syndromed patients, probably because these families fulfill more daily needs and recognize the addictive ailment as a medical disease.
Descriptors: Organic brain syndrome (Korsakoff's syndrome), familial relations.

469. Bailey, M. B.; Haberman, P. W.; and Alksne, H. The epidemiology of alcoholism in an urban residential area. Quarterly Journal of Studies on Alcohol, 1965, 26, 19-40.
Extensive analysis presented on the public health dangers of alcoholism in urban residential areas. Public-health approaches to disease stress identification of vulnerable groups in the population, the estimation of treatment needs, and etiologic clues leading to further research. Household surveys made of New York residents show the peak prevalence of alcoholism lies in the 45 to 54 age range. Most vulnerable are elderly widows (10.5 percent). Implications of these data for adopting population surveys over the Jellinek alcoholism estimation formula are discussed.
Descriptors: Public-health, demography, urban culture.

470. Bainton, B. R. Drinking patterns of the rural aged. In C. L. Fry (ed.), Dimensions: Aging, Culture, and Health. New York: Praeger Publishers, 1980.
Cultural drinking patterns described in this chapter outline the context out of which elderly drug abuse emerges. Statewide survey of 600 households in rural counties reveals two basic conclusions. First, the principle sociodemographic correlates of drinking are not different from those found in the general population. Second, two factors greatly associated with aging and deterred drinking are increased religiosity and failing health. The majority of elderly also change their drinking patterns insofar as reducing the average quantity of absolute alcohol consumed daily. Discussed in brief are policy considerations in the isolation of rural drinking problems.
Descriptors: Rural drinking patterns, religion, socio-economic factors.

471. Barry, D. Substance Abuse Among the Elderly. (Report no. NCAI-063853). Rockville, MD: National Institute on

Alcohol Abuse and Alcoholism, 1980.

Study examines substance abuse among elderly residents of New Jersey. Information obtained through interviews and direct mail survey of service providers indicates the over-65 group most commonly abuses prescription and over-the-counter medications. Potential drug effects, especially from mixing alcohol with prescribed medication, are poorly monitored by health care professionals. Recommended is that physicians be educated about medication misuse and how cultural factors within the elderly's surroundings easily lead to polydrug abuse.

Descriptors: Prescription medication, cultural patterns, drug-drug interactions.

472. Berger, A.; Wrober, T.A.; and Lycaki, H. Levels of basic personality factors in a psychiatric population. Journal of Clinical Psychology, 1980, 36, 378-382.

Diverse factors appear in substance abuse pathology associated with psychiatric hospitalization. Examined are 400 psychiatric patient records based on ratings of 14 criteria. Several factors indicative of depression, anxiety, and social maladjustment in middle-aged patients derive from Eysenck's three-factor model of personality at the universal or general level. A fourth factor is interpreted in behavioral dimensions and includes family and socio-interpersonal orientation. These data further imply psychosocial disorders in the geriatric population and viable forms of intervention.

Descriptors: Psychiatry, hospitalization, personality factors, drug patterns, Eysenck's three-factor model.

473. Bergin, J.W. Report to the Department of National Health and Welfare on Canadian Research on Psycho-social Aspects of Cigarette Smoking, 1960-1972. Ottawa: Department of National Health and Welfare, 1974.

Epidemiologic changes are reported on the number of cigarette smokers since 1965 and the relationship of smoking patterns to sex and age. Decreasing habits in persons aged 20 to 64 and low and stable use in persons over 65 years is proportionally greater than consumption rates in adolescent ages. Still, elderly groups are designated as high-risk groups in need of education to reduce smoking and develop effective stress management systems. Questioned are the validity of smoking cessation programs and alternative uses of behavior modification employing aversive stimuli and self-control techniques.

Descriptors: Canada, Cigarette smoking demography, behavior modification.

474. Bergmann, H.; Holm, L.; and A'Gren, C. Neuropsychological impairment and a test of the predisposition hypothesis with regard to field dependence in alcoholics. Quarterly Journal of Studies on Alcohol, 1981, 42, 15-23.

Explored is the hypothesis that field-dependent persons (elderly) are prone to alcoholism while suffering from medical and social deterioration. Two groups of Swedish inpatient alcoholics ("more deteriorated" and "less deteriorated") ranging from 45 to 62 years

old have drinking histories known for at least ten years.   IQ tests and neurological tests administered to both groups reveal significantly better performance by the less deteriorated group.   Test of field dependence show no differences between groups, suggesting that field dependence may precede rather than follow alcoholism.
Descriptors: Field-dependence, nursing homes, drug-related pathology, alcoholism.

475.   Blaney, R. , and Radford, I. S.   The prevalence of alcoholism in an Irish town.   Quarterly Journal of Studies on Alcohol, 1973, 34, 1255-1269.
Interviews are conducted on 181 male and 179 female residents of Northern Ireland, varying percentages of whom are drinkers.   Abnormal drinking patterns did not correlate significantly with religion, social class, or number of years since the first drink. Diagnostics, such as the Preoccupation with Alcohol Scale, raise questions about which evaluation tool is most accurately representative for cross-cultural comparisons.   Advantages of this preoccupation scale for social research are noted.
Descriptors: Northern Ireland, drinking patterns, Preoccupation with Alcohol Scale.

476.   Block, M. R. ; Davidson, J. L. ; and Grambs, J. D.   Women over Forty: Visions and Realities.   New York: Springer Publishing Company, 1981.
This volume explores and dispels many twentieth-century myths about aging women as perceived by American culture.   Myths and stereotypes that affect self-image play a role in the socialization process, physiological process, and in the determination for types of therapy such as estrogen replacement therapy.   Medical conditions (hysterectomy, osteoporosis, breast cancer, etc.) are discussed in relation to stress, depression, suicide, drug abuse, and alcoholism.
Descriptors: Ageism, mental health, socio-cultural patterns.

477.   Bozzett, L. P. , and Macmurray, J. P.   Drug misuse among the elderly: A hidden menace.   Psychiatric Annals, 1977, 95, 99-103; 107.
Provides discussion on the various dimensions of drug abuse among senior citizens, with a critique of the medical profession's response.   Noting the dearth of accurate sociologic prevalence data on elderly drug misuse, the authors call for a broader definition of misuse to include inappropriate drug use, adverse drug reactions and interactions, and drug dependence.   Considered through this definition are (1) the nature of drug misadventures among aged, (2) how adverse drug reactions occur, (3) the gravity of alcohol abuse, and (4) how discrimination and ageism may magnify substance abuse disorders.
Descriptors: Conceptual definitions, sociocultural patterns, medical practice.

478.   Brenner, B.   Alcoholism and fatal accidents.   Quarterly Journal of Studies on Alcohol, 1967, 28, 517-528.

Studies the relationship between alcoholism and accident mortality among 1,343 San Francisco Bay area alcoholics. Age- and sex-specific death rates for area residents indicate over 2,651 residents being 50 years or over. Circumstances of death would suggest the elevated rate of accident mortality reflects not only immediate effects of alcohol but also life patterns, personality, and types of care received when elderly are ill or injured.

Descriptors: Auto accidents, alcohol-related pathology, accident prevention.

479. Brody, E. M. , and Ward, M. The Physical History Form. Philadelphia, PA: Philadelphia Geriatric Center, 1966.

Reports the application of the Physical History Form as part of a study exploring specific treatment for mentally impaired, and institutionalized elderly. Baseline evaluations collected on cognitive, emotional, and physical level of functioning are then categorized by topic (major complaints, surgical history, family history, etc.) into the history form. Also included is a physical examination outline by which physicians can perform a medical examination and list diagnosed symptoms in different categories. Noteworthy is that the scale's convenient categorization system allows for a more rapid diagnosis of prominent symptoms and appropriate treatment.

Descriptors: Physical history form, demography, diagnosis.

480. Busto, U. ; Kaplan, H. L. ; and Sellers, E. M. Age- and sex-related differences in patterns of drug overdose and abuse. Social Science and Medicine, 1981, 15, 275-282.

Prospective examination of cases describe the occurrence of drug poisoning (overdose) among children and older adults. Statistics showing that this prevalence is due to particular sex factors engender questions about the sociocultural conditions involved in substance abuse. Victimization of elderly persons on both prescribed and "borrowed" medication is considered an increasing problem in this Ontario study.

Descriptors: Demography, sex factors, drug overdose.

481. Chafetz, M. E. Problem of Alcoholism in the United States. Paper presented at the International Symposium on Alcoholism and Drug Addiction, Zagreb, October 1971.

Demographic data cover the various problems and costs of alcoholism to social welfare. Fact areas surveyed include (1) the number of alcoholics statistically shown in the United States, (2) deaths by traffic accidents, by homicide, and by suicide owing to alcoholism, (3) the lack of proper funding for research, (4) the annual cost of alcoholism, (5) life expectancy for alcoholics, (6) problem drinking among youth and elderly, (7) the isolation of health and social workers due to poor communication about alcoholism, (8) industrial alcoholism, (9) environmental circumstances leading to alcoholism, and (10) the incidence of alcoholism among Native Americans. Examination of topics also considers the recent federal and state alcoholism legislation and urgency toward national and international collaboration.

Descriptors: National trends, demography, alcoholism prevalence.

482. Chien, C. P.; Townsend, E. J.; and Ross-Townsend, A. Substance use and abuse among the community elderly: The medical aspect. Addictive Diseases, 1978, 3, 357-372.
Drinking parameters are analyzed in 242 aged persons interviewed about their drinking consumption patterns. Largest majority of interviewees are nonusers (47 percent), and only 9 percent take about one drink per day. Those respondents with confessed alcohol problems are already in "sobering-up" stations. Underlying these results is the contention that medical intervention is sufficient for initial alcohol rehabilitation programs.
Descriptors: Medicine, drinking patterns.

483. Cohen, S. Drug abuse in the aging patient. Lex et Scientia, 1975, 11, 217-221.
Observes that the covert overuse of drugs by the aged may be as important a problem as drug addiction in youth. Cases of drug abuse from depressants, such as alcohol and sedatives, represent a means of escape from stress intensified by socioeconomic problems. Addiction in the elderly is described as predominately (1) medical or iatrogenic dependencies through use of analgesic medication, or (2) dependencies on sedative or tranquilizer agents prescribed originally for anxiety. Recommendations for considerably more cautious use of drugs include entry into resocialization programs and improved channels of communication between physician and patient.
Descriptors: Age comparisons, iatrogenic disease, prescription medication.

484. Cluff, L. E.; Thornton, G. F.; and Seidl, L. G. Studies on the epidemiology of adverse drug reactions. Journal of the American Medical Association, 1964, 188, 976-983.
Epidemiologic techniques provide an analysis of untoward reactions to therapy and predisposing variables to adverse drug reactions. With rare exception, the exact incidence of adverse reaction to any one drug is not known. Most often the adverse reaction is not severe, but the predictability of severity is not always possible. A community alert to mechanisms in the culture highly amenable to judicious or injudicious administration of drug therapy represents an initial step in establishing closer physician contact with patients on prescriptive medication. Physical symptoms typically mistaken for adverse effects are also considered.
Descriptors: Adverse drug reactions, prescription medication, epidemiology.

485. Colbert, J. N.; Kalish, R. A; and Chang, P. Two psychological portals of entry for disadvantaged groups. Rehabilitation Literature, 1973, 34, 194-202.
Examines responses by employers and real estate agencies about mentally ill, blind, aged, crippled, alcoholics, mentally retarded, drug addicts, prison parolees and welfare recipients. Housing acceptance and employability of most groups depend on feelings toward how "responsible or irresponsible" the disadvantaged persons are, although the extremely low rank for drug addicts raises additional concern. Goals in rehabilitation for vocational recovery might

be more difficult. Employment acceptance also shows a decreasing order along different ethnic backgrounds. Discussion follows on the predictable problems of normalization for those groups ranked low on the scale.

Descriptors: Attitudes, disadvantaged groups, employment, housing.

486. Crooks, J., and Stevenson, I. H. Drugs and the Elderly: Perspectives in Geriatric Clinical Pharmacology. Baltimore, MD: University Park Press, 1979.

The aging process itself produces profound effects in terms of the pharmacological action of therapeutic substances. This volume takes as its major focus the development of aging and pharmacologic problems inherent in drug therapy and, to this extent, covers drug prescribing with reference to aging processes in animals and man. Computer techniques for diagnostic analysis as well as symptoms of dementia represent the wide range of current (treatment) perspectives on prescriptive and nonprescriptive practices in geriatric medicine.

Descriptors: Geriatric medicine, pharmacology, animal research.

487. Cseh-Szombathy, L. Internalization of deviant behavior patterns during socialization in the family. Sociological Review Monograph, 1972, 17, 207-216.

Interviews carried out on middle-aged men during the period 1968-69 make it possible to narrow the role of orientation factors. Psychological battery of three projective tests (PFT, Luscher, TAT) also help to determine if alcoholic men model their behavior on alcoholic fathers. Results show this hypothesis to have some validity; 10.5 percent of the fathers are excessive drinkers, 19 percent are alcoholics, and 40 percent drink regularly but moderately. Alcoholism of the father is still a questionable predictor of the offspring's inebriety, and familial drinking practices are not entirely causal. However, findings do show the male (alcoholic) offspring experiences some degree of internalization of norms which favor excessive drinking. Later manifestation of these internalized norms (i.e., onset of drinking) is possibly due to both family and socializational factors.

Descriptors: Orientation factors, familial relations, norms.

488. Dobbie, J. Substance abuse among the elderly. Addictions, Fall 1977.

Critical evaluation presents pros and cons on why elderly abuse of alcohol and other drugs receives improper attention from local, state, and federal sources. Prevalence issues regarding the etiologic and psychologic reasons for the vulnerable elderly are contrasted with a backdrop of concerns in the medical profession for regulation and review of prescription services.

Descriptors: Demography, prescription medication, social rejection.

489. Douglass, R. L.; Hickey, T.; and Noel, C. Study of the Maltreatment of the Elderly and Other Vulnerable Adults. (Report no. NCAI-049931). Rockville, MD: National

Institute on Alcohol abuse and Alcoholism, 1980.

Final report outlines the need for continual investigations into characteristics of neglect and abuse of aging populations. Personal interviews with over 250 professionals--police officers, physicians, nurses, clergy, social workers, nursing home administrators, nurses, and aides--indicate reasons for the inability of caretaker families to meet the needs of dependent adults. Among these include (1) lack of sensitivity, (2) lack of training, (3) lack of understanding or knowledge of community resources, and (4) alcohol abuse by caretakers, rendering them incapable of competent performance. Characteristics of the social etiology and domestic violence responsible for physical and psychological abuse are discussed, with suggestions for direction in the field.

Descriptors: Neglect and abuse, domestic violence.

490. Douglass, F. M. , and Khavari, K. A. A major limitation of the percentile index of overall drug use indulgence. International Journal of the Addictions, 1982, 17, 283-294.

Examines the prolific availability of street and psychotropic drugs to different age groups. Substance abuse potential in adolescence and after 65 is exceedingly pronounced by the increased cases of misdiagnosis and medication errors. Methods to better assess the population's increasing consumption of drugs in relation to socioeconomic factors are offered.

Descriptors: Drug consumption, diagnostic errors.

491. Douglass, F. M.; Khavari, K. A.; and Farber, P. D. Three types of extreme drug users identified by a replicated cluster analysis. Journal of Abnormal Psychology, 1980, 89, 240-249.

Discusses differential features in the personality of drug users. Space-time clustering is the analysis used for identifying the elderly and younger medicine recipients as highest risk populations, in whose personalities there are tendencies toward drug reliance. Social conditions effectively instrumental in combatting substance dependency (for both genders) include family and external (nonfamilial) relationships.

Descriptors: Drug-risk population, epidemiology.

492. Douglass, F. M.; Khavari, K. A.; and Farber, P. D. Limitations of scalogram analysis as a method for investigating drug use behavior. Drug and Alcohol Dependence, 1981, 7, 147-155.

Investigates functional utility of the scalogram analysis for diagnosis of drug user personalities. It is a procedure for constructing attitude scales and supports conclusions about the development of drug patterns. Applications of the scalogram reveal three possible limitations. First, drug usage patterns are not always generalizable to drug users. Secondly, drug use patterns are questionable when patients are on psychotropic medicine. Third, measures of "unidimensionality" are at times equivocal and don't confirm actual unidimensional drug use patterns. Re-evaluations of these data and future research using the scalogram are suggested for alternative

analytical procedures.
Descriptors: Scalogram, drug user patterns.

493. Drug Takers in Scotland. Scottish Medical Journal, 1971, 16, 342-344.
Reviewed is that the drug abuse problem in Scotland is less serious than that of alcoholism. Growing is the significant middle-aged group of neurotic barbiturate-dependent addicts. Amphetamine abuse is also considerable and competes with the social controversy surrounding the use of marijuana and LSD. Reasons for this abuse stem largely from urbanization, noting there is a greater route of accessibility through a metropolis. Drug control actions to be taken against these routes are briefly reviewed.
Descriptors: Scotland, demography, barbiturates, amphetamines, urbanization.

494. Dunlop, J.; Skorney, B.; and Hamilton, J. Group treatment for elderly alcoholics and their families. In M. Altman and R. Crocker (eds.), Social Groupwork and Alcoholism. New York: Haworth Press, 1982.
Treatment motivations for elderly drug-using patients are usually difficult to identify. This demonstration project, funded by NIAAA, determines (1) the extent of problem drinking in age 60 and over populations, (2) types of training and information serviceable to the community about alcohol and drug consumption, and (3) effective treatment modalities for the elderly. Treatment groups described here are for alcoholic counseling and consist of aftercare groups, couples' counseling, and family counseling. Noted in comparative reviews between types of counseling interventions within this project is that the elderly respond better to group counseling. Critical characteristics unique to geropsychology and problem drinking are provided.
Descriptors: Treatment, motivation for elders, social casework.

495. Dunlop, J.; Skorney, B.; and Polefka, D. Family Involvement in the Treatment of Older Alcoholics. Paper presented at the NCA Forum, Los Angeles, April 1981.
Implications from a local survey of older drinkers determine the development and implementation of guidance programs. Several factors contributing to the underestimation of alcoholic problems among the elderly relate to low priority for treatment of this group. Alternative treatment programs run through three phases: (1) motivational counseling, (2) intensive inpatient treatment, and (3) aftercare counseling. Clinical issues also address the need for family involvement, education, and the alleviation of negative emotional effects of alcoholism.
Descriptors: Psychotherapy, motivation, epidemiologic survey.

496. Edwards, G.; Chandler, J.; and Hensman, C. Drinking in a London suburb: I. Correlates of normal drinking. Quarterly Journal of Studies on Alcohol, 1972, 6, 69-93.

A quantity-frequency index of drinking patterns is used on 928 London residents. Demographics on males and females with respect to frequency of drinking and religion suggest that more Roman Catholic men are heavy drinkers. Extraversion scores, in addition, are higher for both men and women heavy drinkers (cf. Eysenck Personality Inventory). Historical determinants likely to have etiologic significance further explain personality differences and enable a discussion on prevention.

Descriptors: Demography, London, drinking patterns.

497. Effects of Retirement on Drinking Behavior. (Report no. NCAI-032279). Rockville, MD: National Institute on Alcohol Abuse and Alcoholism, 1977.

Drinking patterns of older residents of New York City cover the social context of alcoholism. Selected dimensions of the impact of retirement on alcohol and old age include perceptions, drinking norms, and common practices. Limitations inherent in the research design are also probed, noting methodological constraints on demographic studies with elderly samples. Directions suggested by the patterns of elderly drinking are explored.

Descriptors: Drinking patterns, socioeconomic status, retirement.

498. Ehrsam, J. L. Issues Involving Aging and the Aged. Paper presented at the Conference on Aging, Hershey, PA, April 1977.

Presents general background concepts and facts about aging and the invasion of alcohol abuse among elderly. Estimates of over 128,000 alcoholics aged 65 and over in Pennsylvania indicate the growth of this problem over the last two decades. Boredom, loneliness, and feelings of rejection brought on by retirement all contribute to initial interests in drinking, as do economic reasons. Stress is also upon yearly expenditures for OTC drugs and prescribed medication. In nursing homes, for instance, medications are occasionally dispensed for the convenience of the staff. Other prevailing drugs and their potential hazardous interactions are described in reference to national statistics.

Descriptors: Drug patterns, demography, etiology, aging.

499. Eisenstadt, S. N. Comparative Social Problems. New York: The Free Press, 1964.

Social and community networks interfacing with the health and illness problems of urban and rural areas are part of the large spectrum of cultural events explored in this book. Poverty, welfare, stress, suicide, tribalism, unemployment, and medicine enter as predictors of family stability problems involving drug abuse and alcohol. Conflict values in European and non-European cultures also depend on age-related pathology developing because of physical diseases or mental illness. How cultures deal with addiction and other similar problems are put through a functional analysis and consequently a model for understanding cultural processes is addressed.

Descriptors: Sociological models, demography, cultural aging.

500. Encel, S.; Kotowicz, K. C.; and Resier, H. E. Drinking patterns in Sydney, Australia. Quarterly Journal of Studies on Alcohol, 1972, 33, 1-27.
    Details the contemporary prevalence of alcoholism in Sydney, Australia through survey questionnaires of 373 males and 447 females. Sample respondents are broken down into heavy drinkers (48% of men, 15% of women), moderate-frequent drinkers (19% and 12%), moderate-infrequent (7% and 13%), light-frequent (6% and 14%), light-infrequent (11% and 29%) and abstainers (9% and 18%). Noteworthy are heavy and moderate drinking patterns for ages 50 to 59 (74% and 35%, respectively), and over age 60 (58% and 60%, respectively). Data organized for education, occupation, income, social class, marital status, and religious affiliation generally indicate that heavy drinking is normative and socially acceptable. The social context of Sydney evocative of alcohol drinking is discussed with respect to prevention and treatment.
    Descriptors: Australia, demography, drinking patterns.

501. Epstein, L. J.; Mills, C.; and Simon, A. Antisocial behavior of the elderly. California Mental Health Research Digest, 1970, 8, 78-79.
    Law enforcement issues relative to elderly problems, particularly for alcoholism, are examined. Very few persons aged 60 or older are arrested or enter the judicial system unless alcoholism is the primary diagnosis. Recommended is that attention be given to effective methods for handling the alcoholic elderly and that diversion programs similar to those applicable for juvenile delinquents be employed.
    Descriptors: Law enforcement, alcoholism.

502. Feuerlein, W. Epidemiology of Alcoholism. Schleswig-Holsteinisches Aerzteblatt, 1981, 3.
    Classification problems in the epidemiologic diagnosis of alcoholism entail such variables as life-expectancy, morality, and alcohol-related pathology in elderly persons. Methodological problems in determining the number of alcoholics in a population, consumption rates by youth, hospital admissions, and distributions by sex, profession, and social class are enumerated. Specifically, however, the risk factors predictive of alcoholic (elderly) persons provide a basis for several different directions in the definition of alcoholism.
    Descriptors: Classification-definition of alcoholism, demography, correlation matrix.

503. Fillmore, K. M. Drinking and problem drinking in early adulthood and middle age: An exploratory 20-year follow-up study. Quarterly Journal of Studies on Alcohol, 1974, 35, 819-840.
    Descriptive account of 20-year follow-up on 109 men and 97 women who receive treatment during their college years. Measurements taken on quantity and frequency of current drinking habits show there is a tendency toward moderate levels with aging. Few respondents are heavy drinkers and over half drink at least twice a

week. In further analyses, quantity and frequency of drinking 20 years ago seems causally indicative of mild or moderate drinking patterns at the time of interviews. Conclusions support the hypothesis that problem drinking is significantly attributable to earlier drinking history and maladjustments in behavior still unresolved since college.

Descriptors: Follow-up, demography, alcoholism, drinking patterns.

504. Fishburne, P. M.; Abelson, H. I.; and Cisin, I. National Survey on Drug Abuse: Main Findings 1979. (Report no. NCAI-049853). Rockville, MD: National Institute on Alcohol Abuse and Alcoholism, 1980.

Statistical results of the sixth national survey on drug abuse drawn from household populations of the United States are presented. Measurement of drug prevalence provides trends across the seventies for inhalants, hallucinogens, phencyclidine, cocaine, and heroin, as well as for licit substances (e. g., psychotherapeutics, alcohol and tobacco). Tabulations from 7,224 interviews conducted between August 1979 and January 1980 involve a variety of perspectives from youth, young adults, and older adults. Besides the demography itself, summaries attempt to describe how the drug phenomenon spreads and becomes instilled in the social milieu.

Descriptors: National survey, demography, epidemiology, licit and illicit substances.

505. Glantz, M. Prediction of elderly drug abuse. Journal of Psychoactive Drugs, 1981, 13, 117-126.

Theories explaining the onset of alcoholism typically offer a factor analysis between environmental and behavioral variables. Review of the literature discusses drug and alcohol use, misuse, and abuse by elderly, implying that a more viable model for prediction lies with antecedent and consequent changes. Adolescent drug abuse compares to elderly abuse within this model, which suggests there is an equivalent pattern in the genesis of psychoactive dependency. Application of behavioral theories to elderly drug abuse is explored.

Descriptors: Psychological models, treatment, adolescence.

506. Glatt, M. M. Experiences with elderly alcoholics in England. Alcoholism Clinical and Experimental Research, 1978, 2, 23-26.

Reviews studies conducted by the author on alcoholism in England. Correlations of age, sex, drinking patterns, type of drinking, and complications of excessive drinking appear for 200 patients, 159 of whom are under psychiatric care. Causality between psychological and socioeconomic variables observed in the geriatric patients raise several possible directions for etiology. One conclusion is that such common geriatric problems as self-neglect, falls and confusion are due to alcohol abuse rather than senility or irreversible dementia. Organic pathology usually related to chronic alcoholism among elderly is also considered relative to England.

Descriptors: England, geropsychology, etiology, drinking patterns.

507. Goodwin, D. W.; Shulsinger, F.; and Hermansen, L. Alcohol problems in adoptees raised apart from alcoholic biological parents. Archives of General Psychiatry, 1973, 28, 238-243.
    Compares drinking practices, problems, and other life experiences of male adoptees with the history of alcoholic biological parents in a matched control group. Higher incidence of alcoholic potential and psychiatric illness correlates significantly with having an alcoholic biological parent. Adoptees given a positive healthy environment during their biological and psychological growth, although the offspring of alcoholics, have less risk toward indulgence. Nature and nurture dichotomy is explored to explain this apparent discrepancy in the predisposition to alcoholism.
    Descriptors: Offspring, demography, male adoptees.

508. Gorwitz, K.; Bahen, A.; Warthen, F.; and Cooper, M. Some epidemiological data on alcoholism in Maryland: Based on admissions to psychiatric facilities. Quarterly Journal of Studies on Alcohol, 1970, 31, 423-443.
    Study focuses on longitudinal patterns of care and effects on mortality rates among alcoholics. Samples are 6,432 persons registered as having been under psychiatric care for diagnosis of alcoholism, 357 of whom are now dead. Noteworthy distinctions between the general Maryland populace and sample subjects are the age at drinking onset, number of treatment episodes on record, and age ranges (from 14 years to elderly). Strikingly similar, however, are the educational levels between both groups.
    Descriptors: Alcoholism, demography, Maryland, psychiatry.

509. Gurland, B. J., and Cross, P. S. Epidemiology of psychopathology in old age. Some implications for clinical services. Psychiatric Clinics of North America, 1982, 5, 11-26.
    Exploratory study examines community health services and entire organizational structure involved in health service needs. Events relative to life changes, depressive and neurotic disorders, substance abuse, suicide, schizophrenia, dementia, and social isolation require special provisions most care facilities are unprepared to offer. Cross-sectional studies indicating the urgency for alternative programs designed for diverse cases of psychopathology in the elderly are discussed.
    Descriptors: Epidemiology, social casework, mental health, psychopathology.

510. Guttman, D. Individual adaptation in the middle years: Developmental issues in the masculine mid-life crisis. Journal of Geriatric Psychiatry, 1976, 9, 41-59.
    Masculine mid-life crisis is interpreted as being a constructive or destructive consequence of personal and cultural circumstances. A TAT card (defining heterosexuality) is administered to men of four different cultural groups, including Navajos, lowland and highland elderly in Mexico, and elderly in the Middle East. Results of the study indicate homogenous transitions in aging regardless

of the culture, and that urbanized man experiencing a middle-age crisis turns to alcoholism, psychosomatic illness, and reactive disorders.

Descriptors: Middle-aged males, cross-cultural, demography, TAT.

511. Guttman, D. Patterns of legal drug use by older Americans. Addictive Diseases, 1978, 3, 337-356.

Survey analysis describes personalities of 447 elderly Americans selected from a larger sample in the greater Washington, D. C. area. Daily alcohol use (18. 6 percent) and infrequent use (24. 6 percent) compare with 11. 6 percent who drink beer and distilled spirits. Among the users, nearly 80 percent give social and psychological reasons for drinking rather than attribute it to habit. Corollaries to income, knowledge of community resources, and degree of life satisfaction all impact on the likelihood of alcohol use.

Descriptors: Licit drugs, drinking patterns, demography.

512. Haberman, P. W. , and Baden, M. M. Alcoholism and violent death. Quarterly Journal of Studies on Alcohol, 1974, 35, 221-231.

Studies the incidence of alcoholism and controllable drinking on death in 1,000 decedents ranging from 18 years to old age. Registered deaths involving alcoholism comprise 25 percent for accident victims, 8. 6 percent for suicides, 26 percent for homicides, and 25 percent for those dying of narcosis. Blood and brain alcohol concentrations found in 33. 3 percent accident victims and 42. 2 percent suicides are . 10 percent or over. This finding significantly confirms the high association between alcoholism and violent deaths and suggests alcoholism is underreported on several instances.

Descriptors: Drinking-related deaths, drinking patterns, demography.

513. Hannenman, G. J. , and McEwen, W. J. Use and abuse of drugs: An analysis of mass media content. In R. E. Ostman (ed.), Communication Research and Drug Education. Beverly Hills, CA: Sage Publications, 1976.

Explores impact of mass media on advocating chemical means of coping with life problems. Advertisement and television programming indicative of drug promotions are hypothesized to carry explicit drug messages. By contrast, antidrug messages are rare exceptions to the philosophy underlying commercials broadcasted during prime-time network shows. Recommendations are that policy makers and broadcasting groups be warned of abuse potentials.

Descriptors: Mass media, television, sociology.

514. Hinkle, L. E. ; Robinson, T. ; Varma, A. O. ; and Hayes, J. G. Prevention of Acute and Fatal Cardiovascular Disease. (Report no. 1HL 18776 2). Washington, DC: U. S. Department of Health, Education and Welfare, 1976.

Examines precursors of sudden cardiovascular deaths and major disabling illnesses. The analyses, covering men aged 20 to 65, follow through initial examinations and tape recordings of electrocardiograms. Risk factors explored include social disorders, high

alcohol intake, and carbohydrate metabolism imbalances. This computer-assisted analysis pioneers the development of a 24-hour diagnostic approach. Implications for chronicity of addictive disorders are discussed.
>Descriptors: Alcohol-related pathology, cardiovascularity, diagnosis.

515. Hjortzberg, N. H. Abuse of alcohol in middle-aged men in Gosteborg: A social-psychiatric investigation. Acta Psychiatrica Scandinavica, 1968, 44, 55-127.
Investigates personality correlates predictive of social and cultural factors in 390 fifty-year-old males in Göteborg. Psychasthenic traits predominate personality profiles and correlate high with drinking arrests and various social maladjustments. Early alcohol abusers also live in lower standard dwellings, earn lower incomes or are unemployed, and receive less education. Societal programs aimed at preventing abuse are reviewed within an anthropological model, noting obvious pitfalls with the long- and short-range objectives.
>Descriptors: Personality factors, anthropology, demography, alcohol.

516. Hochauser, M. A chronobiological control theory. National Institute on Drug Abuse Research Monograph Series, 1980, March, 262-268.
Etiologic and psychological views are presented on the pharmacodynamics in amphetamine and barbiturate abuse on humans and nonhuman organisms. Antidepressive agents producing toxic drug effects and consequential symptoms of depression and circadian rhythms largely comprise the research into biological reactions. Naloxone compounds are examined in view of recent findings supportive of periodicity.
>Descriptors: Amphetamine, barbiturate, etiology, circadian rhythms.

517. Hodkinson, H. M. Common Symptoms of Disease in the Elderly. London: Blackwell Scientific Publications, 1980.
Alterations in symptomatology in adults and in particular the elderly reflect a combination of disease states, or polymorbidity. Fever, pain, or leucocytosis, for instance, may unexpectedly be absent while mental symptoms could be the prominent manifestation of physical disease. Diagnosis and treatment confusions largely stemming from this complicated matrix of symptoms are unraveled in different chapters that focus primarily on treatable conditions. Specific guidelines to provide simpler detection of pathology and etiology are related in comprehensive detail, allowing the maximal distinctions between childhood, adulthood, and elderly physiology. Underlying this technical theme is the presentation of beliefs regarding the stoically uncomplaining elderly who readily attribute undiagnosed symptoms to mere old age.
>Descriptors: Aging, etiology, polymorbidity, diagnosis.

518. Horn, J. L. , and Wandberg, K. W. Symptom patterns related to excessive use of alcohol. Quarterly Journal of Studies

on Alcohol, 1969, 30, 35-58.

Survey of intercorrelations among social and psychological dimensions of alcoholic personality is conducted on 2,300 of the 2,331 patients admitted to a mental health center between 1961 and 1964. A 69-item questionnaire containing items about drug history are factored to produce 13 first-order factors. Among these include (1) broad severity of distilled-spirits drinking, (2) social beer drinking, (3) advanced stages--beverage-substitute severity, (4) physical symptoms, and (5) sustained binge drinking. Extrapolated from these findings is the conclusion that differentiation is greatest along racial and ethnic dimensions, with varying demographics highlighted in hierarchical order.

Descriptors: Cultural patterns, mental health hospitals, drinking.

519. Hyman, M. M. Extended family ties among alcoholics: A neglected area of research. Quarterly Journal of Studies on Alcohol, 1972, 33, 513-516.

Family and kinship among alcoholics is examined from clinical files of 68 male patients treated during the 1950s. Nearly half of the patients not living with a spouse live with their parents or siblings. Unmarried patients who live with kin are financially dependent on their families and border on severe destitution. Evidence from these data strongly identify extended family ties as emotional supportive groups for rehabilitation; they strongly influence decisions regarding abstinence. Modified home arrangements and familial involvement in inpatient and outpatient recovery (aftercare) programs are discussed.

Descriptors: Family and kinship, treatment.

520. Jelen, J. Injuries and deaths following abuse of alcohol. Problemy Alkoholizmu, 1972, 7, 1-4.

Analysis of 296 alcohol-related injuries provides a panoramic review of head and brain accidents associated with uncontrolled alcohol. Subjects from the ages of 21 to 40 are usually male and manual workers for whom the frustration and daily monotony of unresolved stress leads to drinking. Cases of multiple injuries and the considerations relevant to reliable prognosis are outlined through concept comparisons.

Descriptors: Injuries, alcohol-related pathology.

521. Jick, H. Drugs--remarkably nontoxic. The New England Journal of Medicine, 1974, 291, 824-828.

Data taken on the acute and long-term toxicity of most drugs used in adult medicine are extrapolated for implications for the American population. Drug reactions in their totality clearly afflict many persons later in need of hospitalization. Deaths from drug effects number in the tens of thousands. However, evidence suggests that rates and severity of adverse drug reactions are low in relation to a drug's pharmacologic properties and to its potential destructive effects. Concern for the high prevalence of extensive drug use and polymorbidity among differently aged recipients should be considered as two separate issues rather than mutually causative.

Descriptors: Drug effects, demography.

522.   Johnson, L. A. , and Goodrich, C. H.   Use of Alcohol by Per-
       sons 65 and Over.   Upper East Side of Manhattan.   (Re-
       port no. HSM-43-73-38NIA).   New York: Mount Sinai
       School of Medicine, 1974.
       Health survey reports on 322 persons aged 62 years and
over who are interviewed twice within a three-year latency period.
Interview results indicate that drinking is, at times, associated with
perception of one's health and frequently by persons with good health.
Social activity and general psychological satisfaction are no different
for heavy and moderate drinkers than for abstainers, depending on
socioeconomic indicators, such as employability, income, and reactivity to the general residential area.
       Descriptors: Manhattan, New York, drinking patterns,
       demography.

523.   Kandel, D. B. ; Adler, I. ; and Sudit, M.   The epidemiology of
       adolescent drug use in France and Israel.   American Jour-
       nal of Public Health,   1981, 71, 256-265.
       Urban samples of adolescent and adult (aging) groups are
comparatively examined along dimensions of culture, gender, religion,
and socioeconomic factors.   Cross-cultural comparisons show that
adolescents residing in France and Israel differ significantly in use
of alcoholic beverages, cigarettes, and illicit drugs.   Lifetime and
current prevalence of substance use is higher in France, but the
ranking of prevalent drugs is identical between the two countries and
also with that of Americans.   Socioeconomic differences are rare.
Religiosity only affects the rate of drug use in France and nonalcoholic substances consumed in Israel.   Qualitative values reflected in
the culture of concern to drug use potential are organized into the
discussion.
       Descriptors: France, Israel, drug-taking patterns, demog-
       raphy.

524.   Kearney, M.   Drunkenness and religious conversion in a Mex-
       ican village.   Quarterly Journal of Studies of Alcohol, 1970,
       31, 132-152.
       Examines the prevalence of drunkenness endemic to the
Zapotec-mestizo town of Ixtepeji in Mexico.   Ixtepeji drinking develops
in middle-aged men and causes extremely pervasive personality and
behavioral changes.   The epidemiology of this "Ixtepeji" syndrome
explores several folk beliefs and ritualistic practices condoned by the
culture that are perpetuators of moral and religious conversion.   Con-
verts perceive religiosity as a means of social escape from institutionalized patterns compelling abstainers to drink.   Suggested is that
underlying the motivation to drink are emotional experiences negatively perceived by villagers who resist their geographic environment.
       Descriptors: Mexico, religiosity, epidemiology, folk be-
       lief, conversion, rituals.

525.   Keeley, K. A. , and Solomon, J.   New perspectives on the
       similarities and differences of alcoholism and drug abuse.

Currents in Alcoholism, 1981, 8, 99-118.

Reviews similarities and differences of alcoholism and drug abuse from a biopsychosocial perspective. In biology, the emerging role of endorphines and isoquinolines is contrasted against traditionally recognized clinical drug abuse disorders. Such psychological themes as addictive personalities and success of prevention strategies are assessed with respect to treatment innovations. The legal, political, and social climate largely responsible for cross-cultural differences upon age-related chemical use and abuse are noted concerning the biological and civil rights issues of users. Biopsychosocial causes relative to etiology represent a rational synthesis of present knowledge that is universal. Drug dependency examined through this theoretical model integrates newer developments of pharmacology with widely accepted interpretations in both sociology and psychology.

Descriptors: Theoretical model, psychology, sociology, pharmacology, review article, demography.

526. Kiev, A. , and Slavin, J. R. Life Crisis Inventory. New York: Cornell Program in Social Psychiatry, Cornell Medical Center, 1970.

A device called the "Life Crisis Inventory" yields information significant to the clinical management of patients of drug abuse, alcoholism, and interpersonal distress. Preliminary use of this inventory instrument for nondirective interviews shows it can cover drug behavior, suicidal ideations, and clearly display a spectrum of psychosocial factors predictive of life-style adjustments. Diagnostic decisions rely upon this combination of questions and ratings, containing 51 items of multiple-choice, ranks, and essay replies. Age-specific diagnosis is another area it expects to serve.

Descriptors: Life Crisis Inventory, diagnosis, psychosocial history.

527. Kola, L. A. , and Kosberg, J. I. Model to assess community services for the elderly alcoholic. Public Health Reports, 1981, 96, 458-463.

Revision of an earlier conference paper, this article presents planning and implementation stages of elderly alcohol prevention programs within a community model. Conceptually, the nature of client problems should govern the design of network of services. Identified are three directions client care should focus on: (1) client level, (2) agency level, and (3) community level. On each level the required analysis and evaluatory process determines involvement by the following sociocultural factors: demand, current resources, adequacy of community resources, general gaps and problems, recommendations, target groups, objectives, personnel, budget costs, sources of financing, and priorities. Prevention programs also directly absorb the responsibility to assess the agency's continual level of service delivery along eight areas of competence: policy, treatment philosophy and practice, continuity of care, record-keeping, manpower, knowledge and training, accessibility of resources, and funding. Community awareness generated by prevention programs is seen to include varying ethnic, racial and age-related populations

prone to drug abuse.
Descriptors: Community prevention, social casework.

528. Lamy, P. P. Misuse and abuse of drugs by the elderly. In
      R. Faulkinberry (ed.), Problems of the 70's: Solutions for
      the 80's. Lafayette, LA: Endac/Print Media, 1980.
      Discusses the expansive problems with elders misusing
drugs. Author contends that fear of drug misuse and determination
to prevent misuse clearly leads to situations where drugs are with-
held inappropriately. Research documenting the therapeutic effects
of, for instance, alcohol, challenge this traditional sanction on potentially addictive substances. Also noted are misassumptions created
by the medical establishment that greatly interfere with treatment
decisions.
      Descriptors: Physician attitudes, medication regimen,
      cultural attitudes.

529. Law, R., and Chalmers, C. Medicines and elderly people:
      A general practice survey. British Medical Journal, 1976,
      1, 565-568.
      Comprehensive survey interviews 151 patients of 75 years
and over regarding their health and management of medication. Most
respondents are responsible for their own medication but leave them
exposed in unsafe places or are uncertain about how to dispense un-
wanted drugs. Number of drug prescriptions is three times the
number prescribed for the general population, with women taking
twice as many drugs as men. Discouragement by pharmacist and
physician to self-medicate and the common confusions arising from
miscommunication are observed.
      Descriptors: Prescription medication, physician-patient
      relationship, demography.

530. Leuthold, C. A.; Matthews, C.; Berg, L. P.; and Harley, J. P.
      Halstead Test Responses in an Elderly Male Population.
      (Report no. ZO-2321710). Washington, DC: U. S. Veterans
      Administration, Department of Medicine and Surgery, 1976.
      Comprehensive report traces the demography and neuro-
psychological test results of 193 older VA patients. Conclusions are
generally that (a) changes in overall test performance level are a
function of increasing chronological age, (b) differential rate of decline across chronology appears in specific categories of adaptive-
psychological abilities, and (c) neuropsychological inferences can be
drawn regarding the degree of cerebral impairment. Measures of
neuropsychological patterns revealed by the Halstead Test undergo
comparisons between the scores of alcoholic and nonalcoholic patients.
Indications from this comparison for developing a neural diagnostic
profile are discussed.
      Descriptors: Neuropsychology, Halstead Test, alcoholism.

531. Linn, M. W. Attrition of older alcoholics from treatment.
      Addictive Diseases, 1978, 3, 437-447.
      Study examines attrition rate in an inpatient alcoholism
treatment unit and compares results against the backdrop of national

demographics. Questionnaires distributed to 44 patients (mean age is 59) classifies moods and attitudes indicative of reasons for drop-out. Age indicators correlate with drop-out rates on three critical dimensions: (1) older drop-outs perceive less spontaneity among patients and between patients and staff, (2) they have less involvement in program, and (3) they feel less encouragement toward autonomy. Implied is that interventions tend to favor younger patients and, seen from a national perspective, create serious drawbacks for motivated elderly abusers.

Descriptors: Treatment, national trends, alcoholism.

532. Linsky, A. S. The changing public views of alcoholism. Quarterly Journal of Studies on Alcohol, 1970, 31, 692-704.

Household survey conducted in Vancouver, Washington, explores attitudes of drinking and chronic alcoholism. Completed interviews by 305 residents (mixed-age groups) generally show approval of alcohol beverages by those with more education and exposure to mass media (e. g., newspapers, magazines, radio, TV). Responses regarding methods of alcohol control name the professions of psychology and medicine as primary servicers, with other choices including will-power, religion, and legal control. Opinions about etiology show theories based on biological causes to receive less approval (16 percent) than both theories based on personality (29 percent) and psychological reactions to stress (27 percent). Attitudinal changes, the authors contend, largely reflect the waning influences of the Protestant Ethic in American culture.

Descriptors: Addiction theories, attitudes, surveys.

533. Looney, J. G., and Gunderson, E. K. Longitudinal Health Patterns Among Career Naval Personnel. (Report no. ZO-N 477092 2). Washington, DC: U. S. Department of Defense, Navy, 1977.

Data on hospitalizations and morbidity among naval service personnel undergo a retrospective analysis over a nine-year period. Illness patterns tend to cluster periodically in an individual's life and by predicting this pattern it improves medical screening in occupational health programs. Demographic and service history information drawn from computer tapes details the extent of single or multiple episodes of illness. Influenced by illness (and vice versa) are factors such as duty assignments, service status changes, and manifested psychiatric disorders. Examined closely is the impact of naval career changes on middle-aged personnel.

Descriptors: Navy, occupational hazards, hospitalization, demography.

534. Lutterotti, A. de. L'aspect social de l'alcoolisme dans la vieillesse. Revue de l'Alcoolisme, 1969, 15, 49-57.

Exploratory analysis of the working class community as it passes through the metamorphosis of unemployment and retirement. Retirement is an important turning point when moderate drinkers turn to heavy drinking simply because daily occupational demands are absent and replaced by cultural invitations to enjoy this new freedom. Assessed are the potential psychological frustrations experienced by working persons who in their alcoholism neglect familial and financial responsibilities.

> Descriptors: Working class, retirement, frustration (emotion).

535. McCuan, E. R. Social Variables of Geriatric Alcoholism. Paper presented at the NCA forum, Washington, DC, May 1976.

> Briefly reviews many complex interrelationships between aging and alcoholism. Social dimensions of treatment outcome and causation factors relative to the client's history and current level of functioning add to an understanding of alcoholism in general. Elderly alcoholics kept in isolation experience dehumanization by society and risk the development of physical diseases that worsen drinking. Structural stresses prompting alcoholism are contrasted with favorable social changes in a safer environment wherein elderly may grow old with dignity. Community applications toward this goal are cited.

> Descriptors: Aging, dignity, sociocultural factors, treatment.

536. Mandolini, A. The social contexts of aging and drug use: Theoretical and methodological insights. Journal of Psychoactive Drugs, 1981, 13, 135-142.

> Carefully examines the genesis of drug addiction within various social settings. Industrial and residential contexts greatly differ from the iatrogeny of medical (prescription) abuses. Occurrences of substance abuse from prescriptive and nonprescriptive preparations also vary by the methodology used to report or analyze them. Sociological models helpful in reducing artifact bias in research are noted for future studies.

> Descriptors: Sociology, industry, research, methodology.

537. Massachusetts Department of Public Health. The wayward elderly. New England Journal of Medicine, 1972, 287, 1096-1097.

> Describes features about the homeless or hostel-residing male elderly in the center of Boston, containing the largest known reservoir of communicable tuberculosis. These transient persons are generally past middle-age, alcoholics, and largely unresponsive to normal methods of treatment or persuasion. Through self-neglect, organic vulnerability to illness continues to worsen. Moreover, hospital records show that typically these elderly leave the hospital against medical advice or receive early discharges due to lack of cooperation or aggression. Community resources integrating with medical care units have a responsibility to develop street programs wherever men are likely to gather. Implications of this recommendation for Boston homeless are discussed.

> Descriptors: Boston, economically disabled, tuberculosis, prevention.

538. Matsubara, T. Mental hygiene in diminishing population areas. Australian and New Zealand Journal of Psychiatry, 1976, 10, 111-113.

> Discusses mental problems in Japan in response to the

population growth of industrial sections and diminishing population in rural mountain areas of isolated villages. Mental disorders frequently arise in families unable to adapt to crowded, noisy, and unfamiliar surroundings. Older family members who return to their native villages live alone, unassimilated to the social mainstream. Prolonged isolation from family and community results in the high alcoholism and suicide rates. Alternatively, suggestions offer direction for helping newcomers better adjust to the strange city environment and recognizing the advantages over village life.

Descriptors: Japan, mental health, demography, industry.

539. Ottenberg, D. J. , and Madden, E. E. (eds.). Substance Abuse: The Family in Trouble. Eagleville, PA: Proceedings of the 13th Annual Eagleville Conference, May 1980.

Papers, seminars, and training modules presented at this conference address such topics as program sensitivity to minority services, medical perspectives of substance abuse and the family, theories of family substance abuse, and sexuality and substance abuse. Family disintegration is the underlying problem responsible for violence, sexual abuse, and reactional maladjustments due to ethnic patterns or economic disadvantages. Historical background information on the development of the Eagleville hospital and rehabilitation services places the theme into perspective of practical solutions for change.

Descriptors: Family, sexuality, socioeconomical patterns.

540. Pearlin, L. I. , and Radabaugh, C .W. Economic strains and the coping functions of alcohol. American Journal of Sociology, 1976, 82, 652-663.

Coping functions evocative of emotional and behavioral adjustments to economic strain are explored by means of survey results in urban areas of Chicago. Scheduled interviews with persons aged 18 to 65 yield patterns of coping strategies and basic stresses which are antecedent to alcoholism. Interconnections are shown to exist between economic hardships, anxiety, and drinking for relief of distress. Results also suggest that onset of heavy drinking in persons having low self-esteem may stem from feelings deeply rooted in the family and social organization.

Descriptors: Family, emotionality, personality, stress, economics.

541. Peck, D. G. Alcohol abuse and the elderly: Social control and conformity. Journal of Drug Issues, 1979, 9, 63-71.

Argues that the failure to systematically study alcohol misuse by the aged establishes an urgency for a working model of treatment and prevention. Social control theories offer one possible direction, proposing that deviant acts result from a weak or broken bond between individual and society. Critical elements focused on by this theory include social norms, commitment to conformity, involvement of conventional activities, and beliefs about obedience to rules. Factors related to ethnicity, religiosity, social class, and level of drug consumption assist in the categorization of deviant symptoms. Moreover, authors distinguish between aging alcoholics

and geriatric alcoholics.
> Descriptors: Aging, alcohol misuse, social control theory, demography.

542. Perrow, C. B.   The Dynamics of Short Run Social Change. (Report no. 1MH 20006 4).   Washington, DC: U. S. Department of Health, Education and Welfare, 1974.
Continues a study on short-run indicators of social change in the U. S. from 1948 to 1972.   Issues and changes in major institutions are examined by coding the synopses of stories in the New York Times Index.   Examined have been ethnic groups, drug abuse, peace movements and agricultural workers, whereas pollution, prison revolts, and selective consumerism lead the majority of new issues still under consideration.   Interactive dynamics of special groups--"insurgent groups"--that enter into the decision-making process of cultural institutions play a drastic role in the heating and cooling periods of American revolutions.   These same revolutions, when applied to the growth of drug use and abuse, indicate reasons for the spread of abuse among different age groups.   Government structure is discussed with respect to these cultural changes.
> Descriptors: Social issues, insurgent groups, consumerism, social behavior.

543. Petersen, D. M.   Introduction: Drug use among the aged. Addictive Diseases, 1978, 3, 305-309.
Epidemiological findings endemic to elderly abuse of alcohol and drugs are discussed.   Findings from previous studies which correspond to or dispute the author's hypothesis that abuse is due to societal reasons offer background information for developing treatment recommendations.   Alcoholic typology is examined within the context of public attitudes and social prejudice.
> Descriptors: Epidemiology, cultural attitudes.

544. Petersen, D. M. , and Whittington, F. J.   Drug use among the elderly: A review.   Journal of Psychedelic Drugs, 1977, 9, 25-37.
Widespread use and misuse of drugs is descriptive of a serious phenomenon reviewed here in detail.   References to drug abuse problems among the aging are abundant but clearly sorted differences in effects on this age compare only with young users rather than with age cohorts.   This article summarizes relevant literature and research showing age cohort comparisons.   Furthermore, it identifies gaps in the existing knowledge and synthesizes conceptual interpretations of use and misuse.   Recommendations for warranted research are enumerated.
> Descriptors: Review, drug use and misuse, research, cultural patterns.

545. Peterson, W. J. , and Heasley, R. B.   Study of the Effectiveness of Advertising in Changing Attitudes Toward Alcoholism in Nine Alaskan Communities.   (Report no. NCAI-030821).   Rockville, MD: National Institute on Alcohol Abuse and Alcoholism, 1977.

A survey beginning in 1974 to test effects of a statewide multimedia campaign on attitudes toward alcohol is reviewed. Survey questionnaires circulated around the state suggest the populace is aware of the growing statistic of alcoholism. Attitudinal shifts are particularly visible in rural areas of native Alaska, where traditional village life predominates the drinking rituals. Estimates show another 20 percent of the respondents being more conscious of alcohol pathology and concerned with treatment opportunities. That this media campaign can reach urban and rural residents indicates its potential for longitudinal effects.

Descriptors: Alaska, public attitudes, media.

546. Pflanz, M.; Basler, H. D.; and Schwoon, D. Use of tranquilizing drugs by a middle-aged population in a West German city. Journal of Health and Social Behavior, 1977, 18, 194-205.

Sociological research gives the strong impression that consumption of tranquilizing agents is entirely due to sociocultural variables assailable through national surveys. This study's aim is to document these theoretical claims in a questionnaire survey in Germany between 1970 and 1972. Random selections of 1,251 subjects born in 1920 who answered the questionnaire show that 14.7 percent men and 27 percent women take tranquilizers regularly. Relationships are drawn between mental health and subjective indicators of physical status during the subjects' lifetime. Relatively strong interest in the sociologic analysis of drug use is ultimately challenged and replaced by a psychiatric-medical model. Analysis of the medical model and its legitimation against scores of criticism (e. g. , Szasz) is elaborated.

Descriptors: Medical model, Germany, sociocultural patterns.

547. Poe, W. D. , and Holloway, D. A. Drugs and the Aged. New York: McGraw-Hill Book Company, 1980.

The threatening economy of drug abuse and its degenerative effects on aging come together under a single umbrella which explores the topic closely. This book claims to be a logical extension of the authors' years of experience and work in natural laboratories. Pharmacologic determinants of drug abuse, prescription practices, and the sociodemographic posture largely imposed on elderly Americans provide an instructive direction for practitioners, and patients themselves. Collaborative insights by both authors clarify several false assumptions in the field of drug addictions.

Descriptors: Pharmacology, prescription practices, aging.

548. Phoon, W. O. The implications on behavioural patterns of health and social changes. Tropical Doctor, 1980, 10, 32-37.

Constituents of social change emerging from accidents, substance abuse, and negligible health in general are explored. Family planning incentives for mothers help to anticipate infant mortality or maternal mortality. Public housing instructions greatly reduce homeless or hostel living and the growing rate of evictions.

Social change analysis also considers the communicability of venereal and other diseases highly ostensible in industrial and urban cities. The role of social institutions in health behavior is additionally considered.

Descriptors: Sociocultural patterns, public housing, family planning, mental health.

549. Porche, M. Alcohol Abuse Concerns and Needs of Minority Populations. Paper presented at the National Council of Alcoholism 29th Annual Forum, New Orleans, April 1981.

Societal moralistic attitudes prevail largely in minority populations in whose cultural heritage there are drinking traditions. Populations examined within this model include Blacks, females, teenagers, elderly, Spanish-speaking persons, and Native Americans. Exploring their unique demography enables some predictions about incidents and outcomes, needs and concerns, preventive measures, and prospective research findings. Treatment programs aimed at serving minority Americans must adopt a completely different philosophical posture and be aware of their individualistic life-styles.

Descriptors: Minorities, demography, treatment.

550. Quirk, B. Substance Abuse Among the Elderly: Current Studies and Issues. (Report no. NCAI-055667). Rockville, MD: National Institute on Alcohol Abuse and Alcoholism, 1980.

Reports on the current status of a study conducted by the Task Force on Aging, Alcohol and Other Drug Abuse in Dane County, Wisconsin. Outlines a brief chronologic history of the Task Force and problem areas identified for intervention. Five major substance abuse problems include (1) illicit drug use (2) over-utilization of drugs, (3) under-utilization of drugs, (4) polypharmacy, and (5) alcohol abuse and alcoholism. Noteworthy are several issues during the study regarding methodology and ideology that compete with the goals of comprehensive assessment and evaluation.

Descriptors: Community evaluation, surveys, social casework.

551. Rathbone-McCuan, E. Elderly victims of family violence and neglect. Social Casework, 1980, 61, 296-304.

Intrafamily abuse involves several tacit distinctions rarely made in the literature. Barriers to intervention, marriage and family aspects influencing intergenerational patterns, and the relative disinterest by society all contribute to unrecognized symptoms of geriatric abuse. Representative case studies present intrafamily violence and note characteristic personality traits of offenders (alcoholism, retardation, psychiatric illness, etc.). Introduction of protective and preventive strategies for aged victims includes those community services and resources available for consultation.

Descriptors: Elderly violence, intrafamily abuse, drug abuse victims.

552. Renker, K. Details of calculating and estimating harmful influences and impairments and their causes on the world

scale. Zeitschrift für die Gesamte Hygiene und Ihre Grenzgebiete, 1981, 27, 258-270.

Child, preschool, and middle-age disease abnormalities are examined in view of their etiologic and epidemiologic foundations. Evaluates the occurrence of pregnancy complications, accidents, wounds and injuries, and communicable diseases transmitted through cultural practices and from deprivation of proper medical and nutritional services. Handicapped persons worldwide suffer greatest from polymorbidity because of both unsuitable treatment conditions and poor channels for entering into the social mainstream. Causes of socially-induced disability relative to genetic and adventitious disorders (e. g., drug abuse) are reviewed.

Descriptors: Sociodemographics, mental health, public health, etiology.

553. Rhoades, E. R.; Marshall, M.; Attneave, C.; Echohawk, M.; Bjorck, J.; and Beiser, M. Mental health problems of American Indians seen in outpatient facilities of the Indian Health Service, 1975. Public Health Reports, 1980, 95, 329-335.

Community mental health centers oriented toward North American Indians are examined regarding utilization and types of symptomatology seen on an outpatient basis. Mental disorders frequently range from neurosis to psychotic and personality dysfunctions. Among the latter categories are several cases of substance abusers apparently having chronic abuse histories. The extent to which these local public health services attend to the rate of incidence is closely observed along dimensions of organizational structure, personnel, management of services, and treatment outcome.

Descriptors: Native Americans, public health, mental health.

554. Robertson, J. A. Optimizing legal impact--A case study in search of a theory. Wisconsin Law Review, 1973, 5, 665-726.

Studies the effect of a Massachusetts law authorizing pre- and post-trial diversion for drug defendants. Implications of this ruling question the ability of law to alter behavior and initiate social change. Defendant groups studied consist of adult drug cases before and after the law's enactment. Comparative patterns reveal the following ways that legality can affect behavior. First, accurate identification of a problem can alter decisions. Second, communication of law to those responsible for its implementation affects outcome. Third, the structure to motivate positive or negative attitudes can inspire desired action and counteract inertia, resistance, and hostility. And fourth, existence of organizations with official or non-official mandates can direct and better monitor the implementation process.

Descriptors: Age-related drug crimes, diversion programs, law.

555. Robertson, N. C. The relationship between marital status and the risk of psychiatric referral. British Journal of Psychiatry, 1974, 124, 191-202.

Reports survey results of patients in northeast Scotland that female and male divorcees have higher risk of psychiatric referral. Single males, more often than those married, and ages 25 to 60 show early signs of psychoses and alcoholism. Single females, by contrast, show signs resembling those of schizophrenia. Etiologic indicators of psychiatric disorders in the Scottish culture help to explain the connection of behavior with marital status.

Descriptors: Marital status, Scotland, psychiatry.

556. Robins, L. N.; Murphy, G. E ; Woodruff, R. A.; Taibleson, M. H.; and Herjanic, B. Epidemiology of Achievement and Psychiatric Status. (Report no. 1MH 18864 5). Washington, DC: U. S. Department of Health, Education and Welfare, 1975.

Examination of young black men, school and police records, depression, and prior war experiences in relation to tendency toward alcoholism. Identifiable causal sequences are visible in the childhood deviance during school years. Regarding records, the parents' arrests and police record are powerfully predictive of subsequent delinquency in offspring. Traced records of police arrests of blacks and whites for alcohol-related crimes also reflect juvenile involvement. To assess current pathologic potential, five psychiatric diagnosis screening interviews are run on areas of hysteria, alcoholism, depression, anxiety neurosis, and antisocial personality. Information about drugs, alcohol, and concurrent reactions to depression offer a valid prognosis to determine liability to readdiction in receovering narcotic addicts.

Descriptors: History, psychopathology, personality, cultural patterns.

557. Royce, J. E. Special groups. In J. E. Royce, Alcohol Problems and Alcoholism: A Comprehensive Survey. New York: The Free Press, 1981.

Racial and ethnic groups largely comprising the inebriates of minorities and military personnel are compared by age distinctions. Elderly and young Blacks, Indians (male and female), and typical "skid-row" inebriates differ by the societal pressures and responsibilities upon them. Alcoholism, furthermore, is not synonymous with "drinking" and could clarify much overlap attributed to cases where moderate drinkers become heavy drinkers. Adult and elderly drinkers prone to severe physical incapacity are also seen in view of occupational problems and their impact on military services.

Descriptors: Racial groups, ethnic groups, alcoholism.

558. Royer, F. L.; Gilmore, G. C.; and Gruhn, J. J. Normative data for the Symbol Digit Substitution Task. Journal of Clinical Psychology, 1981, 37, 608-614.

Chronicity of brain damage is assessed in relation to substance abuse using the Symbol Digit Substitution Task. Administrations of three forms of this test are on subjects (16 to 80 years) who are normal, schizophrenic, and members of other hospitalized groups. All forms vary in difficulty and measure visual information-processing ability from which a clinical diagnosis is derived. Symbolism, being the chief variable, creates a stimulus array perceptible in varying dimensions, which is predictive of general cognitive complexity and reasoning ability.

Descriptors: Wechsler scales, Symbol Digit Substitution Task, mental health, psychometry.

559. Schernitzki, P.; Bootman, J. L.; Likes, K.; Hughes, J.; and Byers, J. Acute drug intoxication at a university hospital: An epidemiological study. Veterinary and Human Toxicology, 1980, 22, 235-236; 292; 238.

Exploratory study of academic medical centers in Arizona that treat different cases of chemical toxicity. Drug abuse seen in preschoolers, adolescents, and elderly is frequently due to poisoning or overdose. Risk factors ignored by those patients most amenable to abuse, such as the elderly on multiple prescriptions, account for a large portion of cases, whereas second to this problem are complex cultural pressures on youngsters. Gender and epidemiologic factors are examined as being necessary areas for patient education and also for directives to community agency services.

Descriptors: Chemical abuse, preschoolers, adolescence, education.

560. Schmidt, W., and De Lint, J. Causes of death of alcoholics. Quarterly Journal of Studies on Alcohol, 1972, 33, 171-185.

Examines mortality rates of 6,478 alcoholics treated from 1951 to 1964. Ratio of observed to expected deaths varies between males and females and among age differences. Excess mortality is highest among younger patients, but older patients react to organic and social stresses with less recovery. While 70 patients died within the first year after admission, subsequent mortality rates of 40 to 56 are largely attributed to combinations of cancer, alcoholism, arteriosclerotic heart disease, pneumonia, liver cirrhosis, peptic ulcers, accidents and suicide. Alcohol-related pathology is also due to smoking habits, uncontrolled emotional states, and difficult life-styles.

Descriptors: Mortality, alcohol-related pathology, gender differences.

561. Schneider, K. A. Neglected Ministry: Alcohol, Pills and Older Adults. Paper presented at the 29th Annual Meeting of the Alcohol and Drug Problem Association, Seattle, September 1978.

Anecdotes and involvement of spiritual belief in alcoholic recovery already comprise several approaches to treatment, the most popular being Alcoholics Anonymous. Alcoholics Anonymous delegates the alcoholic disease to the drinker and forms an obligatory commitment between drinker and sobriety. With the influx of medication, pills are consumed and misused at faster rates than reported incidences of alcoholism. Argued is that religiosity is absent in medication abuse treatment and is critically lacking behind the national statistical trends. The urgency for religious participation in treatment intervention is particularly stressed for older Americans.

Descriptors: Religion, Alcoholics Anonymous.

562. Schuckit, M. A.   Geriatric alcoholism and drug abuse.   The Gerontologist, 1977, 17, 168-174.

Reviews literature and presents critical data on alcohol and drug problems in older Americans.   Opiate addicts, inadvertent drug misusers, and deliberate abusers comprise a large percentage of this population.   Individuals drinking alcohol in excess after age 40 invariably develop chronic alcoholism well into their early retirement years and experience societal pressures due to unsympathetic rejection of the need to treat elderly.   Current findings regarding etiology and treatment options are also discussed.

Descriptors: Sociocultural patterns, opium, addiction.

563. Schuckit, M. A.   A theory of alcohol and drug abuse: A genetic approach.   National Institute of Drug Abuse Research Monograph Series,   1980, 297-302.

Comparative study allows for an analogue analysis of genetic traits having strong impact on the etiology of alcoholism.   Social environmental variables are commonly the reasons for antisocial personality, and familial disruption.   Substance abuse and alcoholic factors unexplained by environment or learning theory are the ubiquity of certain habits within one ethnic group such as an intergenerational spread of addiction.   A factor analysis run on aspects of psychological disorders lends support to the hypothesis that elderly addiction is inheritable, but remains dormant until provoked by socially hostile circumstances.

Descriptors: Genetics, addiction, environmental theory.

564. Schuckit, M. A. , and Pastor, P. A.   Elderly as a unique population: Alcoholism.   Alcoholism: Clinical and Experimental Research, 1978, 2, 31-38.

Critical evaluation of the shortcomings of existing studies on elderly and alcoholism.   Hypothesis presented generally supports the theory that elderly alcoholics have fewer social than physical problems compared to younger cohorts.   Drinking patterns in older people show a steady increase in daily use, but the consumption per occasion is less than for younger drinkers.   Consequently, health care needs of older alcoholics greatly surmount the average incidence of aging polymorbidity, plus their medical disorders place financial demands on a typically inadequate income.   Estrangement of elderly drinkers who either cannot or will not pay for medical services creates a serious drawback for both casefinding and the containment of this problem.

Descriptors: Social isolationism, economics, medical health.

565. Shader, R. I ; Salman, C. ; Greenblatt, D. J. ; Kochansky, G. E. ; and Harmatz, J. S.   Drug Studies with Women, the Elderly, and Groups.   (Report no. 1MH 1227912).   Washington, DC: U. S. Department of Health, Education and Welfare, 1977.

Basic goals of this laboratory investigation are to develop rational approaches to psychopharmacological treatment for specialized minority groups (women and elderly).   Pharmacokinetics of chlordiazepoxide and other benzodiazepines in the treatment of anxiety require a careful reappraisal. These agents also alter metabolism and clearance in elderly physiology and may bear functional relationship to early symptomatic signs of senile deterioration. Methods for rating this dementia as well as memory dysfunction and depression are considered. Emanating from this research are specific guidelines for practitioners, students, and professionals.

Descriptors: Pharmacokinetics, chlordiazepoxide, metabolism, drug-related pathology, cognition.

566. Siassi, I.; Crocetti, G.; and Spiro, H. R. Drinking patterns and alcoholism in a blue-collar population. Quarterly Journal of Studies on Alcohol, 1973, 34, 917-926.

Surveys blue-collar workers aged 60 and over on familiar drinking patterns. Of those who drink, 10 percent of men and 20 percent of women do it for social escape purposes while the remainder identify strictly physiologic or family reasons. Explanations regarding adjustment are measurably similar to other socioeconomic groups working in industrial urban areas. Implications for lifestyle reconstruction and prognosis are suggested.

Descriptors: Blue-collar, socioeconomic demography, personality patterns.

567. Slater, P. E., and Kastenbaum, R. Paradoxical reactions to drugs: Some personality and ethnic correlates. Journal of the American Geriatrics Society, 1966, 14, 1016-1034.

Pharmacological reactions are complex interactions between chemical agent and individual organism. In the last decade or so investigations of both parts of this interaction have been systematic and show impact on personality traits. Here the concern rests with personality correlates to drug responsivity. Differential reactions to a stimulant, a tranquilizer, and a placebo are observed in geriatric groups. Knowing expected effects of drugs, the authors hypothesize that the tendency to respond expectedly or unexpectedly to drug agents is correlative both to coping mechanisms for stress and also to the method of administration of the drug itself.

Descriptors: Expectancy effects, stimulants, tranquilizers, personality factors.

568. Smith, C. J. Global epidemiology and aetiology of oral cancer. International Dental Journal, 1973, 23, 82-93.

Reliable morbidity and mortality statistics are available for international comparisons on oral cancer. Explored are possible causes of oral cancer developing from pipe smoking, cigarette smoking, cigar smoking, tobacco chewing, snuff dipping, and inhalants. Incidence of oral cancer varies across different populations, for gender, or in terms of precipitant oral diseases. For instance, oral precancerous lesions, primarily leukoplakia and submucosa fibrosis, show an increased susceptibility to oral cancer than non-diseased tissue. Etiological factors already recognize these variations and, through future research, may possibly identify hazards of nonaddictive agents orally consumed.

Descriptors: Oral cancer, inhalants, cigarette smoking, pathology.

569. Smith, J. W. ; Seidl, L. G. ; and Cluff, L. E.   Studies on the
      epidemiology of adverse drug reactions.   Annals of Internal
      Medicine, 1966, 65, 629-640.
           Adverse pharmacologic effects or allergic reactions pro-
duced by drugs depend on the drug itself and those who take it.   Several personal and clinical variables also determine this reaction and
make it possible to predict which patients are prone to adverse effects.   Examined are epidemiological studies showing that such clinical factors predispose patients to untoward effects of drugs.   Observations report the number of drugs given, severity of illness,
adverse reactions, infection, and renal function forming from variation between drugs.   In view of the culture, these epidemiologic observations speak for future methods of patient management and predictability.
           Descriptors: Pharmacology, allergies, adverse drug
      effects, epidemiology.

570. Spencer, C. , and Navaratnam, V.   Patterns of drug use
      amongst Malaysian secondary schoolchildren.   Drug and
      Alcohol Dependence, 1980, 5, 379-391.
           Representative sample sizes of 16, 166 secondary school
children from two states of Malaysia are surveyed regarding their
experiences with drug use.   Of the total, 11 percent indicate some
experience.   Predominance of cannabis and sedatives are for older
students and only few report early progression of drug use to heroin.   Steady and rapid drug migration is to a large extent due to
availability of drugs and local tradition of smoking or inhaling rather
than injecting opiates.   Youthful abusers also undergo indoctrination
of cultural practices by elders who, themselves, are frequent users.
Known consumption among young and old Malaysians contributes,
in part, to country-wide epidemic and highly routine demands of the
local market forces.
           Descriptors: Malaysia, cultural patterns, school chil-
      dren.

571. Spencer, C. , and Navaratnam, V.   Social attitudes, self-
      description and perceived reasons for using drugs: A
      survey of the secondary school population in Malaysia.
      Drug and Alcohol Dependence, 1980, 5, 421-427.
           Continues the examination of secondary school children from
Penang and Selangor (Malaysia).   Known to this research team is that
Kelantan (another state) has essentially similar drug use patterns
reported.   Youthful drug use is most clearly due to precocious self-
assertion, plus many beliefs and attitudes about drug-taking behavior.
Unrelated are indicators of social deprivation or personal problems.
Consequently, conclusions hold that adolescent development in Malaysia inherits the traditions of older cultures and also more uni-
versally familiar norms of sociopsychological growth.
           Descriptors: Adolescence, attitudes, Malaysia, school
      children.

572. Steur, J. , and Austin, E.   Family abuse of the elderly.
      Journal of the American Geriatrics Society, 1980, 27,
      272-276.

Intrafamily abuse affecting disabled elderly persons is widespread in America.   Reviews 12 cases of family abuse with the majority being against older women.   Abusing caretakers include spouses, children, siblings, or other relatives typically alcoholic, affected by financial concerns, or reactive to long-term family conflicts.   Most common forms of neglect are physical abuse sometimes resulting in decubitus ulcers and vermin infestation.   Disruptions of medical therapy and psychological abuse take on the following forms: derogation, infantilization, threats of institutionalization, abandonment, and homicide.   Recommendations include ideas for protective management of abusive families.

Descriptors: Family abuse, medicine regimen, caretakers.

573.   Stevick, C.P.   Some demographic and diagnostic characteristics of a geriatric population in a state geriatric facility. Journal of the American Geriatrics Society, 1980, 28, 426-429.

Hospitalization of geriatrics during psychiatric and alcoholic recovery permits an analysis of certain personal demography.   Modern psychiatric treatments for schizophrenia and depressive illness should greatly reduce long-term residency for many inpatients.   However, large number of beds for inpatients with irreversible organic brain damage due to cerebrovascular disease continues unabated. Studied are 124 men and 152 women (mean age: 81.6 years) with diagnosed alcoholic dementia and hospital durations lasting from 4 to 29 years.   Alternative mechanisms for adjustment after discharge are considered in view of the affective disorders, length of care, and previous psychotherapy.

Descriptors: Demography, psychiatry, hospital, dementia.

574.   Trott, L.; Barnes, G.; and Dumoff, R.   Ethnicity and other demographic characteristics as predictors of sudden drug-related deaths.   Quarterly Journal of Studies on Alcohol, 1981, 42, 564-578.

Analysis regards mortality-related findings of drug-induced accidents.   Involvement of substance abuse in suicides, homicides, and accidents (both traffic and other) varies across different ethnic groups, with North American Indians shown as the most at risk. Age factors predictive of mortality concentrate primarily on adolescence and older persons.   Occupational predictors and sex factors also determine the extent of potential drug toxicity problems in ethnic, racial, or family groups.   Characteristic differences in cultural practices leading to accidents are also reviewed.

Descriptors: Mortality, drug-induced, age factors.

575.   Tymowski, A.   The living conditions of wage- and salary-earners' families in Poland.   The Polish Sociological Bulletin, 1974, 1-2; 27-28; 69-75.

Indicators of family income relevant to measures of "prosperity" help the Polish government compute annual income per family member.   Statistical curves reflecting prosperity rates include occupations (farming and forestry), family size, marital status, and several other demographics.   Equally significant are types of expenditures except on alcohol and tobacco. High expenses are for transportation, communication, education, and recreation. Quality differences determined by age show that middle-aged persons spend most money on medication, food, and medical services disproportionate to their income levels.

Descriptors: Poland, socioeconomics, income, prosperity.

576. Vincent, M. D. Physicians after 65. Canadian Medical Association Journal, 1979, 120, 998-999.

Findings from a senility study conducted at a private psychiatric hospital show that drug dependency is a major contributing factor in 18 of 32 physicians aged 65 and over admitted during 1960 to 1977. Inpatients treated for chronic organic brain syndromes without other complications have barbiturate and alcohol abuses typically combined with emotional disturbances. Drug addiction and affective disorders occur more frequently than dementia and require professional training programs within the hospital itself to educate staff about this occurrence.

Descriptors: Physicians, hospitalization, addiction.

577. Vener, A. M.; Krupa, L. R.; and Climo, J. J. Drug usage and health characteristics in non-institutionalized Mexican-American elderly. Journal of Drug Education, 1980, 10, 343-353.

Theories claiming that polydrug addiction among elderly provokes negative public attitudes is examined within the Mexican-American culture. Minority group stigmas are surveyed in a questionnaire study of 32 retired Mexican-Americans (mean age: 69). Attitudes toward physicians, medicine, and physical health contrast with perceptions of life-style. By determining daily intake of drugs, estimates show there is general satisfaction with life-styles and minimal interest in drinking for psychological or medical reasons.

Descriptors: Mexican-Americans, drinking patterns, minority.

578. Volpe, A., and Kastenbaum, R. Beer and TLC. American Journal of Nursing, 1967, 67, 100-103.

Study reveals that a major improvement is noted in previously difficult geriatric patients given larger amounts of beer, group activities, music, and social stimulation. Indications are that sedative effects of beer mixed with social attention is an effective alternative to psychotropic schedule.

Descriptors: Beer, hospital, demography.

579. Wallace, J. G. Drinking and abstainers in Norway: A national survey. Quarterly Journal of Studies on Alcohol, 1972, 33, 129-151.

Interviews cover 3,954 Norwegians in regard to their drinking within the past year. Beer, wine, and distilled spirits are three beverages drunk by 79 percent of men and 62 percent of women. Drinkers more frequently are young people in higher income brackets and with more educational background who live in large communities where purchase of liquor is least restricted. Identified as viable

predictors of alcoholism are religiosity, parents' abstinence, and gender. Largest proportion of drinkers, for instance, have no abstaining parents or family members 40 years and older either in treatment or alcoholic.
Descriptors: Norway, beer, wine, distilled spirits, religion.

580. Waller, J. Alcohol and unintentional injury. In B. Kissin and H. Begleiter (eds.), Social Aspects of Alcoholism. New York: Plenum Press, 1976.
Chapter probes cases of unintentional injury resulting from drug-related accidents and the nature of this relationship. Types of individuals involved and countermeasures to combat accidents are explored with respect to drinking and driving, traffic injury, and prevention issues. Alcohol itself is seen as contributory to fatalities more often than it is to less severe injuries. Protective measures employ an epidemiologic systems model in developing guidelines for practitioners and service recipients.
Descriptors: Drunk driving, accidents, injury, prevention.

581. Wechsler, H.; Thum, D.; and Demone, H. W. Social characteristics and blood alcohol level: Measurements of subgroup differences. Quarterly Journal of Studies on Alcohol, 1972, 33, 132-147.
Biological data on blood-alcohol concentrations (BAC) in 6,266 adults are examined during admission to hospital emergency services. BACs of 0.05 percent and above are found mostly for men and women between ages 46 to 65. High BACs also appear in Protestant native-born whites, in Italian Catholics, in Jews, and in other Protestants. Demography identifying correlations between religious, cultural, and ethnic groups are further compared to marital status and age-integrative communities.
Descriptors: Medicine, hospital, demography, blood-alcohol concentration.

582. Welsh, R. P. Investigation of the Alcohol-Related Problems of the Elderly in Ottawa. Paper presented at the Futuraction '77 Conference, Winnipeg, July 1977.
Surveys Ottawa's social service workers to determine societal attitudes about drinking patterns. Workers indicate a large percentage (14 percent) of their clients have alcohol-related problems due to social isolation and loneliness. Prolonged alienation from family members and poor adjustment to increasing economic instability after retirement lowers the elderly's tolerance for abstinence. Treatment programs specializing in geriatric recovery are recommended with detoxification and alcohol rehabilitation services. Drinking parameters of the Ottawa elderly community indicative of the need for program development are discussed.
Descriptors: Treatment, Ottawa (Canada), alcohol-related problems.

583. Wolff, S., and Holland, L. A questionnaire follow-up of alcoholic patients. Quarterly Journal of Studies on Alcohol,

1964, 25, 108-118.

Follow-up studies yielding reliable information about treatment outcome tend to involve a laborious process. In this investigation the use of direct questionnaires help to determine (1) characteristics of patients who replied as compared with nonrespondents, and (2) outcome relative to a number of prognostic factors. Patients receiving intensive psychotherapy in an alcoholic hospital in 1959 and administered disulfiram (antabuse) after discharge are contacted by questionnaire, letter, or telephone through a relative or doctor. Outcome results of this group are relatively poor and support the hypothesis that patients belonging to the Dutch Reformed Church have significantly higher relapse rates than patients with other religious affiliations.

Descriptors: Follow-up, religion, hospital, treatment.

584. Yamamuro, B. Alcoholism in Tokyo. Quarterly Journal of Studies on Alcohol, 1973, 34, 950-954.

Treatment of alcoholism in mental hospitals in Japan is reported by per capita statistics and number of admissions in 1969 by persons 20 years and older. Admissions between ages 40 and 60 comprise nearly 50 percent of the total, with 21 percent accounting for patients 60 years and over. Over 70 percent of inpatients show combinations of cardiovascular, liver, respiratory, gastric, and venereal diseases. Organic brain disorders, psychopathology, schizophrenia, and feeblemindedness largely are proportionally less frequent. Conclusions show the total of yearly admissions to be increasing rapidly.

Descriptors: Tokyo, alcohol-related pathology, psychopathology.

585. Zax, M.; Gardner, E. A.; and Hart, W. T. Public intoxication in Rochester. Quarterly Journal of Studies on Alcohol, 1964, 25, 669-678.

Several reports document cases where excess drinking leads to arrest and incarceration. Records of 5,524 of the 5,555 arrests for public intoxication in Rochester, New York, during 1961 are examined for characteristic patterns in demography. Non-white men show higher rates of arrest than white men at all ages, and most of these crimes cluster around the central business area. Dispositions of the cases by five judges presiding in the city court are noteworthy for their uniformity. Judges seem more reluctant to imprison women than men. Future studies on the nature of alcoholics arrested, particularly those older than 40, are hoped to shed further light on treatment and preventive efforts.

Descriptors: Arrests, New York, judges, prison, racial groups.

5. EPIDEMIOLOGY: PUBLIC POLICY FACTORS

586.   Aged clients (60 and over) Treated in NIAAA Funded Programs,
       Calendar Year 1977. (Report no. NCAI-038709). Rock-
       ville, MD: National Institute on Alcohol Abuse and Alco-
       holism, 1979.
          Reviews data on clients over 60 years treated in NIAAA-
funded facilities in 1977. Patterns determined in referral, treatment, and aftercare services are drawn from 21,000 clients compared
according to program activity and drinking patterns. Majority of
aged clients are white males and heavy drinkers. Self-referrals are
the most frequently documented source of referral into treatment for
elderly. Moreover, evidence supports beliefs that aged clients show
a higher abstinence rate after entering treatment than younger ones.
Demographic factors regarding income, household conditions, and
employability further describe the recovery and treatment information.
          Descriptors: NIAAA programs, referral, treatment.

587.   Alcohol abuse and alcoholism. Mental Health Digest, 1970,
       1-7.
          Reviews extensively documented efforts to combat levels of
alcoholism through training and development of research programs.
New divisions within the National Institute of Mental Health are described as focusing on the eradication of community alcoholism. Noted
is that an adequate conceptualization of alcohol addiction must encom-
pass a wide variety of biological, psychological, and social factors
analyzed by an interdisciplinary model. Extramural and intramural
programs of this new NIMH division thus strive for holistic services.
Clinical and epidemiological studies reflecting this approach offer
applications for policy development.
          Descriptors: NIMH, mental health, alcoholism.

588.   Borkman, T. Where are older persons in mutual self-help
       groups? In A. Kolker and P. I. Ahmeds (eds.), Aging.
       New York: Elsevier Biomedical, 1982.
          Policies for the gerontologic treatment of alcoholism form
distinctive types of programs. Community involvement in programs
known as "self-help" groups (e. g. , Alcoholics Anonymous) establish
unique support systems that are typically unavailable to most elderly.
Mutual self-help groups derive from voluntary human service associations in which consumers with a common problem organize to
define and resolve problems through experiential learning. Policy
and goal setting are functions inherently administered in these groups

and may satisfy needs of older people. Views of contemporary gerontology toward elderly involvement in self-help groups are examined.
Toward this end, public attitudes about aging in general are considered as a potential obstacle.

    Descriptors: Self-help groups, experiential learning, Al-
coholics Anonymous.

589. Christmas, J. J. Delivery of Alcoholism Services: Meeting
      Whose Needs? Paper presented at the Seminar on Alco-
      holism Treatment in Prepaid Group Practice, Group Health,
      Boston, February 1977.

    The hidden emergence of elderly alcoholics in need of
treatment has created a demand by human service systems for third
party reimbursement. Complex limitations facing these systems are
reviewed in relation to women's uses of tranquilizers and teenage
drinking. Sociocultural aspects of alcoholism which determine entry
into care systems and the caretakers are also criticized for contributing
to health maintenance programs. Further, recommendations are that
alcoholism services be linked to social service agencies, rehabilitation centers, and educational facilities.

    Descriptors: Care systems, social casework, third party
reimbursement.

590. Cohen, C. I. , and Sokolovsky, J. Social networks and the
      elderly: Clinical techniques. International Journal of
      Family Therapy, 1981, 3, 281-294.

    Group psychotherapies represent one, among many, chan-
nels for social interaction in cases of geropsychological disorders.
Authors describe a social network analysis to an elderly population
living in single occupancy hotel rooms in New York City. This analysis lends itself to clinical interpretations of agency planning decisions and possible interventions for the elderly. For instance, in
social relationships, the development of indigenous leaders (within the
hotel) greatly narrows the gap between personnel and resident. Several other social configurations center on alcohol use and prevention,
gambling, and card playing.

    Descriptors: Social networks, social casework, agency
planning, prevention.

591. Coppin, V. E. H. Life styles and social services on skid row.
      A study of aging homeless men. Dissertation Abstracts
      International, 1974, no. 74-28430.

    Studies eight aging homeless men living in Los Angeles,
California. Similarities and differences are compared with respect
to race, occupational role, drinking habits, and services available.
Most clients seeking services are from broken homes and never
achieve occupational roles. Attitudes toward social services viewed
from a rehabilitative standpoint consider the needs of skid row residents, but are oblivious to chronic alcoholism.

    Descriptors: Social services, Skid Row, occupations.

592. Dominick, G. P. Community programs for the treatment of
      alcoholics. In R. E. Tarter and A. A. Sugerman (eds.),
      Alcoholism. Reading, MA: Addison-Wesley, 1976.

Discusses community programs by differentiating those which provide services to persons unbiased to creed, color, or ability to pay. Federal, county, state, and local groups funding these programs evidently determine the policy structure and extent of multidisciplinary involvement. Known limitations in Georgia treatment agencies are examined as the foundation for eight assumptions upon which most treatment philosophies should be based. Largely evolving from these assumptions are components of comprehensive service, emergency care systems, inpatient care, and the treatment process. Important elements of outreach, education and prevention alternatives are entertained.

Descriptors: Multidisciplinary programs, discrimination, government, and prevention.

593. Ferrigno, R. A.; Robbins, D. S.; Erickson, W. L.; Yoffie, N. E.; and Naucke, D. A. Selected Human Services: Needs, Costs and Forecasts for the State of Missouri. (Report no. HUD-CPA-MO-1023). Kansas City, MO: Missouri Office of Administration, Division of Budget and Planning Department, 1976.

Pilot project assesses the level of need of sixteen selected human service programs sponsored by the State of Missouri. Forecast estimates on programs serving alcohol and drug abuse, the economically disadvantaged, family planning, and mental health outline the nature and extent of major problems in the social service network. Methodological problems using forecast models in the prediction of adult and elderly consumption of services are substantive and require more accurate profiles of the cost analysis and public health systems.

Descriptors: Missouri, forecast estimates (research), mental health.

594. Gabelic, I. Geriatric service and geriatric club. Anali Klinicke Bolnice Dr. M. Stojanovic, 1971, 10, 221-226.

Article calls for scientific research to push toward establishing a relationship between alcoholism and the involutive age, aligning itself with increased awareness of psychopathological patterns. Research attention is also lacking on the prophylactic effect, the process of aging, and on work productivity after recovery from alcoholism. Critical evaluation is offered on strategies to integrate community service groups and agencies toward this improvement in research.

Descriptors: Research, psychopathology, occupation, social casework.

595. Gold Award: Mental health services for rural counties. Hospital and Community Psychiatry, 1971, 22, 298-301.

Kings View Hospital is the administrative center of a network of mental health facilities serving five counties and responsible for outpatient and aftercare programs. Local projects established by the facility for school counselors and welfare department workers, and in methadone and nursing programs, have been for short-term patient evaluation. Geriatric patients, in particular, utilize these

resources. Local program units receive financial support from the hospital, but are free to construct and implement methods and services relevant for their community. Orientational aspects of this system are compared to service delivery systems in other states.
Descriptors: Mental health, outpatient and short-term programs, evaluation, hospital.

596. Harris, H.; Errion, G. D.; Farabee, D.; and Ramirez, R. R. Development of Standards for Community Mental Health Centers. (Report no. 1MZ 806 1). Washington, DC: U. S. Department of Health, Education and Welfare, 1974.
Organizes a methodology for the systematic development of sound standards and selected survey procedures for evaluation and accreditation of community mental health centers. These standards aim to quantify (a) accessibility of program to potential clients, (b) continuity of care through referrals, (c) consultation and education services, (d) capacity in meeting mental health needs of the patient, (e) self-appraisal of staff mechanisms, (f) interrelationship between community mental health (CMH) and other mental health programs, and (g) clinical and medical training experience. Nature and extent of tests, laboratory work, and examination dynamics all undergo evaluation. Physical care is especially concerned with the geriatric population in connection with addictive disorders.
Descriptors: Community mental health, evaluation, standards.

597. Human Services Planning, Finances and Delivery in Virginia (Vol. III): Legislative Resources of Human Service Delivery. Springfield, VA: Virginia Division of State Planning and Community Affairs, 1974.
A directory describes legislative information and federal funds. One part presents abstracts of the major human services, listing the legislation passed by Congress. Second, a federal legislative tracking guide details accounts of certain services and how to use those services. Valuable resource tool when doing research on federal governmental services.
Descriptors: Human services, government, federal grants.

598. Isbister, J. D. Statement by the Administrator of the Alcohol, Drug Abuse and Mental Health Administration Before the Subcommittee on Alcoholism and Narcotics (Hearings Report no. NCAI-040974). Rockville, MD: National Institute of Alcohol Abuse and Alcoholism, 1976.
Critically evaluated are studies regarding drug use pattern among the elderly and their behavior toward alcohol. Studies largely funded by NIAAA and the National Institute on Aging are reviewed for pitfalls unresolved by current research. Elderly problem drinkers face a synergistic effect of aging and alcohol abuse rarely treated in a holistic approach but rather as two distinctive etiologies.
Descriptors: Alcoholism, NIAAA, National Institute on Aging, holistic treatment.

599. Lazar, I. Community Service Implications of Public Law PL-92-603. (Report no. GY 65286.) Albany: New York

State Government, 1976.

Offers recommendations to the State of New York for supplemental payment levels, service needs, and strategies in the evaluation and management of service agencies. Inventories surveying consultants, the aged and blind, physically handicapped, and totally and partially handicapped indicate different demands for cost and quality of service delivery systems. Estimates of cost distributions and availability of New York agencies are given in proportion to populations at risk and impediments to service. Fiscal implications also consider the normalization and social competencies of afflicted groups.

Descriptors: Minority, government, handicapped, social casework.

600. Martincevic, L. R. Organization and development of gerontological-geriatric services in the clinic for neurology, psychiatry, alcoholism, and drug addiction. Anali Klinicke Bolnice Dr. M. Stojanovic, 1973, 12, 351-357.

Organization and development of gerontologic services includes special sociomedical care for persons older than 40. Current health care systems reviewed are inadequate because they focus on treatment of acute disease. Alternative phases of rehabilitation for elderly involve (1) staff recognition, (2) welfare approach, and (3) professional training on the job or through rehabilitation workshops. Approaches taken by the Geriatric Clubs in the area of psychosocial rehabilitation, scientific research, diagnosis, prophylaxis, and treatment for regenerative therapy are indications that health care networks require greater awareness by the community.

Descriptors: Community service, rehabilitation, geropsychiatry.

601. Nashalook, H. Unalakleet Community Development Association. (Report no. 1AA 1361, 1). Washington, DC: U. S. Department of Health, Education and Welfare, 1974.

A community development association run by the village council and other activist groups (Mother's Club, Sewing Circle, etc.) organizes small contributions for purchasing office materials needed for voluntary training programs. Discussed are the community centers' planning objectives that cover elderly drug abuse and alcoholism, learning of native culture, and recreational facilities for both young and old residents. Progress in these sponsored programs depends on recruitment of community funds and motivation by participants to expand the current resources.

Descriptors: Community center, training programs, volunteers.

602. Noble, J.; Widem, P.; and Solarz, A. Alcoholism Services Grant Program in Medicare and Medicaid. Paper presented at the Division of Special Treatment and Rehabilitation, New Orleans, April 1981.

Program implementation for inpatient and outpatient services, halfway houses, and detoxification units is presented before panel reviewers. Criticism focuses primarily on the impact of Medicare and Medicaid coverage to alcohol treatment programs and

evaluatory strategies by which programs are assessed. Instructions for panel reviewers evaluating this proposal are noted.
Descriptors: Medicare and Medicaid, rehabilitation, evaluation.

603. Report Required by P. L. 95-210 on the Advantages of Extending Medicare Coverage to Mental Health, Alcohol, and Drug Abuse Centers. (Report no. NCAI-038572.) Rockville, MD: National Institute on Alcohol Abuse and Alcoholism, 1978.
Health insurance status for elderly recipients in mental health and alcoholism treatment programs impacts the decisions of extended Medicare coverage. Discussed are the limitations of Medicare coverage thought to discourage outpatient alcoholism services in favor of more costly services. Lack of professional training rated especially high on insurance evaluations is examined with respect to geriatric treatments. The reluctance of elderly to seek psychiatric services also contributes to this poor evaluation. Argument is that restrictive Medicare service places unnecessary burden on professional team and patient compliance. Advantages and disadvantages spoken on this issue are considered and the recommendation either to terminate or extend Medicare is unresolved.
Descriptors: Medicare, professional training, psychiatry.

604. Results and synthesis of the psychiatric care policy. Bulletin d'Information sur l'Alcoolisme, 1981, 146, 13-17.
Hospital admission and discharge statistics reviewed from 1960 to 1980 are indicators of psychiatric care policies regarding the treatment of psychosis, alcoholism, and other mental health disorders. Recorded morbidity data show the organizational shift in France during these years as moving from resistance to acceptance of minority populations into general, public, and private mental hospitals. Prognoses for the young, foreign, and elderly are carefully contrasted with cases in 1960 and interpreted for epidemiologic changes.
Descriptors: France, hospital, policy changes, psychiatry.

605. Sackin, C. Youthful and aged alcohol abuse: Some policy implications. Journal of Alcohol and Drug Education, 1980, 26, 69-75.
Responsibility of service providers in the identification and delivery of treatment to polydrug abusers and those diagnosed as mentally ill is viewed in retrospect to changes in national policies. Among the findings are clinical distinctions between elderly and youth addictive habits. Drinking problems are relative to contextual life stages, reactivity to prevention policies instituted in schools, and the establishment of false attitudes toward policy planners. Decision makers are advised to re-examine primary prevention as it perceives elderly and youthful abusers being prone to depression, suicide, and alcoholism.
Descriptors: Youth, national policies, prevention, lifestyle.

606. Sanchez, R. B.; Anson, R.; Meneses, C.; and Stavros, P. Cossmho's National Task Force on Mental Health. (Report

no. 1MH 25411 4). Washington, DC: U.S. Department of Health, Education and Welfare, 1977.

A national organization serving mental health and human service needs of Spanish-speaking groups (COSSMHO) is explained. It helps members work together and develop research and training in fields of health, prevention and treatment of developmental disabilities, alcoholism, drug abuse, youth opportunities and gerontologic disease. Funded by NIMH in 1973, COSSMHO's continual expansion is largely due to its integration of many autonomous mental health agencies from the Mexican-American minority. Membership represents over 150 agencies, organizations, and institutions able to consolidate issues of mutual concern on contemporary problems facing mental health systems.

Descriptors: Mexican-American minority, mental health, gerontology, NIMH.

607. Smith, C.M. Mental health developments in Saskatchewan. Canada's Mental Health, 1970, 18, 15-20.

Reviews prevalent changes in the Saskatchewan mental health network from 1960 to 1969. Normalization programs seeking alternative outpatient care represent the major psychiatric plan proposed during these years. Community involvement is another instrumental development. The recruitment, retention, and training of qualified personnel in childhood psychology, mental retardation, forensic psychiatry, alcoholism, and nonmedical use of drugs for the aged has been fully successful in supplying more complete mental health service. Implications for services to the aged are discussed.

Descriptors: Saskatchewan, psychiatry, community services, social casework.

608. Social Work Practice, 1971: Selected Papers, 98th Annual Forum. (The National Conference on Social Welfare). New York: Columbia University Press, 1971.

Selected papers from the conference cover topics on organizational ways to combat racism, faulty advocacy groups, and interfamily and alcohol problems. Private foundations and social welfare programs intimately involved in implementation of new mental health delivery systems see drug abuse treatment programs for Blacks, elderly, and prisoners indicative of contemporary community action. Voluntary agency involvement is discussed in relation to its paraprofessional role with social work and social service agencies.

Descriptors: Welfare, racism, minority, volunteers, prisoners.

609. Volunteers in Community Mental Health. (Report no. PHS-2071). Washington, DC: National Institute of Mental Health, 1970.

This booklet is about volunteer accepted programs in operation around the nation. Nine different types of activities described in this booklet stress helping relationships with children, adults, elderly, and resources through which this help is provided. Helping the elderly, for instance, involves volunteers in households and assuring that elderly neighbors finish daily chores or visit friends and keep appointments. Community programs, citizen action on drug abuse programs, and community service programs emphasize skills on telephone instruction, counseling, and reaction to emergencies.

Descriptors: Volunteers, community programs, policy structure.

6. EPIDEMIOLOGY: MENTAL HEALTH AND GERIATRICS

610. Apfeldorf, M., and Hunley, P. Comparability of ACL ratings by self and others in older institutionalized subjects. Gerontologist, 1970, 10, 44.
Using MMPI alcoholism scales, personality correlates of alcoholism are observed in patients in a Veterans hospital. Older residents (243 samples) identified by the Macandrew and Holmes scales reveal a record of problem drinking (e. g. , N = 94). Psychometric advantages in examining personality of veteran alcholics are considered regarding the effects of prolonged hospitalization in mental health systems.
Descriptors: Veterans, MMPI, mental health.

611. Ayd, F. J. The treatment of anxiety, agitation and excitement in the aged. Journal of the American Geriatrics Society, 1957, 5, 92-96.
Pharmacologic management of psychiatric disorders in elderly challenges the therapeutic decisions of physicians. Article reviews tranquilizing agents potentially beneficial for anxiety relief, introducing the positive effects of trilafon. Drugs are not the final answer to troublesome emotional problems of senescence, but clearly assist in nonmedical interventions. Validity tests on trilafon are administered to diagnosed neurotics, paranoid psychotics, schizophrenics and for several agitational depressive disorders. Rapidly active, trilafon calms psychomotor excitement and has little effect on endogenous depression.
Descriptors: Trilafon, psychiatry, depression, neurosis.

612. Ayd, F. J. Panel discussion of tranquilizing drugs in the clinical management of mental disease in geriatric patients. Journal of the American Geriatrics Society, 1958, 5, 379-396.
Moderator Frank J. Ayd leads a panel discussion on current uses of tranquilizing drugs in management of mental illness. Physicians with extensive clinical experience note repercussions from exclusively relying on drug maintenance. Advantages noted are the ability to restore the elderly's psychological balance sufficiently for domestic adjustment. The analysis of drug compounds in institutional settings and outpatient care is drawn from observations of drug interactions, aging physiology, and contraindications relative to certain emotional or psychiatric disorders. Developed from this panel

163

are preliminary frameworks for understanding the mechanisms of drugs and elderly.
Descriptors: Drug maintenance, drug-related pathology, institution.

613. Ayd, F. J.   Tranquilizers and the ambulatory geriatric patient.
Journal of the American Geriatrics Society, 1960, 8, 909-914.
Discusses the plethora of major and minor tranquilizers produced in the pharmaceutical industry.   Several of them are already obsolete and few, such as the phenothiazine derivatives, remain actively prescribed in psychiatry.   Treating the ambulatory geriatric with phenothiazines requires knowledge of its structure, action, and dosage recommendations.   Phenothiazine preparations reserved for symptoms such as anxiety, tension and psychomotor excitement have additional advantages for physically healthy elders.   Explanation of these advantages explores the categories of (1) piperazines, (2) chlor-promazines, and (3) piperidines.
Descriptors: Phenothiazine, pharmacology, anxiety.

614. Barnes, R. F. , and Raskind, M. A.   DSM-III criteria and the clinical diagnosis of dementia: A nursing home study.
Journal of Gerontology, 1981, 36, 20-27.
Dementia symptoms demonstrable in 64 out of 70 elderly nursing home patients meet DSM-III criteria in a clinical evaluation.   Diagnostic criteria are reviewed for primary degenerative dementia, multi-infarct dementia, or alcoholic dementia.   Alcoholic dementia, in particular, derives from a disorder involving behavioral and intellectual deterioration following a long history of chronic alcoholism.   Etiologic significance of DSM-III for detecting dementia rests on the premise that psychiatric disorders related to cognitive dysfunction are frequently attributed to arteriosclerotic cerebrovascular pathology.   Definitions of DSM-III categories and criteria help to distinguish physical from psychological symptomatology.
Descriptors: DSM-III, etiology, alcohol dementia.

615. Barnes, R. F. ; Veith, R. C. ; and Raskind, M. A.   Depression in older persons: Diagnosis and management.   Western Journal of Medicine, 1981, 135, 463-468.
Examines clinical role of alcohol in depression and medical illness associated with diagnosis and treatment intervention.   Case evaluations observe that alcohol is a major contributor to depressive symptoms, the onset of which tends to worsen treatment prognosis.   Forms of drug therapy to replace psychotherapy are reviewed concerning the affective disorders, stress, conflict, and anxiety.   Management prospectives in clinical drug therapy are also covered.
Descriptors: Alcoholism, depression, drug therapy.

616. Benson, R. A. , and Brodie, D. C.   Suicide by overdoses of medicines among the aged.   Journal of the American Geriatrics Society, 1975, 23, 304-308.

Reviews current literature on suicide by medicinal overdose among elderly living in United States and Britain. Older white males rank high among national trends showing that drugs prescribed for treatment are misused for suicide. Common preparations of barbiturate and psychotherapeutic agents dispensed by pharmacists are considered in relation to the exposure of the elderly patient to potentially lethal drugs. Suicide is usually a serious consequence of unresolved depression, emerging from declining income, prestige, and loss of mental and physical powers. Recommended is an attitude change toward elderly mental health to reduce societal rejection of high risk medication problems.

Descriptors: Mental health, prescription medication, barbiturates and psychotherapeutics.

617. Blazer, D. , and Williams, C. D. Epidemiology of dysphoria and depression in an elderly population. American Journal of Psychiatry, 1980, 137, 439-444.

Epidemiologic investigation of geriatric symptoms of dysphoria and depression in 997 persons with known histories of alcohol abuse. Inebriates shown to relapse into affective disorders and depression in cyclical episodes reveal medically related alterations in attitude, behavior, and cognitive complexity. Complications deriving from the cultural impact of economic and social isolation are explored.

Descriptors: Epidemiology, dysphoria, depression.

618. Bond, D.; Braceland, F. J.; Freedman, D. X.; Friedhoff, A. J.; Kolb, L. C.; and Lourie, R. S. The Year Book of Psychiatry and Applied Mental Health. Chicago, IL: Year Book Medical Publishers, 1971.

One of a series on practical medicine, this volume presents the working essence of outstanding recent international medicoscientific literature in annotations. Articles cover neurophysiology, psychology, psychophysiology, biochemistry, psychiatry, adolescent psychiatry, delinquency, genetics, learning and memory, psychosomatic medicine, geriatric psychiatry, and several subcategories related to therapeutic interventions. Alcoholism and drug addiction, and suicide draw from current demographic studies, medical research, and developments attained in the application of theory and technology. Important subject and author indexes are provided for reference.

Descriptors: Reference, medicine, geropsychiatry.

619. Bron, B. Recent aspects of the suicide problem. Fortschritte der Neurologie-Psychiatrie, 1980, 48, 556-568.

Problems of suicide generate not only from psychiatric and psychological causes but also from sociological, ethical, legal, and theological ones. Interpretation here holds that psychoanalytic aspects of suicide reflect a conflict between aggression and narcissistic crisis, descriptively titled "presuicidal syndrome." Structural analysis of this suicidal typology shows it has striking frequency among adolescents, the aged, drug addicts, dipsomaniacs, and alcohol addicts. Issues of suicide prevention are, the author notes, difficult to resolve since the goals should be to correct the inner attitude of the

person and change conditioning factors in the social environment.
Preventive measures therefore tax the therapist's resources and
make suicidal urges a mental disorder highly prone to misdiagnosis.
Descriptors: Suicide, prevention.

620. Bron, B. The suicidal patient. Incidence, special suicidal
syndromes, therapeutic possibilities and problems. Fortschritte der Medicin, 1981, 7, 648-653.
Complications recognized in the legislative and psychological examination of suicide are expounded. Juridical thoughts typically
consider that psychological disturbance goes hand in hand with suicide and psychiatric illness. Majority of "sick" patients attempting
or committing suicide are also known to "stick" to their intentions.
By contrast, special suicidal syndromes particularly observable in
the elderly emanate from incurable diseases, psychosis, drug addiction, and derogation of self-esteem. Because suicidal action is increasing, the difficulty in describing systematically the complex
reasons for it weakens prevention measures and the legal control exercised through courts.
Descriptors: Suicide, courts, law, mental health.

621. Brown, B. , and Fuller, T. E. International Collaboration in
Mental Health. Rockville, MD: NIMH, 1973.
Summarizes the international cooperation between fields of
mental health developments funded through NIMH. Research projects
cover different topics such as schizophrenia, mental health networks,
and utilization factors in psychotherapeutic drug therapy. Heredity
and social factors upon which the analysis of psychologic pathology
is based include criminality, suicides, drug abuse and alcohol, and
organic disorders indigenous to aging. Laboratory methods offer new
perspectives on the direction of applied and experimental research
for future international collaborations.
Descriptors: International mental health systems, crime,
suicide.

622. Cadoret, R. Depression and Alcoholism. Paper presented
at the Annual Meeting of the National Council on Alcoholism, Washington, April 1973.
Etiologic study focusing on hospitalized alcoholics looks at
personality correlates to depression and suicidality. A heterogenous
group of 259 male and female alcoholics of varying adult ages are
examined for psychiatric indicators of primary or secondary classifications of depression. Frequent among depressives are males who
have a history of suicide attempts. This concept of depression is
regarded as useful for predicting suicidal behavior and amenability
to age-related drug addiction.
Descriptors: Personality, etiology, suicide, psychiatry.

623. Carrasco, S. ; Carrasco, G. J.; and Alonso, A. Suicide attempts: A study of a group of 4 attempted suicides. Ar-
chivos de Neurobiologia, 1970, 33, 131-169.
Describes psychiatric aspects of suicide attempts of 94 patients (between 11 and 74 years old) admitted to a Spanish Social

Security General Hospital. Analysis shows middle age as high risk
for suicide potential, explainable by (a) the culturally determined demand factors, and (b) conditions of physical or social reversibility.
Noted in family and individual case histories are alcoholism, drug
dependency, homosexuality, and predominate motivations toward suicide. Argument is that suicide attempts are often unavoidable reactions to irreversible situations and independent of one's own con-
sciousness or personal motivations.
> Descriptors: Socioeconomic status, suicide, Spanish-
> speaking, family.

624. Ciompi, L. Late suicide in former mental patients. Psychi-
      atria Clinica, 1976, 9, 59-63.
      Results are shown of long-term follow-up studies indicating
the incidence of suicide in old age. Former mental patients in Swiss
hospitals show considerably higher suicide rates than the average
populace, especially for depressions, alcoholism, and neurotic and
psychopathic personality disorders. Involvement of aftercare programs to prevent suicide potential is considered for expansion follow-
up projects.
> Descriptors: Suicide, mental health, Switzerland, neurosis,
> depression.

625. Cala, L. A. , and Mastaglia, F. L. Computerized axial tomog-
      raphy in the detection of brain damage: 1. alcohol, nu-
      tritional deficiency and drugs of addiction. Medical Jour-
      nal of Australia, 1980, 23, 193-198.
      Radiographic analysis of the complex neural and psycholog-
ical pathology associated with substance abuse complications is reviewed in some depth. Cerebral cortex and other brain disorders
brought on by anorexia nervosa, alcoholism, and drug addiction depend on the age of patients and can be assessed properly by cranial
computerized axial tomographic scans. Investigations of this scan in
240 alcoholics compared to 115 normal volunteers who are either
total abstainers or light, infrequent drinkers show that atrophy is
the most frequent pathology. Scan replications are also on addicted
patients and on patients with anorexia nervosa.
> Descriptors: Anorexia nervosa, CAT scan, atrophy,
> radiography.

626. Curlee, J. Alcoholism and the "empty nest." Bulletin of the
      Menninger Clinic, 1969, 33, 165-171.
      Reports on 100 women treated in an alcoholism center.
High percentage of the group experience middle-age identity crisis
sometimes referred to as "empty-nest" syndrome. The trauma
triggers their alcoholism and changes perspectives of their roles as
mother, wives, and females. Similar to adolescent identity crises,
this syndrome coincides with menopause, the loss of loved ones
(spouses), and children's departure into their single lives. Etiologic
links to familial disruptions are explored as secondary causes to the
crisis.
> Descriptors: "Empty-nest" syndrome, alcoholism, men-
> opause.

627. Epstein, L. J. , and Alexander, S.   Organic brain syndrome
      in the elderly. Geriatrics, 1967, 22, 145-150.
      Examines 534 persons 60 years and older admitted to a
psychiatric screening ward during 1959. Proportionally, about one
in three observed patients drink to excess or possess addictive tendency toward increased medication or alcohol abuse. Organic disorders largely developing from continuous degeneration of physiology
and aggravated by chemical or substance dependence are recognized
as having obscure symptoms or symptoms also apparent in nonorganic
diseases.
      Descriptors: Organic disorders, alcoholism, psychiatry.

628. Evans, R. L. ; Werkhoven, W. ; and Fox, H. R.   Treatment of
      social isolation and loneliness in a sample of visually im-
      paired elderly persons. Psychological Reports, 1982, 51,
      103-108.
      Experimental study explores the effectiveness of outreach
programs for 42 isolated elderly veterans who are legally blind.
Treatment alternatives involve a form of group therapy conducted by
telephone that emphasizes determinants of depression, loneliness,
interpersonal relations, agitation, alcohol, and drug abuse. Pre-
treatment and post-treatment tests on these determinants indicate
that (1) significant decreases in loneliness and increases in activity
level rely on the telephone intervention, (2) interpersonal and agitation scores are insensitive to intervention, and (3) alcohol and drug
use is least problematic. Communicational methods using the telephone to establish treatment goals and effective behavior change in
impaired elderly are found to offer wider accessibility to those who
are "psychosocially" at risk and unlikely to enter a helping agency.
      Descriptors: Telephone therapy, visual impairment, de-
pression.

629. Felix, R. H. , and Clausen, R. A.   The role of surveys in ad-
      vancing the knowledge in the field of mental health.   Public
      Opinion Quarterly, 1953, 17, 62-70.
      Outlines contemporary research and needed research in
planning stages of mental health care.   Intensive training is especially called for by the proliferation of "folklore" responses by consumers to medical emergency needs, such as consulting clergymen for
counseling.   Information on educational programs for clergy and
methods to alter public attitudes toward medical establishments stress
the areas of drug and alcohol abuse, child-rearing, services for the
aging, morbidity trends, and intrafamily mental illness.   Suggested
directions are regarding the family's role in transmitting public
health information and the rejection of false advertising about public
health services.
      Descriptors: Public health, mental health, clergy.

630. Freemon, F. R. , and Rudd, S. M.   Clinical features that pre-
      dict potentially reversible progressive intellectual deterior-
      ation. Journal of the American Geriatrics Society, 1982,
      30, 449-451.

Age factors apparent in deteriorational diseases, such as Alzheimer's, and atrophic diseases are examined in this comparative study of organic and affective disorders. Radiographic analyses on the pathologic structure of cerebral cortex and neural areas in general conclude that complications are possibly irreversible for cryptococcosis, some dementia, hydrocephalus, encephalitis, hematoma, and organic mental disorders diagnosed largely around middle age. Substance abuse effects on intellectual deterioration are less precise regarding the etiology but will combine with neural losses.

Descriptors: Neuropsychology, age factors, Alzheimer's disease.

631. Fruensgaard, K. Withdrawal psychosis: A study of 30 consecutive cases. Acta Psychiatrica Scandinavica, 1976, 53, 105-118.

Thirty consecutive patients (ages 20 to 74) are studied for withdrawal psychosis during hospitalization. Drug withdrawal cases consist mostly of females, whereas male patients make up the majority of alcohol withdrawal psychoses. Since cessation of drug use follows immediately upon hospital admission, neuroleptics replace predelirium treatment or this treatment is omitted altogether. Instead, indications of using benzodiazepines and dextropoxiphene for instances of withdrawal psychosis manifested after 14 days are discussed.

Descriptors: Withdrawal syndrome, psychosis, benzodiazepine, dextropoxiphene.

632. Garetz, F. K. Common psychiatric syndromes of the aged. Minnesota Medicine, 1974, 57, 618-620.

Reveals psychiatric syndromes commonly seen in elderly, their treatment, and differential characteristics for diagnosis. Noted are chronic and acute brain syndromes, depression, psychogenic thought disorders, and alcohol and drug abuse. Etiologic patterns underlying the early and late onset of senile dementia either related to or independent of cerebral arteriosclerosis and depression are contrasted to current theories and research. Implications draw from the collection of physiologic-psychologic integrated syndromes arising with advancing age.

Descriptors: Organic syndromes, aging, depression.

633. Gittleson, N. L. Psychiatric emergencies. Practitioner, 1981, 225, 1144-1149.

Discusses importance of diagnosis in middle-age mental disorders with respect to the judicial and psychiatric ramifications of an emergency. Commitment of the mentally ill in psychiatric emergencies is a difficult decision usually influenced by factors predictive of suicide, substance abuse, puerperal disorders, and schizophrenia. Mental disorders complicated by pregnancy place constraints on the immediate need for drug therapy and may also be confused with symptoms of manic disorders. Precautionary guidelines are encouraged in preparing diagnosticians to differentiate between emergency and nonemergency decisions.

Descriptors: Mental health decisions, emergencies, pregnancy.

634. Gonzales, M. G. On the problem of alcoholic paranoia. Actas Luso-Españolas de Neurología y Psiquiatría, 1970, 29, 79-102.

Catamnestic work by G. W. Schimmelpenning on paranoid psychosis is extended for a relationship between schizomorphs and chronic alcoholic psychosis. Alcoholic habits characterized by frequent remissions, constant concomitant somatic symptoms, and presence of psychoorganic syndromes are similar to the paranoid psychosis of aged. To determine the extent of resemblance, chronic alcoholic psychotics and nonalcoholic paranoids are observed over ten years indicating a prepoderance of gamma and delta types noted among the alcoholic psychotics, whereas the beta types are noted for the paranoids. Psychodiagnostic results of this study add to the growing conception of organic and nonorganic paranoid psychosis in mature adults.

Descriptors: Paranoia, alcoholism, psychosis, diagnosis.

635. Gross, B.; Kearney, G.; and Jurgensen, L. Grief Work Model. Paper presented at the NCA Meeting, Denver, April 1974.

Workable models for the interpretation of grief, stress, conflict, and anxiety are examined in terms of advantages and disadvantages. Depression and guilt are both a process leading to alcoholism unless prevented. Typical reactions within this process are denial of depression, starting new relationships, drinking to ease organic or stressful pain, and avoidance of grief process. Formulated is a model through which affective responses are treated in different cycles of depression and by positive reconstruction of belief systems. Distinctions between the grief work model and available geriatric theories stress the improvement with a holistic approach.

Descriptors: Depression, grief, stress, affective responses.

636. Gross, G. A study of longevity in mental patients. Schweizer Archiv für Neurologie, Neurochirurgie und Psychiatrie, 1971, 108, 125-143.

Surveys hospitalized patients over 80 years old and determines that the majority largely have schizophrenia and character disorders. Prognostic implications are that potential for recovery depends on the patient's acceptance of symptomatology and cooperation in treatment. Minority of patients showing alcohol or drug abuse problems are subject to the same prognosis. But because of frequent remissions, fewer patients would require long-care treatment. Noteworthy are classifiable distinctions the author draws between the organic and character disorders.

Descriptors: Schizophrenia, character disorders, hospital, diagnosis.

637. Haberman, P. W., and Baden, M. M. Alcoholism and violent death. Quarterly Journal of Studies on Alcohol, 1974, 35,

221-231.
Studies incidence of alcoholism and drinking patterns prior to death in 1,000 decedents aged 18 years and over. Records established by informants (relatives, friends, etc.) for the Chief Medical Examiner in New York City show that 297 of the sample are alcoholics. Deaths are traceable to life maladjustment and accidents, suicides, homicides, and narcotism. Principal activities of decedents during their last year is employment and taking drugs which confirms the high assocation believed between drinking and violent death. Noted is the extent to which alcoholism is underreported by informants or fails to appear on both death certificates or post-mortem examinations. Demography correlative to these findings offers a basis for distinctions among ethnic and racial groups.
Descriptors: Autopsies, violence, alcoholism, suicide, ethnic groups, racial groups.

638. Hamilton, L. D. Aged brain and the phenothiazines. Geriatrics, 1966, 21, 131-138.
Phenothiazine derivatives shown to manage the mental disorders of the aged are in danger of misprescription unless precautions are observed. Individualization of drug dosage relative to certain symptoms or a client's case history depends not only on a knowledge of drug action but also on a knowledge of those physical or mental changes concomitant to the aging process. Altered body functions due to aging cause variability in the clinical response to phenothiazines and increased sensitivity to desired actions. Considerations of biological aging in the treatment are essential to safe and effective drug uses.
Descriptors: Prescription medication, dosage, pharmacology, phenothiazines.

639. Hedri, A. Suicide among the aged as a preventive medicine problem. Therapeutische Umschau, 1969, 26, 571-573.
Observes national trend in Switzerland from 1961 to 1965 regarding the age of suicide victims. No reported suicides are by persons older than 65 years, most of whom have physical infirmities accompanied by psychoses and isolation. Among the women, local suicides largely stem from inadequate reaction to stress, depression, and dependence upon others. Provisional forms of prevention considered are to increase treatment of diseases, reduce depressive states, increase socialization, increase housing arrangements, and devise structure for hospital treatment of elderly alcoholism. Mechanisms for the preventive medicine model applicable in Switzerland are enumerated.
Descriptors: Switzerland, suicides, prevention, medicine.

640. Hochauser, M. Learned helplessness and substance abuse in the elderly. Journal of Psychoactive Drugs, 1981, 13, 127-133.
Factor analysis draws from the prevalence of behavioral theories on learned helplessness and alcoholism. Concepts advanced in the substance abuse field are the focus in developing a model of

psychosocial factors related to stress, conflict, and anxiety. Temporal perception of psychologic and physiologic dependency relies, to a large extent, on the person's ability to foresee escapable or avoidable routes from addiction. Toward this analysis, specific topics address learned helplessness and life events, substance abuse and coping dynamics, and substance abuse and self-destructive reactions (mostly suicide). Motivational functions inherent in the learned helpless process are explored.

Descriptors: Learned helplessness, stress, suicide.

641. Hospital detoxification patient attempted rape on female geriatric patient. United States v. Bell, 505, F. 2D 539 (Illinois) U. S. Court of Appeals, Seventh Circuit, November 11, 1974. Mental Health Court Digest, 1975, 19, 1.

Legal brief annotates the court decision that affirmed the conviction of assault with intent to commit rape on a female geriatric patient. Psychiatric testimony heard that the female victim has a mental disease and is incapable of forming a reasonable apprehension of bodily harm is overturned based on ethical codes exercised within a Veterans hospital. The defendant's participation in the detoxification unit for alcohol and drug addiction makes him a responsible agent entitled to privileges possibly denied to patients on other wards.

Descriptors: Law, rape, mental disease, detoxification.

642. Jacobson, S. B. Accidents in aged. Psychological and psychiatric viewpoint. New York State Journal of Medicine, 1974, 74, 2417-2420.

Psychological factors identified in the accidental injury of organic systems are especially ostensible for elderly. Accident proneness is categorically split into emotional antecedents and mental-organic antecedents. Emotional antecedents considered are unconscious motivation, accident proneness, and the influences of functional mental illness and transient and chronic emotional states. Psychophysiologic functions of the central nervous system associate with the mental-organic factors, comprising most of the iatrogenic causes of accidents and extensive adverse effects of drugs.

Descriptors: Accidents, emotionality, psychophysiology.

643. Jellinger, K.; Koeppen, D.; and Rossner, M. Long-term treatment of depressive syndromes with Psyton. Wiener Medizinische Wochenschrift, 1982, 132, 183-188.

Examines experimental administration of Psyton (nomifensine/clobazam) in 23 patients exhibiting anxious-depressive symptoms. Benzodiazepine tranquilizers in general are critically compared through physical and laboratory investigations of weight, pulse rate, blood pressure, EKG, ophthalmology, blood, urine analysis and liver function tests. Drug tolerance to Psyton is relatively good with minimal side effects (seen in 39 percent of patients) occurring within four weeks after onset of treatment. Placebo comparisons further support the nonaddictive quality of the drug during treatment and after discontinuation of Psyton, indicating its potential utilization for long-term control of anxious depressive syndromes in middle age patients.

Descriptors: Psyton, benzodiazepines, research, anxiety, depression.

644. Lajama, R. J. Grief and depression. Journal of Geriatric Psychiatry, 1974, 7, 26-47.
Carefully assesses the contemporary social and psychological role of bereavement and depression on clinical changes in both older and younger persons. Observations contrasting normal from pathological grief patterns explore dimensions of narcissism and relation to trauma. The more acutely bereaved are vulnerable to mental and physical disorders of drug abuse and suicide. To illustrate, a case history of a 57-year-old Jewish widow traces her personality structure and readjustment following personal loss and its effects on the outcome of mourning. Reactional stages during and after death are variable depending on age-related mental stability or instability.
Descriptors: Grief, religion, narcissism, personality patterns.

645. Kaplan, O. J. Psychopathology of Aging. New York: Academic Press, 1979.
Presents topics concerning current views in geriatric psychiatry. Research into the etiologies of mental disorders that accompany aging include (1) genetic aspects of psychopathological disorders, (2) acute and reversible psychotic reactions, (3) psychological testing of seniles, (4) manic-depressive illness, (5) depression, (6) older schizophrenic, (7) neurosis and mental retardation, (8) alcohol and drug abuse, (9) criminality and deviant sex behavior, (10) sociopathy, and (11) suicide. Exploratory accounts of effective treatment strategies and public positions on aging and mental health recur in each chapter.
Descriptors: Psychiatry, mental health.

646. Klerman, G. L. Introductory statement: A view from the alcohol, drug abuse, and mental health administration. In N. Miller (ed.), Clinical Aspects of Alzheimer's Disease. New York: Raven Press, 1981.
Notable statement made at the Second International Conference on Alzheimer's Disease and Senile Dementia is on the organizational structure of systems devoted to alcohol, drug abuse, and mental health. Bifurcations between clinical and basic research create an artificial boundary between the biomedical and behavioral sciences concerned with geriatric care. These distinctions are difficult to maintain and they ignore fundamental needs within the field of gerontology to address the pseudodementias of depression versus true dementias. Efforts toward a viable rapprochement in administrative applications are suggested.
Descriptors: Administration, mental health, Alzheimer's Disease.

647. Lettieri, D. J. Empirical prediction of suicidal risk among the aging. Journal of Geriatric Psychiatry, 1973, 6, 7-42.
Analyzes formula for the empirical prediction of suicidal

risk among aging, drawn from four basic suicidal death prediction scales. Statistical selection of final scale items allows for more prognostic reliability. Items aim at gaining theoretical or descriptive understanding of suicide phenomena and of underlying variables that discriminate suicide in other age groups. By combining this scale with other diagnostic methods, results yielding both theoretical and applied information can offer direction for counselors. Attached appendixes consider the efficacy of these suicidal death scales and describes instructional procedures for their implementation.

Descriptors: Suicide, diagnosis, theory.

648. McCord, J. A Longitudinal Study of Adult Antisocial Behavior. (Report no. 1MH 26779 2). Washington, DC: U.S. Department of Health, Education and Welfare, 1976.

Study traces developmental changes in subjects from childhood to middle age during the period between 1939 and 1945. Social workers recorded observations of life-style change and compared them to a control group. Case records for the 510 subjects include evidence of criminality, admission into mental hospitals, alcoholism, and deviancy stemming from marital or social relationships. Cultural factors indicative of adult-life patterns are further explored through the later use of interviews and questionnaires. Links between childhood and adult antisocial behavior independent of cultural indoctrination and medical illness are among the considerations viewed.

Descriptors: Childhood and adulthood, culturalization, personality.

649. McKenna, G. J. Psychopathology in drug dependent individuals: A clinical review. Journal of Drug Issues, 1979, 9, 197-204.

Developed is a single unifying theory to explain the phenomenon of drug dependence experienced by varying age groups. Typically the theory focuses on psychoanalytic or ego functions, socioeconomic factors, and physiologic effects of drugs examined independent of behavioral reactions. Pathology in addicts is alternatively viewed through emphasis on psychiatric disorders that predispose and accompany drug dependence. Being a multi-etiological phenomenon, drug dependency apparently undergoes a series of psychiatric-related transitions before becoming a biochemical problem. Explored are the various transitional phases and predispositional disorders identified in the dependency process.

Descriptors: Theory, drug dependency, aging.

650. Manson, M. P., and Engquist, C. I. Adjustment of eighty discharged geriatric-psychiatric patients. American Journal of Psychology, 1960, 117, 319-325.

Popular beliefs hold that many older patients encumbered with severe physical and psychological illnesses have little chance of returning to family and community unless provided with careful and continual professional assistance. Validity of this claim undergoes investigation in a study of discharged veterans ages 26 to 82 years and formerly diagnosed psychotic, brain syndromed, and with various cardiopulmonary and addictive diseases. Discharged patients spend an average of 21. 7 months in the hospital and the majority have histories of hospitalization. Encouraging data suggest the adjustment potential for living outside the hospital is greater than anticipated by popular belief. Discharge and mortality correlations are examined with respect to recidivism.

     Descriptors: Normalization, hospitals, veterans.

651. Masserman, J. Handbook of Psychiatric Therapies. New
      York: Jason Aronson, 1973.

     Overviews recent developments in psychiatric therapies since 1960, with chapters on suicide, the aged, drugs, addiction, and institutional therapy, among other related topics. Such prominent contributors as Rollo May and Milton Greenblatt equip the book with relevant reference material.

     Descriptors: Psychiatry.

652. Maultsby, M. C. , and Carpenter, L. Emotional self defense
      for the elderly. Journal of Psychedelic Drugs, 1978, 10,
      157-160.

     Articulates the current research into drug abuse and alcoholism as a coping strategy for emotionally distressed elderly. Treatment use of rational behavior therapy and self-counseling are contrasted with drugs and medication for the removal or temporary relief of involuntary activity, losses, feelings of abandonment, loneliness, and anticipation of death. Societal norms favor the pharmacological orientation of having prescribed or OTC medicaments, but this approach largely impairs psychological recovery. In view of the learned nature of drug use, treatment should instead focus on inaccurate perceiving and habits of irrational thinking and emotional responses. Conducted is an exploratory study comparing effects on elderly in both a psychotropic drugs group and rational emotive therapy group. Implications for wider acceptance of behavior therapy in addiction research are discussed.

     Descriptors: Behavior therapy, rational-emotive therapy, medication.

653. Mental Health Program Reports. Washington, DC: U. S. Gov-
      ernment Printing Office, 1968.

     Comprehensive review of reports presented by the various programs on NIMH grants. Studies reviewed include (1) the role of learning in narcotic addicts, (2) training and mental health, (3) psychology and biochemistry of depression, (4) geriatric mental health, (5) narcotic influence on body, and also several studies incorporating occupational or recreational activities into a workable treatment regimen. These proceedings provide an available source of reference material for research agencies interested in exploring prior NIMH supported projects. Noteworthy are the increasing volumes of NIMH grants funded for the examination of gerontologic factors pertinent to drug abuse.

     Descriptors: NIMH studies, reference.

654. Mental disturbance of the aged. Kokoro No Kenko Series,
     1969, 5, 18-27.
     Discusses mental disturbance and physiological indicators
of disease among the elderly.   Etiologic confusion typically arises
when there are multiple disease states interactive on the cognitive
or behavioral process.   Disturbances due to arteriosclerosis, senile
dementia, schizophrenia, manic-depression, progressive paralysis,
chronic alcoholism, and neurosis are considered.   Because they
interrelate, psychiatric symptoms which foster common characteristics of mental illness take a long time for recovery.   Chronicity
of psychological pathology in relation to the older person's overall
health is explored.
     Descriptors: Mental health, psychiatry, etiology.

655. Milliren, J. W.   Some contingencies affecting the utilization
     of tranquilizers in long-term care of the elderly.   Jour-
     nal of Health and Social Behavior, 1977, 18, 206-211.
     Study explores a secondary analysis of data concerning
the utilization pattern of drugs in long-term care facilities for the
elderly.   Concentrates on the social contingencies effective in the
organization of medical care and responsible for the administration
of major tranquilizers.   Definitions elaborate the concept of "anxious"
or "depressed" patients in need of drug therapy and this helps establish the hypothesis that when social contingencies are known, physicians can more readily diagnose disease and accurately prescribe
tranquilizers.   Observed patterns reveal that females are more likely
than males to receive major tranquilizers and be defined as "anxious."
Sex-role distinctions affecting the clinician's decisions about diagnosis and treatment lend support to the hypothesis in question.
     Descriptors: Prescribing practices, attitudes, sex-roles,
     anxiety.

656. Mo, S. S. , and Kersey, R.   Prior time uncertainty reduction
     of foreperiod duration in schizophrenia and old age.   Jour-
     nal of Clinical Psychology, 1977, 33, 48-52.
     Examines 20 college students diagnosed into categories of
psychosis and alcoholism and judged on reactivity to varying stimulus
dimensions.   Experimental modifications in sound, intervals between
onset of warning signal and the stimulus, and judgments about duration comprise the foreperiod observation.   Estimates for foreperiod
durations are indistinguishable between schizophrenics and nonschizo-
phrenics, although receptivity of prior information associated with
time is unique to schizophrenics.   Variability in estimated scores
is compared for different age groups (between 22 and 72 years).
     Descriptors: Foreperiod durations, psychoses, stimulus
     dimensions.

657. Muller, C.   Spezielle alterspsychiatrie.   In Alterspsychiatrie.
     Stuttgart: Georg Thieme, 1967.
     Exploratory account of psychogenic diseases in the aged in-
cludes addiction to drugs or alcohol.   Advancing age brings on deterioration of several sensory mechanisms and slows down metabolism
and absorption functions working on consumable substances.   Reduced

malleability accompanies the loss of memory, perceptual acuity, and adaptive performance of daily tasks that require muscular coordination. Further damage increased the elderly's vulnerability to addictive medicine.
Descriptors: Psychophysiology, addiction.

658. Osgood, N. J.   Suicide in the elderly: Are we heeding the warnings? Postgraduate Medicine, 1982, 72, 123-130.
Asks the question whether social deviance among older people is preventable or diagnosable in clinical services.   Case illustrations show that the elderly endure loneliness, depression, and increased susceptibility to suicide.   Warning signs of potential suicide are changes in sleeping pattern, weight loss, extreme fatigue, increased alcohol consumption, mood or behavioral changes, and sudden interest or disinterest in religion.   Because most elderly commit suicide shortly after visiting their physician, responsibility lies with physicians to identify some essential suicidal cues.   Family and physician comprise a social network of interchange between the elderly and potential events leading to suicide.   Methods of family prevention of suicide and depression are elaborated for application.
Descriptors: Suicide, prevention.

659. Parkinson, S. R.   Aging and amnesia: A running span analysis. Bulletin of Psychonomic Society, 1980, 15, 215-217.
Alcohol-related pathologies endemic to loss of memory and Korsakoff's psychosis are observed in young university students, elderly volunteers, and amnesic alcoholic Korsakoff patients.   All subjects undergo a memory test battery under passive listening instructions.   Interestingly, results show that storage and retrieval deficits in aging and amnesia are limited to secondary memory and that memory impairment in young and elderly groups is more extensive than research frequently indicates.   Details pertaining to prevention of memory deficits are discussed.
Descriptors: Memory, amnesia, Korsakoff psychosis.

660. Parsons, O. A.; Pishkin, V.; Jones, B. M.; Callan, J; R.; Bertera, J. H.; Jenkins, R.; and Blackburn, M. R.   Neuropsychological Changes in Alcoholics and Brain-Damaged Patients. (Report no. ZO-38641 1). Washington, DC: U. S. Veterans Administration, Department of Medicine and Surgery, 1977.
Purpose of reserach is to investigate neuropsychological changes in alcoholic and brain-damaged patients on experimental problem-solving tests.   Older alcoholics showing pronounced deficits in retention and visual-spatial abstracting and general test difficulty compare with significantly better performance by younger alcoholics. Duration of drinking is not necessarily predictive of performance on these tasks (tests), whereas chronology proves to be the discriminating variable and confirms the hypothesis of premature aging in the brain of alcoholics.
Descriptors: Neuropsychology, premature aging.

661. Pearson, M. M.   Middle-aged male crises.   Medical Aspects

of Human Sexuality, 1968, 2, 6-13.
Probes the decline in overall pattern of activities and sexual interest that recurs in a vicious cycle because of frequent expression of emotional problems. Although not as physically strong, energetic or aggressively competitive as in younger years, men still tend to display symptomatic signs of resistance to age. In addition to menopausal reactions, important cultural factors increasing the male's vulnerability are less opportunity for social prestige, insecurity, and uselessness. Rapid in onset, this middle-aged crisis, called "pseudo-climacteric crisis" syndrome, is characteristic of the depression and sexual failure lasting for years. Indications are that because sexual performance is achievable well into the eighth or ninth decade of life (providing there is an active partner and relatively good health), sexual failure is due to a sudden realization of aging. Mental illnesses likely to aggravate this syndrome are certain organic diseases, alcoholism and drug addiction, and manic-depressive reactions.
Descriptors: Male menopause, sexuality, depression.

662. Petrilowitsch, N. Die problemkreise alternder menschen im lichte der suizidalen kranken. In Probleme der Psychotherapie Alternder Menschen. New York: Karger, 1968.
Chapter surveys nonpsychotic older patients with a record of attempted suicide. Suicide potential is traced to cultural deprivations of familial and marital relations and the onset of chronic alcoholism arising from anxiety and depression. A symptom of unresolved personal problems, the escape to alcoholism represents a major precursory warning signal to suicide.
Descriptors: Suicide, alcoholism.

663. Pilet, C. Catamnestic study on the frequency of psychoorganic deterioration in aged mental patients. Schweizer Archiv für Neurologie, Neurochirurgie und Psychiatrie, 1974, 114, 367-396.
Psycho-organic deterioration studied in 398 male and 392 female hospital patients is re-examined in their old age about 20 to 30 years later. Degree of deterioration in diagnosed and undiagnosed groups of patients shows, by and large, that damage increases with old age, although differences between sexes are absent. Lowest degree of deteriorational activity is in the general population with psychogenic disorders, as compared to the highest degree found in groups with effects of organic origin. Post-treatment follow-up methods and the epidemiologic concerns associated with longitudinal research are discussed.
Descriptors: Organic deterioration, psychophysiology, research.

664. Porjesz, B.; Begleiter, H.; and Samuelly, I. Cognitive deficits in chronic alcoholics and elderly subjects assessed by event-related brain potentials abstract. Drug and Alcohol Dependence, 1980, 6, 87.
Experiment focuses on a visual event-related potential

(VERP) to assess information-processing deficits in long-term alcoholics. Alcoholic groups compared to geriatric and matched control
groups are shown responding to rarely occurring (or "novel") stimuli.
Results from the geriatric group are that subjects display significantly delayed latencies when compared to both alcohol and control groups
for all conditions. Electrophysiological brain dysfunction is also
manifested by both alcoholic and elderly groups, but without a clear
explanation for it. Nervous system damage that is collateral to
cognitive process may explain, in part, the periodical or irreversible cases of intellectual impairment.
　　　　Descriptors: Cognitive process, nervous system, visuality.

665. Post, F. Management of senile psychiatric disorders. Brit-
　　　　ish Medical Journal, 1968, no. 5631, 627-630.
　　　　Discussion analyzes the management of psychiatric disorders
resulting from senile brain changes in the elderly. Senility and cor-
responding onset of dementia are only occasionally attributable to unresolved anxiety and manic-depression. A course of drug and nondrug therapy to restore mental balance and encourage physical withdrawal from drug addiction is outlined.
　　　　Descriptors: Senility, psychiatric disorders, dementia,
alcoholism.

666. Reifler, B.; Raskind, M.; and Kethley, A. Psychiatric diag-
　　　　noses among geriatric patients seen in an outreach program.
　　　　Journal of the American Geriatrics Society, 1982, 30, 530-
　　　　533.
　　　　Community health services attentive to over 2,300 patients
referred to a geriatric outreach program are evaluated for the relationship between (1) referral reasons, (2) referral source, and (3)
age. Middle-aged clients entering the referral system tend to receive a diagnosis of depression or forgetfulness and dementia. Families are most likely to initiate referrals for diagnosed demented patients, whereas apartment managers and housing authorities more
likely refer paranoid patients. Indications of this study show age
factors to decrease diagnosis of dementia and increase diagnoses of
depression, alcohol, and drug abuse.
　　　　Descriptors: Mental health services, referral system,
diagnosis.

667. Reimann, H., and Hafner, H. Mental disorders of the elderly
　　　　in Mannheim: An investigation of incidence rate. Social
　　　　Psychiatry, 1972, 7, 53-69.
　　　　Survey in 1965 examines incidence rate of chronic brain
syndromes in residents 60 years and over living in a West German
Federal Republic. Degenerative processes account for 54 percent;
affective psychoses for 15 percent; acute and chronic brain syndromes,
12 percent; neurotic disorders, 7 percent; alcoholism and addiction,
6 percent; and schizophrenia, 4 percent. Alcoholism and brain syndrome appear greater for men than women, whereas women have a
higher incidence of affective psychosis and neurosis. Interpretations
also stress the sex-specific ability on problem-solving tasks and its

relationship to social status, geographic location, and hospitalization.
Descriptors: Mental disorders, demography, West Germany.

668. Rimmer, J. Psychiatric illness in husbands of alcoholics.
Quarterly Journal of Studies on Alcohol, 1974, 35, 281-283.
Psychological stability in husbands of female alcoholics is observed in 25 men interviewed through a private psychiatric hospital. Diagnosed alcoholism and affective depression in the husbands are known to arise both before and after wife's drinking. Findings offer relative support to the contention that alcoholics choose a spouse having psychiatric disturbances or where disturbance is equivocal. Female drinking greatly limits the selection of mates and requires that he be tolerant of mood fluctuations and sociopathy entering the marital and familial relationship.
Descriptors: Alcoholics' mates, husbands, mental health.

669. Robins, E.; Gassner, S.; Kayes, J.; Wilkinson, R. H.; and Murphy, G. E. The communication of suicidal intent: A study of 134 consecutive cases of successful (completed) suicide. American Journal of Psychiatry, 1959, 115, 724-733.
Phenomena related to the successful (completed) suicide are at times unobservable or studied inadequately by statistical methods from coroners' records, case reports, or hospital records of the suicide. Failure to measurably substantiate the precipitant signals of suicide led to the current investigation. Findings concerning suicidal communication before the actual act are reported from interviews taken of patients who later commit suicide. Forms of signals described are (1) direct statements or indirect allusions to their imminent deaths, (2) frequency (of attempts) or chronology, as later related to the time of suicide, and (3) to whom the communications are made. Relationships between communication or its failure and such variables as sex, clinical diagnosis, marital state, occupation, education, and whether the person leaves a suicide note or lives alone firmly document important aspects of this pathology.
Descriptors: Suicide, communication, warning signals.

670. Salzberger, G. J. Anxiety and disturbed behavior in the elderly. American Family Physician, 1981, 23, 151-153.
Behavior disorders observable in the physician's diagnosis of aging symptoms pose special problems because the elderly are keenly susceptible both to psychological stress and vitamin B12 deficiency. Stress and anxiety arise over the fear of fatal disease or family separation. Uncontrolled tension advancing to alcoholism or substance abuse are reversible and treatable in hospitals. But even hospital admission can disorient the elderly. Management of elderly alcoholics who in turn worsen involves the attention of drug therapy, especially oxazepam and lorazepam (drugs with a short half-life). Indications are that short-acting benzodiazepines are appropriate intervention for the elderly patient unable to relieve persistent distress.

Descriptors: Vitamin deficiency, hospital admission, stress.

671. Scher, J. M.   The collapsing perimeter: A commentary on life, death, and death-in-life. American Journal of Psychotherapy, 1976, 30, 641-657.
Descriptive analysis of human relations in the context of social and personal perimeters focuses on several existential questions. The idea, for instance, of a collapsing social network accounts for the progressive trend toward individual alienation within the culture. Personal space and relationship to others play a major role in mental health and illness and determine one's adaptivity under depression, overpopulation, cultural depression, and varying physiologic passages, such as aging. Notions of perimetric human space for the individual are formed into theoretical postulates and extended to clinical cases.
Descriptors: Existentialism, depression, individual space, society.

672. Schmidt, W. , and de Lint, J.   Causes of death of alcoholics. Quarterly Journal of Studies on Alcohol, 1972, 33, 171-185.
Sociologic analysis reviews the cause-specific mortality of 6,478 alcoholics treated at a Canadian clinic over the period 1951 to 1964. Excess mortality is due, as specified on the death certificates, mainly to cancer of the upper-digestive and respiratory organs, to alcoholism, to arteriosclerotic heart disease, to pneumonia, to liver cirrhosis, to peptic ulcer, to accident, and to suicide. Epidemiology factors regarding the national incidence of alcoholism in comparison with these patients' emotional states, life-styles, and type of addiction are analyzed.
Descriptors: Canada, alcohol-related pathology, mortality.

673. Schoysman, M. F.   Masculine infertility. Boreaux Medical, 1974, October, 2229-2236.
Medical review of oligospermia finds that its etiology depends on excessive alcohol or tobacco consumption, the use of stimulants, or physical exhaustion. Spermatoza deficiency develops largely from congenital or adventitious causes and depends on extent of damage done to the epididymus. If adventitious, then oligospermia may be due to the presence of nitrofurans, high levels of androgens, or from inflammation in the epididymus. Treatment by ligation of the epermatic vein will also depend on the reversibility of drug addiction and its effects on aging sexual organs.
Descriptors: Oligospermia, sexual organs, alcoholism, drug addiction.

674. Schuckit, M. A.   High rate of psychiatric disorders in elderly cardiac patients. Angiology, 1977, 28, 235-237.
Draws a relationship between physical and mental disorders in a group of elderly medical and surgical patients evaluated with respect to history of alcoholism. Diagnosis of alcoholism is made when the following symptoms appear: (1) job layoff or firing, (2)

marital discord, (3) two or more nontraffic arrests, and (4) physician's advice that alcohol was already injurious. Reports of alcoholism in cardiac patients (12 percent) compared with noncardiac patients (8 percent) is significant in that cardiac patients are prone to cardiotoxic effects of alcohol. Alcohol decreases cardiac contractility and increases the incidence of rhythm disturbances. Noted also is that lung patients represent the highest rate of alcoholism and smoking. Recommendations favor the physician's increased awareness of addictive behaviors by elderly patients.

Descriptors: Alcoholism, mental disorders, cardiac patients.

675. Schuckit, M. A. , Miller, P. L. , and Hahlbohm, D.   Unrecognized psychiatric illness in elderly medical-surgical patients.   Journal of Gerontology, 1975, 30, 665-660.

Diagnostic criteria are used in structured interviews with 50 elderly patients to evaluate the presence or absence of unrecognized psychiatric disorders. Mental disorders overlooked in 24 percent of the subjects are predominately depression or alcoholism. Geriatric patients having these disorders are older, widowed, have past jail records, psychiatric hospital experience, and indicate episodic vascular disorders. Taken to task are the research claims that undiagnosable symptoms during a geriatric examination are probably secondary and hence deserve less attention than observable symptomatology. That alcoholism, for instance, can worsen cardiac health if unrecognized indicates the urgency to train physicians to exercise greater caution.

Descriptors: Diagnosis, alcoholism, vascular disorders.

676. Sletzer, B. , and Sherwin, I.   The Differential Diagnosis of Organic Brain Syndrome.   (Report no. ZO-38400 1).   Washington, DC: U. S. Veterans Administration, Department of Medicine and Surgery, 1977.

Clinically evaluated are over 135 patients in a chronic neuropsychiatric facility with suspected diagnosis of organic mental impairment. Evaluations cover a case history, laboratory tests, and complete neurological examination. Neurologic testing includes intellectual assessment and strict criteria for the observation of cognitive and behavioral functions. Majority of patients fall into conventional categories of senile dementia, post-traumatic encephalopathy, and alcohol dementia. More quantitative analysis is necessary to reach conclusions about apraxia, aphasia and constructional difficulty.

Descriptors: Neuropsychiatry, tests, cognition.

677. Sims, M.   Sex and age differences in suicide rates in a Canadian province.   Life Threatening Behavior, 1974, 4, 139-159.

Demographic survey and case reviews on the suicide rates of elders and youth are examined against provincial and national trends. Suicide by poison accounts for the increasing proportion of reported suicides. Violent suicides in persons as old as 59 years typically began from rejection of some antisocial behavior, such as drinking, drug abuse, or infidelity. More men than women drink, but females are greater abusers of prescription medication. Concomitant to suicide attempts are emotional manifestations of grief, guilt, and loneliness. Suicide rates appear in correlation to sex, age, and personality patterns pooled over a 20-year period.

Descriptors: Suicide, alcoholism, Canada, demography.

678.   Simon, A.; Epstein, L. J.; and Reynolds, L.   Alcoholism in the geriatric mentally ill.   Geriatrics, 1968, 23, 125-131.

Part of a series of long-range studies on elderly drug abuse is the examination of 534 first admission psychiatric patients. Alcoholics (28 percent) fall into three groupings: (1) with no chronic brain syndrome, (2) with alcohol chronic brain syndrome, and (3) with senile or arteriosclerotic chronic brain syndrome.   Patients assigned to psychiatric wards show characteristics that are common to nonalcoholics but are of Irish descent, divorced or separated, likely to live alone, and probably dead or hospitalized at the end of two years.   Alcoholic elderly run the risk of misdiagnosis and consequently are denied proper entry into social rehabilitation.

Descriptors: Alcoholism, mentally ill, taxonomy.

679.   Small, G. W. , Liston, E. H. and Jarvik, L. F.   Diagnosis and treatment of dementia in the aged.   Western Journal of Medicine, 1981, 135, 469-481.

Neurologic pathology studied in elderly alcoholics offers a direction for differential diagnosis of dementia.   Discussion outlines the symptoms, diagnosis, and management of primary degenerative and multi-infarct dementia, noting that alcohol abuse is a cause of treatable dementia but commonly overlooked in diagnosis.   Needed are definitions of diagnostic criteria by which symptoms of dementia, drug effects, and pseudodementia can be properly delineated.   Cognitive abilities interfered with by dementia would also enter these clinical syndromes.

Descriptors: Differential diagnosis, dementia, alcohol-related pathology.

680.   Smith, H. , and Smith, L. S.   WAIS functioning of cirrhotic and non-cirrhotic alcoholics.   Journal of Clinical Psychology, 1977, 33, 309-313.

Determines whether cognitive dysfunctions found in chronic alcoholics are more significant for alcoholics with Laennec's cirrhosis than for alcoholics without it.   Administrations of WAIS Verbal, Performance, and Full Scale IQ on 60 Caucasian male patients ages 35 to 64 show stepwise differences.   While groups are similar in age, education, and on vocabularly subtests, major Verbal and Performance distinctions clearly support that the cirrhotic physical condition negatively affects intellectual ability.   Cognitive learning deficits indicative of memory and intellectual problems are explored for aging alcoholics whose physical pathology worsens over time.

Descriptors: WAIS, cirrhosis, cognition.

681.   Starkey, I. R. , and Lawson, A. A.   Psychiatric aspects of acute poisoning with tricyclic and related antidepressants--

a ten-year review.
Scottish Medical Journal, 1980, 25, 303-308.
Antidepressive agents are contributory to accidental and intentional poisoning in adolescents and elders on variable dosage requirements. Incidence of acute self-poisoning with tricyclic and related antidepressant drugs increasing in recent years has accounted for 20 percent of all acute overdoses in patients above age 12 being due to this cause. This study traces a ten-year review of psychiatric aspects associated with the poisoning of 316 consecutive patients admitted to a district hospital. Medical advice is sought prior to the overdosage and usual psychiatric diagnosis following the poisoning attempts to assess relationship of events with the original treatment with antidepressants. Preventive steps in medical diagnosis are discussed for implications to quality of inpatient and outpatient services.
Descriptors: Poisoning, antidepressives, psychiatric diagnosis.

682. Straker, M. Adjustment disorders and personality disorders in the aged. Psychiatric Clinics of North America, 1982, 5, 121-129.
Examines parameters of personality disorders among illustrative case reports and the self-inductive sick-roles manifested during psychotherapy. Adjustment disorders reactive to substance abuse are primarily responsible for hypochondriasis and chronic forms of pseudopathology that make it necessary for a differential diagnosis. Precautionary steps for physicians to take in assessing life change events are advised.
Descriptors: Adjustment disorders, personality, diagnosis.

683. Stromgren, T. R. Prevalence of mental illness among 70-year-olds domiciled in nine Copenhagen suburbs. Acta Psychiatrica Scandinavica, 1975, 51, 327-339.
Studies prevalence of mental disorders and especially personality abnormality among a geographically defined group of 70-year-olds. Total psychiatric morbidity is 15.5 percent, with 6.4 percent suffering from psychoses, and 7.4 percent classified as "neurosis plus personality disorders." Those living in homes with senile or arteriosclerotic dementia never have consulted physicians or been institutionalized. Epidemiologic correlates regarding education, sex differences, and alcoholism parallel findings reported from other studies on Denmark.
Descriptors: Denmark, mental disease, personality, aging.

684. Tardiff, K., and Swillam, A. Assault, suicide, and mental illness. Archives of General Psychiatry, 1980, 37, 164-169.
Sex and socioeconomic factors pervasive in cases of diagnosed aggression and other mental disorders are observed in 9,365 patients admitted to public hospitals over one year. Presence of assaultive or suicidal problems prior to admission appear in relation to sex, age, primary diagnosis, education, race, marital status, prior private care, and source of referral. Middle-aged patients

show high recurrence levels of substance dependence and schizophrenia. However, few significant differences are shown regarding the history of previous psychiatric admissions, veterans status, or history of seizures. Methodologically, these findings offer direction for a routine study of psychiatric problems from a data base of life-threatening behaviors.

> Descriptors: Assaultive (violent) behavior, suicide, hospital.

685. Thauberger, P.C.; Ruznisky, S.A.; and Cleland, J.F. Use of chemical agents and avoidance of ontological confrontation of loneliness. Perceptual Motor Skills, 1981, 52, 91-96.

Psychometric documentation of "choice" of avoidance versus confrontation to the issue of loneliness involves using the Ontological Confrontation of Loneliness Scale. Data reflect 118 males and 183 females (30 years and over) selected from both community and university locations in Alberta and Saskatchewan who report use of medications and hard drugs. Higher scores on the test (avoiders) report less use of tobacco than both medium and low scorers, and less consumption of alcoholic beverages than the medium scorers. Earlier research findings comparing results of the Loneliness Scale and use of various chemical agents conform with the current data. Implications suggest an analysis of avoidance learning by addicts.

> Descriptors: Addicts, Ontological Confrontation of Loneliness Scale, loneliness, avoidance.

686. Weismann, M.M., and Prusoff, B.A. Comparison of CES-D with Standardized Depression Rating Scales in Psychiatric Population. (Report no. 1MZ 860 1). Washington, DC: U.S. Department of Health, Education and Welfare, Public Health Service, 1974.

Independent contractor for the government compares the CES-D (depression) scale with three standard rating scales on 250 patients subdivided into five distinct types. Test scales used include Raskin scale, Hamilton scale, SCL-90, and CES-D. Patient diagnostic groups are arranged as follows: (a) acutely depressed patients, (b) recovered formerly depressed patients, (c) methadone patients, (d) patients treated for alcoholism, and (e) schizophrenics with depression. Analysis of test comparisons indicates advantages versus disadvantages for different subcomponents on each test.

> Descriptors: Test comparison (validity and reliability), diagnosis, patient typology.

687. Whittier, J.R., and Korenyi, C. Selected characteristics of aged patient: A study of mental hospital admissions. Comprehensive Psychiatry, 1961, 2, 113-120.

Exploratory analysis of aged patients investigated in a state hospital shows there are predominate cases of heavy chronic alcoholism. Insufficient diagnostic descriptions of alcoholism, drug abuse, and organic syndromes account for its oversight in primary diagnosis and the treatment plan. Alternatives entail a closer differential diagnosis between symptoms caused by physical morbidity and that caused by increasing substance abuse.

Descriptors: Hospitalization, alcoholism, drug abuse, differential diagnosis.

688. Wilkie, F. L.; Eisdorfer, C.; and Staub, J. Stress and psychopathology in the aged. Psychiatric Clinics of North America, 1982, 5, 131-143.

Psychologic adaptation by aging alcoholics often precedes episodes of psychiatric illness, especially depression and suicide. Poor management of stress due to changing circumstances causes the presence of social and physical mediators that are predictable in later symptoms of intrapunitive personality and alcohol dependence. Individuals determined at risk are those on psychotropic and sedative-hypnotic medications who experience changes in life-events without a spouse or confidant. Risk factors associated with psychiatric illness are specific enough for prevention and intervention programs to begin expansion. Suggestions for this expansion are noted.

Descriptors: Stress, mental disorders, alcoholism.

689. Williams, H. D.; Farrar, N. R.; Tapp, M. G.; and Obana, C. E. A Comparison of PICA Standardization Profiles to Obtained Alcoholic Profiles. (Report no. ZO-34614 2). Washington, DC: U.S. Veterans Administration, Department of Medicine and Surgery, 1976.

Performance comparisons are made between the Porch Index of Communicative Abilities (PICA) and obtained alcoholic profiles for 28 patients diagnosed as alcoholic. Measures of bilateral and unilateral performance as demonstrated by PICA subtest profiles show the lowest scores in verbal subtests. Lowest means are in graphic modality tasks. Noteworthy is that alcoholics performed similarly to mildly aphasic patients on language dysfunction. Overall, PICA demonstrates sensitivity in detecting language and behavioral deficits in alcoholics and is relatively resourceful for future investigations on language profiles.

Descriptors: Language, Porch Index of Communicative Abilities, alcoholism.

690. Wilson, I. C.; Alltop, L. B.; and Riley, L. Tofranil in the treatment of post alcoholic depression. Psychosomatics, 1970, 11, 488-494.

Comparative study examines administration of tofranil (antidepressant) to 40 consecutive female, post-alcoholic and depressed patients of 60 years and less. Tofranil groups compare with groups on pamoate liquid or an equivalent dosage of placebo to evaluate the intensity and variability of depression over a six-week period. Active treatment group evidences more psychological improvement in early weeks of treatment on both the Hamilton Rating Scale and Self-rating Depressive Scale, both of which define patterns of individual symptom improvement. Benefits of tofranil therapy in depression are explored for other emotional disorders.

Descriptors: Tofranil, depression, rating scales, placebo.

691. Zeman, F. D.   Neuropsychiatric symptoms of somatic disorders in the aged.   Gerontologist, 1969, 9, 219-220.
Discusses neuropsychiatric symptoms of somatic disorders manifested from a breakdown in intimate relationships, socio-environmental factions, and polymorbidity.   Attention of the geriatric physician focuses on possible etiologies overlooked by stereotypical beliefs as well as haste in the diagnosis process.   Overreliance on diagnostic techniques insensitive to somatic disorders may reduce detection of asymptomatic disorders, overdosage of drugs, and substance abuse problems.   Emphasis is placed on enhancing physical examinations.
Descriptors: Diagnosis, somatic disorders, neuropsychiatry.

7. DRUGS AND ALCOHOL: EDUCATION AND PREVENTION

692. Abert, J. G.   Case Studies of Evaluation in Health, Education and Welfare.   (Report no. PRS 302).   Washington, DC: Russell Sage Foundation, 1975.
Volume consists of 20 case studies divided in three sections: health evaluation, education evaluation, and welfare education. Extrapolations of case findings offer a twofold focus in each area. First, environmental factors relevant to doing an evaluation are examined.   Second, the subject matter is examined with respect to neighborhood health centers, drug abuse rehabilitation, birth control, blood bank policies, performance contracting in education, immigrant education, upward bound, compensatory education, foster grandparents, rehabilitation research, programs for the aged, child care, and other local and county services.   An introductory chapter describing the evaluation programs in the federal Department of Health, Education, and Welfare outlines the department's underlying philosophy and guidelines.
Descriptors: Education, Department of Health, Education and Welfare, evaluation.

693. Ablon, J.   Al-Anon family groups: Impetus for learning and change through the presentation of alternatives.   American Journal of Psychotherapy, 1974, 28, 30-45.
Describes Al-Anon family groups in a metropolitan area as they provide emotional fellowship for spouses, relatives, and friends of alcoholics.   Al-Anon groups inherently provide self-help education through a nonprofessional modality of group therapy and group education concerning mental health.   Historically this stems from the belief that members would be unlikely candidates ready for intensive psychotherapy.   Most groups therefore stress attitudinal and behavioral changes and the re-establishment of self-esteem and independence from the alcoholic.   Sharing experiences is felt to facilitate difficult self-examinations of emotional reluctance.
Descriptors: Al-Anon, family and marital education, alcoholism, rehabilitation.

694. Acres, D.   Primary health care team.   In G. Edwards and M. Grant (eds.), Alcoholism.   Baltimore, MD: University Park Press, 1977.
Discusses prevention and treatment of alcohol problems practiced in English primary health care teams.   Concept of the

family practitioner and health visitor compares with the American versions of practical nurse and medical practitioner. General techniques and positive attitudes useful in the development of family education of alcoholism are expounded upon.

Descriptors: British primary health care teams, family education, alcoholism.

695. AD-PEP: Alcohol-drug Prevention and Education Program for Senior Citizens. (Report no. NCAI-056356). Rockville, MD: National Institute on Alcohol Abuse and Alcoholism, 1980.

Program evaluation centers on a public information instructional package for teaching elders about mixing alcohol with drugs. The AD-PEP is an educational prevention program designed for people age 55 and over to warn of the dangers of over-the-counter patent medications, prescribed medications, and alcohol. Three lectures comprise a series presented to a sample group of elders and subsequently evaluated through pre- and post-test surveys and followup letters. Indications are that similar public programs open channels of communication between the professional community and patients.

Descriptors: AD-PEP, public program on drugs, evaluation.

696. Anderson, F. E., and Landgarten, H. Survey of the status of art therapy in the Midwest and Southern California. American Journal of Art Therapy, 1974, 13, 118-122.

The question of expanding art therapy in Southern California and through the Midwest is assessed by means of a survey of mental hospitals, special schools, penal institutions, geriatric care homes, and facilities servicing a range of psychological and substance abuse problems. Reported results are that art therapy is unfamiliar in many drug abuse and geriatric clinics.

Descriptors: Art therapy, geriatric clinics, hospitals, education.

697. Bartlett, M. D.; Brennan, M. L.; Gazzaniga, A. B.; and Hanson, E. L. Studies on the pathogenesis and prevention of postoperative pulmonary complications. Surgery, Gynecology and Obstetrics, 1973, 137, 925-933.

Pulmonary complications in the postsurgical patient are frequently due to inadequate spontaneous deep breaths. Voluntary maneuvers taught to the patients preoperatively and used frequently after surgery help to sustain maximal uniform alveolar inflation. Evaluations of this respiratory maneuver involve five normal volunteers, 150 patients undergoing laparotomy, and ten surgical patients with normal pulmonary function. Management of breathing regularity in preoperative and postoperative sessions depends greatly on the location of patient's incision, type and length of operation, time of nasogastric intubation, narcotic dosage, and other concomitants such as heavy smoking and chronic obstructive lung diseases. Spirometers can encourage continuance of this breathing pattern, but only

when pathologic obstructions (especially drug usage) are removed.
Descriptors: Pulmonary responses, prevention, cigarette smoking, aging factors.

698. Bury, R. W. , and Mashford, M. L. Use of a drug-screening service in an inner-city teaching hospital. Medical Journal of Australia, 1981, 7, 132-133.
Urinary drug screening offers a practical safeguard against overdose of antidepressive agents in adolescents and the aged. A screening unit is evaluated over a 12-month period after the introduction of a commercially available thin-layer chromatographic system that expands capacity of service efficiency. Specimens are screened when either drug overdose, abuse, or poor compliance with prescribed medications are suspected. Results show that multiple drug use is frequent in groups where the mean number of drugs taken is two. Retrospective examinations of case histories show that this drug screening system is involved in diagnostic or management decisions for at least 66 percent of patients seen.
Descriptors: Urinary drug screening, diagnosis, prevention.

699. Comprehensive Health Planning. (Report no. 6E 44A GRAI-7619). Sacramento, CA: State Department of Public Health, 1971.
Health planning in organizations concerned with the distribution of medical services for elders is explored vis-à-vis the report presented by the Task Force of the First California State Plan for Health. They identify major barriers to the improvement of environmental and personal health care systems. Population factors are the most critical and typically entail area needs such as the poor and aging, venereal disease, drugs and alcoholism, socioeconomic status, immunizations, and public educational resources.
Descriptors: Public health and education, health planning.

700. Development and Validation of Model Educational Program, "Drug Use and Health" and Informational Materials. (Report no. 1MZ 1417). Washington, DC: U.S. Department of Health, Education, and Welfare, Department of Public Health Service, 1977.
Reports on the effective development and evaluation of educational materials aimed at preventing the misuse of both prescription and nonprescription drugs by the elderly and thereby promoting healthy aging. "Drug Use and Health" represents a series of workshops and discussion groups led by occasional educators and those known from within the elderly community (e. g. , social circles, church, community action groups) that tailors information to the express needs of participants. Various informational materials are brochures, fliers, posters, wallet cards, educational workbooks and reading assignments developed for dissemination beyond the actual course itself. Pre- and post-test surveys to determine efficacy of this program are discussed.
Descriptors: Educational drug program, elderly, aging, community action.

701. Dewdney, I. An art therapy program for geriatric patients. American Journal of Art Therapy, 1973, 12, 249-254.
Art therapy programs for geriatric patients are in psychiatric hospitals and undergoing re-discovery for use in education on drugs and health care. Ten patients diagnosed as depressive neurotic, alcoholic, and manic, with pre-senile and senile dementia, are examined through art therapy projects such as (a) drawing and coloring objects from observation, (b) picture completion, and (c) arrangement of shapes and colors. Pre-senile and senile geriatrics revert to functional skills and, on occasion, recognize their own skill potential. Suggested is that art therapy be held in a room away from the ward to encourage interaction in groups.
Descriptors: Art therapy, education, depression, senility.

702. Dickman, F. B., and Keil, T. J. Public television and public health: The case of alcoholism. Quarterly Journal of Studies on Alcohol, 1977, 38, 584-592.
Social forces indigenous to prevention strategy are usually observable in the media's portrayal of drug abuse and alcoholism. In this study a series of programs on alcoholism are broadcasted statewide on television to stimulate public awareness and corrective action. The campaign attracts viewers comparable to those who normally watch public television. However, the campaign is unable to reach segments of the population most at risk (35 years and older) to heavy alcoholism. Explored for future research are the implications of mass media as effective instruments in the weekly telecast of educational programs.
Descriptors: Media (television,) education, alcoholism, prevention.

703. DiNitto, D.; Lauer, B.; and Storm, L. Improving with Age: Developing a Model for Alcoholism Education and Prevention Among the Elderly. Paper presented at the NCA Annual Forum, New Orleans, April 1981.
Elderly volunteer training programs play a part in community programs on drug abuse. A study reviewing the Florida's Citizens Commission on Alcohol Abuse program focuses on their development, implementation and evaluation of a model educational structure of elderly alcohol abusers. This model plan instructs elderly persons in alcohol abuse facts, about aging, stress, and public speaking skills. Encouraged is the Commission's attempt to interest elderly speakers to accept invitations in geriatric and nongeriatric homes.
Descriptors: Volunteers, prevention and education, alcoholism.

704. For two hospitals safety is a matter of prevention: Drug education for seniors. Hospitals, 1981, 55, 30-32.
Health education planning in a hospital with bed capacity for 300 to 499 patients is explored. Geriatric units, in particular, require training on the safe self-administration of medicine and controlled use of alcohol. Prevention of substance abuse begins on the unit and is hopefully generalizable into community aftercare programs

after discharge. Extent of this educational project in Pennsylvania reflects the increasing awareness by medical personnel to problems of elderly drug abuse.

Descriptors: Health education, hospitals, Pennsylvania.

705. Friis, T., and Aagaard, S. Outpatient group therapy in a psychiatric department. Ugeskrift for Laeger, 1980, 142, 666-669.

Describes the establishment of outpatient services in a hospital psychiatric department treating many neurotic disorders and substance abuse clients. Elderly males comprise a large percentage of outpatients treated in group therapy and through educational courses on alcoholism. Psychotherapy is an alternative explored for the prevention of medicine misuse in middle-aged and older patients.

Descriptors: Psychiatry, prevention, alcoholism.

706. Gaetano, R. J., and Epstein, B. T. Drugs and the elderly: Strategies and techniques for consumer education. In D. Petersen, B. Payne, and F. Whittington (eds.). Drugs and the Elderly: Social and Pharmacological Issues. Springfield, IL: Charles C. Thomas, 1978.

Patient misinformation is a crucial problem in the mismanagement of outpatient medication regimens. Patients are the least knowledgeable members of the health team and must coordinate their own health care. Difficulties that the elderly patient encounters in the medication regimen are resolvable through a consumer drug education program. Input by these programs stress the appropriate use of drugs when they are necessary. People over the age of 65 are among high users and can benefit from an aggressive approach to training. Discussion expands this position to practical steps in early implementation stages.

Descriptors: Educational training, elderly, health team.

707. Golann, S. E., and Eisdorfer, C. Handbook of Community Mental Health. New York: Appleton-Century-Crofts, 1972.

Presents a comprehensive collection of recent findings by behavioral scientists and practitioners on the community's role in prevention and education of mental health problems. Original and unpublished studies report on treatment modules related to areas of drug abuse and alcoholism, suicide, the aged, prevention of disorder, and effects of community training methods applied in different cities. Forty-two selected readings allow for sufficient coverage of contemporary themes in drug abuse information.

Descriptors: Community service, prevention, mental health.

708. Goodstat, M. S. Current Progress and Research in Alcohol and Drug Education. Paper presented at the 11th Annual Conference of the Canadian Foundation on Alcohol and Drug Dependencies, Toronto, June 1976.

Reviews social impact of drug education programs in terms of two distinct models: (1) models based upon assumed knowledge-behavior linkages, and (2) models based upon aspects of values theory. Notable increases in the first model approach to primary prevention have been unfortunately ineffective. Evidence shows that exclusive training of attitudes is short of the prediction of altering behavior as much as training the behavior itself. Weaknesses in current drug education stem from its historical reliance on the first model rather than from an alliance with the social sciences. Recognition of research work in behavioral sciences is one direction for improvement.

Descriptors: Drug education, evaluation, behavioral theory.

709. Grant, M. Access and Influence: The Implications of Professional Education for Primary and Secondary Prevention of Alcoholism in the General Population. Paper presented at the 23rd International Institute on the Prevention and Treatment of Alcoholism, E. Germany, June 1977.

Discussion centers on the role of health professionals, doctors, liquor distribution agents, and recovered alcoholics in the expansion of prevention information. To accomplish this, plans aim to coordinate agencies and media resources that effectively can reach at-risk populations. Professional workers educated in prevention are better able to overcome traditional involvement with diagnosis and disseminate information in greater quantities. Integrative preventive approaches are discussed for community planning.

Descriptors: Professional training, prevention, diagnosis, alcoholism.

710. Gregory, D. Alcohol prevention and education programs in Oklahoma. Alcohol Technical Reports, 1977, 6, 23-29.

Describes current upsurge of alcoholism prevention and education services in Oklahoma. Activities emphasize the coordination of local organizations having a participatory role in community awareness and the creation of a special division on alcoholism. Defined objectives also stress appropriate and inappropriate drinking behavior for specific groups (elders, adolescents) and the need for measurable change in attitude and behavior. Statistical tests run on the evaluation of this program are explored.

Descriptors: Oklahoma, community awareness, educational programs.

711. Gunter, L. M. , and Estes, C. A. Providing health information to the elderly. Gerontologist, 1977, 17, 69.

Presents portions of paper read at the 30th Meeting of the Gerontological Society in 1977. Areas of mental illness, chronic disease, and accidents are covered in regard to aging, management of medication, and drug abuse. Critical to this discussion are the methods and resources described for use in surveys of perceived health needs and status for health information on aging. Potential health needs are translatable into skills and objectives that would serve for educational training on drug abuse.

Descriptors: Public health information, aging, drug abuse.

712. Hagen, C. Effects of speech therapy. Archives of Physical and Medical Rehabilitation, 1973, 54, 454-463.

Following a stroke, recovered communication abilities are

sometimes weak or temporary and improvement ceases after about six months. Spontaneous recovery relates to bilateral processes and is important for understanding the entire speech production mechanism. This study engages treatment and control groups through different speech therapies to determine the level of achieved functioning possible after a year of concentrated training. Reading comprehension, language formation, and speech production greatly vary with patient's history of drug and alcohol abuse, or relative pathologies. Speech therapy also provides a meaningful and immediately useful program attentive to a patient's individual social environment or physical condition. Therapy instruction given for both speech and physical health recovery are explored.

> Descriptors: Speech therapy, communication, physical health, education.

713. Harrison, E. A. Preventive Medicine: Mental Health (Bibliography with Abstracts). Springfield, VA: National Technical Information Service, 1977.

Areas covered by the selected annotation of abstracts include health screening, health care requirements, and health planning. Included in these topics are specific mental health categories such as mental retardation, neuroses, clinical abuse, drug abuse, and other mental disorders (42 abstracts contained).

> Descriptors: Bibliography, preventive medicine, mental health.

714. Hippler, R. Behavior Modification, Disorders and Therapy, 1970-April 1980. Springfield, VA: National Technical Information Service, 1980.

Retrospective collection of annotated abstracts is from reports on behavior disorders, modification, and therapy in human subjects. Citation listing covers both adult and youth problems and topics related to mental illness, alcoholism, drug abuse, arson, suicide, aggression, legality, special problems of aging, physically disabled, and developmental perspective of community education and prevention approaches. Contains 194 citations in total.

> Descriptors: Bibliography, behavior modification, mental health, drug abuse.

715. Hun, N., and Vertes, L. Rehabilitation of elderly alcoholics. Alkohologia, 1980, 11, 199-200.

Excessive alcohol drinkers and diseased comprise the membership of alcohol therapy clubs designed for two treatment modalities. First is the maintenance of abstinence using small doses of antabuse. Secondly, enrollment into this club commits one to rehabilitation viewed in contrast with aversive drug therapies and other rehabilitation programs. Cultural drinking habits considered in these programs are those which influence individual patterns and acceptance by the local community.

> Descriptors: Community clubs, international prevention, aversive drug therapy.

716. Kantor, W.; Hiller, A.; and Thuell, J. Developing an activity program in a welfare hotel. Hospital and Community

Psychiatry, 1974, 25, 520-524.
Discusses an activity program run by occupational therapists for elderly and other residents of a welfare hotel. Tenants consist mostly of prior state hospital patients admitted for alcoholism, drug abuse, and crimes. Interventions stress social and recreational needs of the inhabitants to improve their self-image and participation in social mainstream activities. Encouragement for rehospitalization is offered only after tenants either resume or develop maladaptive responses to demands of daily living. Educational technology in a practical hotel setting is explored.
Descriptors: Education, occupational therapy, hotel tenants.

717. Klaus, D. J.; Bridges, L. M.; Gualtieri, P. K.; and Smith, G. W. Assessment of the State Alcohol Services Demonstration Program (SASDP). Appendix I: Participating and Comparison States. (Report no. NCAI-065229). Rockville, MD: National Institute on Alcohol Abuse and Alcoholism, 1982.
Statistical demographic information prepares descriptive profiles on the structure and operations of alcohol services in the states of Connecticut, Michigan, New Jersey, New York, South Carolina, Arkansas, Colorado, Maryland, Pennsylvania, and Virginia. Brief annotations explain the current status of programs based on visits to each state authority during 1980 to 1981. Participating state offices are visited twice, during which auditors review annual plans, funding documents, and educational materials utilized for commercial purposes. Examined more closely are state comparisons among group psychotherapies, the elderly, racial and ethnic groups, and alcoholic females.
Descriptors: State comparisons, NIAAA, alcohol services.

718. Leigh, D. H. Prevention Work Among the Elderly: A Workable Model. Paper presented at the NCA National Alcoholism Forum, Seattle, May 1980.
Prevention goals and program designs largely constitute the models in social services for distributing drug abuse information to elders. An alternative program is in a 126-inpatient transitional hospital devoted to treatment of alcohol and drug abuse in addicted men and women. The hospital's active role in prevention, beginning around 1978, has been in survey evaluations, and outreach guest presentations at local senior adult centers. Evolving from this motivation is a self-help group called ALERT, consisting of persons who have overcome feelings of loneliness, anxiety, and powerlessness by attending seminars and weekly training. Sessions typically focus on legislative action, assertiveness, holistic health, stress management, communication skills, consumer awareness and interpersonal skills.
Descriptors: Community prevention programs, ALERT, self-help groups.

719. Lesnoff-Caravaglia, G. (ed.). Health Care of the Elderly: Strategies for Prevention and Intervention. New York: Human Sciences Press, 1980.
Book takes as its major focus the explication of health care systems appropriate for gerontological or geriatric education.

Papers drawn from the Sangamon State University Fourth Annual
Gerontology Institute (held in 1978) and published in this book are
on strategies for prevention and intervention. Categorical divisions
are arranged into medical care of the elderly, psychosocial problems
in later life, and components of health care. Demography regarding mortality, life expectancy, and drug withdrawal among older persons is brought to bear on constructive actions toward health problems.

> Descriptors: Health care systems, geriatric education,
> drugs.

720. Levenson, J. Treatment Concept for the Older Alcoholic.
     Paper presented at the NCA Forum, Washington, DC:
     May 1976.
     Reports the results of a 15-month study on drinking pat-
terns of elderly people in Baltimore and describes a proposal for
specialized treatment for alcoholics aged 55 and over. Drinking data
identify major gaps in the current alcoholism and geriatric service
continuum. Specific information on purposes, operations, staffing,
and training activities contrast with the proposed system, in which
the link with local support and consumer services is clear. Community rehabilitation programs are examined for their advances in drug
education.

> Descriptors: Geriatric services, community programs,
> prevention, education, alcoholism.

721. Louria, D. B.; Kidwell, A. P.; and Lavenhar, M. A. Primary
     and secondary prevention among adults: An analysis with
     comments on screening and health education. Preventive
     Medicine, 1976, 5, 549-572.
     Major diseases afflicting adults in the United States and
their susceptibility to primary and secondary prevention approaches
are reviewed. Findings show that only a few of the diseases are
preventable by risk factor modification and that in the majority the
risk factors are alcohol and tobacco. Evidence also indicates that
in very few cases is time of detection significant to outcome. Authors recommend augmentation of health education programs, with
special emphasis on licit and illicit intoxicant use, and a focusing
of patient screening efforts on diseases for which modification by
secondary prevention can be reasonably expected.

> Descriptors: Primary and secondary prevention, medicine,
> outcome.

722. Lynch, M. B.; Namkung, P.; and Wegsteen, B. C. Support for
     Drug-Abuse Control System. (Report no. 1DA 767 2).
     Washington, DC: U. S. Department of Health, Education
     and Welfare, Public Health Service, 1974.
     Overall objectives to this study are to reduce potential for
drug abuse through intervention on adolescents shown to have behavioral problems, and secondly, to determine feasibility of young adult
and senior citizens as para-counselors. Study further delves into
possible counselor-counselee potentials of volunteer citizens. The

validity and reliability of measurement devices used to make decisions about counselor potential are in early stages of development
and open to community input regarding counselor profiles. Advanced
is the belief that para-counseling alternatives encourage addicts to
seek treatment otherwise avoided.

> Descriptors: Volunteers, para-counselors, community
> activism.

723. MacDonald, J. H.; and Sparks, P. D. Employee assistance programs for alcoholism and drug abuse: An industry approach. Industrial Gerontology, 1974, 1, 25-27.

Describes innovative program for alcoholic employees whose
performance deterioration has placed their jobs in jeopardy. Alcoholism and drug misuse confronted in the work setting entails a stepwise approach to ease employee tensions. External treatment aimed at
abstinence accompanies improvements in job performance and, in
most cases, will rely on effective coordination of employer, physician, and counselor.

> Descriptors: EAP, job performance, education.

724. Malfetti, J. L., and Winter, D. J. Development of a Traffic
Safety and Alcohol Program for Senior Adults. (Report no.
NCAI-049858). Rockville, MD: National Institute on Al-
cohol Abuse and Alcoholism, 1978.

Drinking and driving programs excel in many states which
serve high-risk populations. Presented is the systematic development of a program to alert seniors to their vulnerability to traffic
accidents under the influence of alcohol and drugs. Films depicting
simulated situations comprise a large portion of the program. Beyond this, safety precautions are discussed to limit mobility when
taking or mixing alcohol and drugs. Underlying this program is the
assumption that by an awareness of vulnerability and opportunity to
examine attitudes and behaviors in relation to driving or walking in
traffic, seniors might well exercise some restraint. Field tests of
the program using pre- and post-test measures show positive acceptance of the information and willingness to change behavior.

> Descriptors: Alcohol and driving, educational programs,
> films, safety.

725. Miller, L. A., and Alexander, S. F. Substance use and older
persons. ERIC Reports, 1981, 211-876.

A substance-use education package, developed for senior
adults and service providers, contains a three-hour module for training seniors for presentation to senior center participants. Follow-up
materials include the following: (1) a three-part article on the hazards of drug use, (2) center presentation handouts, and (3) a brochure
titled "Be Responsible for Your Own Health." In addition, there is
a four-hour "Alcohol-Awareness" component for presentation to residents and staff in an adult rest home.

> Descriptors: Module training package, education, senior
> centers.

726. National Institute on Drug Abuse. Elder-Ed: Wise Use of
    Drugs for Older Americans. (16 mm film or videocas-
    sette; sound; color; 30 minutes), 1979.
    Movie on prevention of drug abuse presents topics about
getting information from physicians about medication practices. Typical problems of drug use at home and alternatives to these are de-
picted in acted vignettes and through narration by persons working
with elderly in the community and professionally. Movie functions
as supplement in community drug-prevention programs for elders.
    Descriptors: Movie, drug prevention, training, vignettes.

727. Pierotti, D. L. Elderly and Substance Abuse: A Need for
    Education, a Need for Advocacy. (Report no. NCAI-
    055671). Rockville, MD: National Institute on Alcohol
    Abuse and Alcoholism, 1980.
    Advocates the position that physicians and health care pro-
fessionals have a responsibility to older persons to actively educate
them on chemical abuse and psychologic or physiologic conditions
most apt to render the elderly vulnerable. Pharmacists and physicians are key figures in the dispensary system of medicine and
should make available a list of things elderly should do and not do
when taking medications or alcohol. General education programs
that include aspects of drinking parameters are useful adjuncts in
the information process.
    Descriptors: Health care professionals, instruction,
pharmacists.

728. Rodstein, M. The prevention of disability and disease in the
    aged. Geriatrics, 1966, 21, 193-196.
    Chronic conditions in need of comprehensive treatment are
among the many reasons for vast care facilities to prevent disability in aged. Indicated by this analysis is that more meticulous
examinations of elderly persons' symptoms are necessary to identify
pathology causing incapacitation. Evidence of dysfunction of the
heart, brain, kidney, sensory and abdominal organs, and organs of
locomotion is frequently covert unless physicians explicitly look for
such disease. Procedures are recommended that are simple, econom-
ical, and not objectionable to the patient, while remaining thorough.
Outpatient examinations further require that elderly be taught symptomatic cues of distress or physical pathology which are due to medication, alcoholism, or general morbidity.
    Descriptors: Medical prevention, disability, geriatrics.

729. Rosenberg, C. M.; Gerrein, J. R.; Manohar, T.; and Velandy-
    liftik, J. Evaluation of training of alcoholism counselors.
    Quarterly Journal of Studies on Alcohol, 1976, 37, 1236-
    1246.
    Comparative study measures the effects of training on at-
titudes and personality characteristics during didactic instructions,
weekly experience group, and practical training in an alcoholism
clinic. Counselor competency is measured, apart from scores on
inventories, from the ability to retain clients in therapy. Results
show that in spite of careful selection policies, considerable differences

among trainees are accountable for the attrition or retention rate of clients in treatment. Interesting is the absence of correlation between changes in attitude and behavior, and progressive improvement in clinical skills. Criticism notes the drawbacks with paraprofessional education in drug rehabilitation settings. Alteration of counselor attitudes is more promising when trainees possess more experience.

Descriptors: Paraprofessional training, drug abuse, demography of clients versus trainees, drug education.

730. Ryan, V.; Popour, J.; Arneson, A.; and Ruben, D. H. (eds.). Fundamentals of Substance Abuse Counseling. Lansing, MI: ARIS, 1983.

Organized handbook developed by the Specialty Program in Alcohol and Drug Abuse and Office of Substance Abuse Services in Michigan on introductory concepts of alcohol and drug abuse required for the first level of credentialing. Handbook overviews general information on pharmacology, treatment process, patients' rights, ethics, and theories of addictive personality. Eight individual modules have questions appearing at the end to prepare readers for the exam questions. Educational priority of this handbook is to recognize the need for minimal levels of competency in substance abuse counselors in the State of Michigan. Degreed and nondegreed counselors (e. g. , former addicts, elderly, etc.) desiring to obtain this competency and first level of credential ("Apprentice-Counselor Credential") are to pass written exam based directly on the book.

Descriptors: Educational manual, substance abuse counselor.

731. Schaps, E.; Churgin, S.; Palley, C. S.; Takata, B.; and Cohen, A. Y. Primary prevention research: A preliminary review of program outcome studies. International Journal of the Addictions, 1980, 15, 657-676.

Studies the research designs reported in drug abuse prevention program evaluations that employ drug-specific outcome measures. Many of these evaluations assess affective, peer-oriented and multidimensional strategies, with few that are purely informational. Characteristic differences lay in positive versus negative outcomes, and types of patients who participate in the programs. While in preliminary reviews the informational programs split between positive and negative effects, caution is advised in interpreting the scientific rigor with which these results are obtained.

Descriptors: Modality of educational program, methods of evaluation.

732. Schneider, K. A. Alcoholism and Addiction: A Study Program for Adults and Youth. Philadelphia, PA: Fortress Press, 1976.

Community prevention programs are especially important for the education of adult abusers or potential abusers adherent to religious beliefs. This book outlines a program to understand alcoholism as an illness of unknown origin, imparting physical, emotional, and spiritual dimensions. It guides community agencies and congregations on ways to present methods of intervention and information supportive of treatment and aftercare programs. Addiction is viewed mainly in terms of alcohol and drugs but largely because of self-destructive behaviors. Materials for presentation (audio-visual, etc.) help participants through new insights and sensitive matters.

Descriptors: Religious education and prevention.

733. Smart, R. G. Social policy and the prevention of drug abuse: Perspectives on the unimodal approach. In M. M. Glatt (ed.), Drug Dependence: Current Problems and Issues. Baltimore, MD: University Park Press, 1977.

Chapter highlights two approaches to prevention of alcoholism and drug abuse. First is the sociocultural approach, positing that social and cultural factors primarily lead to alcoholism. Second is the unimodal approach, proposing that by reducing drug and alcohol consumption the addiction is relieved. Preference for the second approach is due to the often ignored importance of per capita consumption in preventing alcohol abuse, in that regulations on societal consumption directly interact with individual consumption. Policy implications drawn from this approach are consistent with traditional needs for structure in community prevention programs.

Descriptors: Models of prevention, per capita consumption, demography.

734. Smith, M. C. Issues in planning a treatment program for the geriatric alcoholic. In J. S. Madden (ed.), Aspects of Alcohol and Drug Dependence. Kent, England: Pitman Medical, 1980.

Program plans surround a synthesis of service networks considered in a multidisciplinary approach to the prevention of geriatric alcoholism. Basically, these three areas are of primary concern: (1) epidemiologic issues related to defining alcohol abuse and identifying sub-populations at risk, (2) issues on the design of a treatment model appropriate for the elderly, and (3) problems in establishing the intersystem linkages to assure patient access to the full range of community services. Outreach and aftercare programs are for continuation of preventive training until the patient can manage by himself or herself.

Descriptors: Hospital prevention program, community projects, social networks.

735. Social Groupwork and Alcoholism. New York: Haworth Press, 1982.

This book focuses on several community activism groups helping alcoholics achieve sobriety and return to social stability. Experts in group social work knowledgeable about the interaction of family and alcoholism share their treatment programs and discuss methods jointly run with hospital care units. Programs involving stress management, assertiveness, short-term group therapy, and driver education view spouse and child participation as instrumental to alcoholic recovery. Discussed in detail are various strategies for psychotherapy for elderly, alcoholic females, and children of alcoholic parents.

Descriptors: Community activism, treatment programs, education.

736. Silver, R. J.; Lubin, B.; Silver, D. S.; and Dobson, N. H. The group psychotherapy literature: 1979. International Journal of Group Psychotherapy, 1980, 30, 491-538.
Extensive coverage of yearly research developments in counseling technique and group formation of treatments for community education. Self-help groups emerging in response to demands for paraprofessional and community training offer emotional support and, in many cases, organized structure to reduce hypertension, obesity, spouse abuse, substance abuse, and alcoholism. Relevance of inpatient or privately counseled groups to self-help groups is that it provides a smooth transition to independence. Group educational methods noted to assist this transition cover psychodrama, psychotherapy, and modified forms of psychoanalytic therapy.
Descriptors: Self-help groups, obesity, community support, hypertension.

737. Swisher, J. D., and Vicary, J. R. Prevention of alcoholism and drug abuse. In Perspectives in Alcohol and Drug Abuse: Similarities and Differences. Littleton, MA: John Wright, PSG, 1982.
Primary prevention programs represent major strides in the substance abuse field to acquaint addicts and consumers with knowledge to make responsible decisions. Reviewed are the collective routes of exchange in a program that include input from advertising, media campaigns, traffic safety, occupational programs, DWI programs, referrals, emergency care, EAPs, and specialized groups such as elderly and children. General education typically is a self-developmental process much as are prevention programs, whose aims are to examine realistic cases of substance abuse. However, authors recognize that responsible decisions about abuse rest with the individual in spite of the routes of exchange between a person's needs and the model of education.
Descriptors: Primary prevention, social networks, individual responsibility.

738. Taylor, J. A. Guide for the Development and Provision of Alcohol Treatment Services for the Aging. (Report no. NCAI-062047). Rockville, MD: National Institute on Alcohol Abuse and Alcoholism.
Delivery of competent services is hindered by several barriers to treatment that are either unknown or ignored during initial stages of program development. Guidance is given to community agencies for developing alcohol treatment services for the elderly, thereby anticipating possible barriers. The following are topics of discussion: (1) general characteristics of the elderly population, (2) alcohol misuse and abuse, (3) incidence of alcohol abuse, (4) demography of elderly abusers, (5) barriers to effective intervention, (6) complications in the intervention strategy, and (7) development in integrative network of services. Educationally oriented programs for elderly are both widespread and easily begun by

following these guidelines.
Descriptors: Prevention agency, planning strategy, guidelines.

739. Thorson, J. A. , and Thorson, J. R.   Patient education and the
older drug taker. Journal of Drug Issues, 1979, 9, 85-
89.
Drug misuse and abuse is frequently the result of igno-
rance on the part of drug takers. However, removal of responsibility
for self-administration is an example of role-reversal and is often
perceived as insulting. Because most medications taken by elderly
are self-administered, practitioners have an important responsibility
to develop some semblance of educational programs assuring that
older drug takers will receive accurate and timely dosages. Individual sessions are advised for clinicians to provide effective learning
on the part of the aged. Toward this end, objectives and techniques
for patient drug education are provided.
Descriptors: Physician responsibility, outpatient education.

740. Tucker, J. R.   A worker-oriented alcoholism and "troubled
employee" program: A Union Approach.   Industrial Gerontology, 1974, 1, 20-24.
Exploratory study of a program set up by organized labor
in Missouri to assist the alcoholic worker whose job is in jeopardy.
Union stewards conducting the interviews and referral process have
been through training and apparently informed of precipitant signs of
alcoholism as different from symptoms of general fatigue, aging, and
work-related tension. Problems and solutions to worker-union interactions are among the areas examined.
Descriptors: Union programs for prevention, industry.

741. Tyson, R. F.   State Prevention Coordinator Grant. (Report
no. 1AA 1793 1). Washington, DC: U. S. Department of
Health, Education and Welfare, 1975.
Iowa state plan outlines the coordination of alcoholic education activity through the Department of Public Instruction and the
following agency programs: (a) public safety, (b) drinking drivers
schools, (c) social services--ADC Mothers (emphasis on alcoholism
in females) and senior citizens, (d) health department, and (e) youth
organizations. Utilization of state plan will assist in developing
state curriculum for schools, motivation for use, public media, and
implementation strategies. Teachers recruited from schools, private
and public industry, and community agencies are prospective leaders
for the prevention programs. When these mechanisms are in motion,
statewide prevention promises the best chance of success.
Descriptors: Iowa, state prevention planning, integrative
networks.

742. Yakish, S.   AAA launches alcohol-traffic program for senior
citizens. Traffic Safety, 1978, 78, 21.
Briefly describes a film produced by the Automobile Association of America on their recently instituted program on drinking
and driving. The 11-minute film is shown to senior citizens at 13

locations around the United States and Canada and after preliminary analysis there shows a significant improvement in the seniors' attitudes toward alcohol and traffic safety. Alternative prevention tactics using audio-visual displays complementary to the lecture offer a possible direction for enhancing consumer knowledge.

Descriptors: Highway safety, audio-visual (films), prevention.

743. Yancy, S. R. Systems Approach to Primary Prevention in Alcolism. Unpublished dissertation, University of Massachusetts, 1976.

Theoretical model of alcohol prevention explores a community based approach. Author examines various aspects of mass communication, motivation and persuasion, group dynamics, and social systems. In the demonstration section appears a list of steps for health educators and planners to follow in developing a program in most communities and for specialty populations, such as the elderly and adolescents.

Descriptors: Model of alcohol prevention, specialty populations.

8. INSTITUTIONALIZATION AND DRUG ABUSE

744. Albert, E.   The task of the advisory psychiatrist in a home
for the aged. Zeitschrift für Allgemein-Medizin, 1980, 56,
327-334.

Neurologic pathologies reviewed in 52 patients are seen
during a nine-month period at a home for the aged.   Cases of hal-
lucinosis and neuropathy are as frequent as memory disturbance,
disorientation, and illogical thought patterns.   Duties of the consulting or "advisory" psychiatrist apart from diagnosis move into therapy referral, and medication supervision.   Foreign psychiatric consultants are compared to American psychiatrists in terms of case-
load, orientation philosophy, and prescribing practices of drugs for
the elderly.

Descriptors: Psychiatry, home for aged, medication.

745. Bailey, D. N.   Survey of admission toxicology panels in patients
with multiple hospitalizations.   Journal of the Analysis of
Toxicology, 1980, 4, 204-211.

Number of admissions into hospital show the average patient being a 32-year-old male entering the emergency room a mean
of 2. 2 times following episodes of suspected drug abuse.   Found on
admission toxicology screening are ethanol, barbiturates, opiates or
phenothiazines and one third of these recur on subsequent hospitalization admissions.   Visits are usually separated by intervals of 2. 5
months and frequently repeat in the emergency room.   Drug analysis
on the 65 repetitive admissions suggests that specific drug-oriented
searches may be possible for those with this diagnosis.

Descriptors: Repeat admissions, drug toxicology screening.

746. Bissel, L. C. , and Jones, R. W.   The alcoholic nurse.   Nursing Outlook, 1981, 29, 96-101.

Role of nursing supervisor on alcoholic recovery unit is
explored regarding the type of responsibilities expected.   Institutionalization of adult and elderly alcoholics poorly able to accept decreasing physical capacity and detoxification may lead to suicidal
urges. Nurses involved in these emergencies are advised to watch for
warning signals in verbal and nonverbal interactions.   Particularly
for substance abusers, attempted suicides reflect avoidance of
accepting the addiction or need for counseling.

Descriptors: Suicide, hospitalization, nurses.

747. Brown, M. M. ; Cornwell, J. ; and Weist, J. K.   Reducing the

risks to the institutionalized elderly: Part I. Depersonalization, negative relocation effects, and medical care deficiencies. Part II. Fire, food poisoning, decubitus ulcer
and drug abuse. Journal of Gerontological Nursing, 1981,
7, 401-407.

In homes for the aged the occurrence of institutional or
stereotypical reactions in patients are frequently disregarded. Disorders numbering from one to multiple and affective upon organic or
behavioral structure lead eventually to symptoms of depression,
abuse, and depersonalization. Food poisoning and unmonitored self-
administration of medication is further dangerous because of risks of
substance abuse. Alternatively, recommendations call for closer
nurse-patient relations and patient mobility within the hospital groups.
Descriptors: Neglect, patient deterioration, nurse relations.

748. Bustamente, J. P. , and Ford, C. V. Characteristics of general
hospital patients referred for psychiatric consultation.
Journal of Clinical Psychiatry, 1981, 42, 338-341.
Referral and consulting role of psychiatry largely determines the treatment orientation. Here an analysis of 151 psychiatric consults at a large publicly supported teaching hospital indicates that referral rates are greater from the medical services as
compared with the surgical services. Minorities, elderly, and widowed persons are less often referred than depressed and organic brain
syndromed patients. Moreover, organic brain syndrome is the most
common symptom missed in hospital diagnosis. Utilization of psychiatric consultants within the hospital structure is reviewed.
Descriptors: Psychiatric consults, referral, diagnosis.

749. Chien, C. ; Stotsky, B. A.; and Cole, J. O. Psychiatric treatment for nursing home patients: Drugs, alcohol and
milieu. American Journal of Psychiatry, 1973, 130, 543-
548.
Nursing home patients on doxepin, other psychoactive
drugs, or no medication are either placed on an alcohol regimen in
the ward or assigned to a ward with a "simulated" pub setup. Results of the study show marginal differences between the pub milieu
over the ward milieu, thus suggesting that this form of "treatment"
instead be used in preparation for later stages of alcohol therapy.
Descriptors: Analogue therapy, doxepin, alcoholism, ward
milieu.

750. Crowley, T. J. ; Chesluk, D. ; Dilts, S. ; and Hart, R. Drug
and alcohol abuse among psychiatric admissions. A multi-
drug clinical-toxicologic study. Archives of General Psychiatry, 1974, 30, 13-20.
Hospitalized adult addicts reviewed in a psychiatric ward
have fewer psychotic diagnoses, briefer hospitalizations, and less
elevated MMPI scores than other patients sampled. Alcoholism contributes to 25 percent of admissions, with many alcoholics taking
other drugs. Heavier smokers were noted as having toxicologic

results positive for narcotics, sedative-hypnotics, or antianxiety drugs at admission. Attempts to conceal identity of polydrug use is through heavy caffeine and prescription stimulant use. Patients with complex patterns of drug abuse are therefore subject to variable diagnosis and demand focused treatment. Extensions of this hypothesis for nonaddict inpatients are considered.

Descriptors: Addict inpatients, hospital, polydrug, caffeine, narcotics.

751. Douglass, R. L. Aged alcoholic widows in the nursing homes. Journal of Addictions and Health, 1980, 1, 258-265.
Older women with diagnosed alcohol problems comprise a significant majority of widows residing in Michigan nursing homes. State of current knowledge regarding alcoholism morbidity is that this symptom rarely surfaces even by the third diagnosis for nursing home records. Fourth through eighth diagnoses eventually document alcoholic or drug abuse potentiality. So, too, women alcoholics receive less adequate support of nursing staff or family members and friends than do nonalcoholic patients or those undiagnosed. Brought to the forefront are the mandates for increased sensitivity by nurses to alcoholism and implications this has for policy changes.

Descriptors: Nursing homes, women alcoholics, support systems.

752. Elzarian, E. J.; Shirachi, D. Y.; and Jones, J. K. Educational approaches promoting optimal laxative use in long-term-care patients. Journal of Chronic Diseases, 1980, 33, 613-626.
Drug utilization study is conducted in a long-term care facility determining that, medically, dosage of cathartics preoccupy the medication schedules. Cost analysis figures show elderly spend more money on cathartics than other medicaments, but misuse them or accidentally overuse them resulting in substance abuse. No education about cathartics is avilable for long-term patients and this responsibility rests with nursing team. Medical management issues are regarding aging, hospital prescriptions and nurse-patient communication.

Descriptors: Cathartics, nurses, overmedication.

753. Garb, J. L.; Brown, R. B.; Garb, J. R.; and Tuthill, R. W. Differences in etiology of pneumonias in nursing homes and community patients. Journal of the American Medical Association, 1978, 240, 2169-2172.
Comparisons between 35 elderly patients hospitalized with pneumonia acquired in either nursing homes or the community uncover that 14.3 percent of them are in the community. Community-origin diseases spreading unarrested suggest there is an increasing need for containment of elderly vulnerable to polymorbidity. Preventive methods in nursing homes and implications for extension of prevention into community senior centers are explored.

Descriptors: Community versus institutionalization, nursing homes, pneumonia, alcoholism.

754. Ghose, K.   Hospital bed occupancy due to drug-related prob-
     lems.   Journal of the Royal Society of Medicine, 1980, 73,
     853-856.
     Bed occupancy statistics collected in England reveal that
length of stay for middle-age males is largely due to substance abuse
cases.   Utilization of hospitals by emergency and nonemergency drug
abuse victims is, by comparison to other diseases, more demanding
of nursing attention during longer intervals of time.   Demography
considered in drug abuse admissions are consistent with patient
characteristics shown for neighboring countries.
     Descriptors: Bed occupancy, drug abuse patients, England.

755. Glasscote, R. M.   Seven program descriptions in San Luis
     Obispo County Mental Health Services, San Luis Obispo,
     California.   In The Psychiatric Emergency: A Study of
     Patterns of Service.   Washington, DC: The Joint Informa-
     tion Service, 1966.
     Details emergency psychiatric service in San Luis Obispo,
California.   Mental health expenses are reimbursable under the
Short-Doyle Act, and average length of stay in inpatient (locked ward)
hospitals is ten days.   More than half of inpatients are alcoholics of
varying age, with the remainder diagnosed mainly as depressive and
schizophrenic.   Two salient lacks are the hospital's cooperation with
community mental health and the severe absence of rehabilitative
services.   Noted by contrast is the efficient emergency psychiatric
care offered by the hospital.
     Descriptors: Emergency psychiatric care, hospital, commu-
     nity mental health.

756. Goldstein, S. , and Grant, A.   The psychogeriatric patient in
     the hospital.   Canadian Medical Association Journal, 1974,
     111, 329-332.
     Record reviews of 148 patients over 60 shown to be dis-
charged reveal excessive drinking in 24 percent of men and 7 percent of women.   Those with alcohol problems have shorter stays
than those with affective disorders, except for cases of undifferen-
tiated diagnosis.   Cases of post-discharge alcoholism relating to
iatrogenic etiologies compare with those patients whose readjustment
is inadequately safe without frequent inpatient or outpatient admissions.
Recidivism rates in alcoholics are examined in some detail.
     Descriptors: Hospital records, affective disorders, diag-
     nosis, alcoholism.

757. Greenwald, S. R. , and Linn, M. W.   The younger nursing home
     patient.   Journal of Gerontology, 1972, 27, 393-398.
     Study examines adjustment potential of younger patients
placed in a nursing home setting compared to older residents.   Two
primary findings are that (1) younger patients not considered to have
good prognosis need supportive help in adjusting to the nursing home
placement and (2) unlike older patients, younger ones are more
vulnerable to drinking problems.   Facility treatment plans lack special needs for alcohol prevention and this omission currently creates

a central disjointment in the management of health care.
Descriptors: Nursing homes, age-related adjustment, alcoholism.

758.   Handy, I. A.   The geriatric psychiatric patient: A challenge
       for social workers.   Journal of the American Geriatrics
       Society, 1966, 14, 1067-1071.
       Mental hospitals typically have geriatric psychiatric patients who remain there long after they no longer need intensive hospital care.   Hospitals stand to expect higher percentages of this type of patient unless treatment programs are developed that prepare patients to leave the hospital.   Caseworkers are responsible to recognize this serious problem and avert the injustice being rendered to geriatrics.   Two alternative solutions concern hospital accommodations and social programs.   Beds are needed for acutely ill patients but others should be freed by healthy elderly.   Concurrently, social workers have to approach the development of aftercare rehabilitation for aging patients so they can live within the limits of their tolerance. Resistance of social workers to face this problem and their obligation to its alleviation are explored.
       Descriptors: Length of geriatric hospital stay, social workers, aftercare.

759.   Harrington, L. G. , and Price, A. C.   Alcoholism in a geriatric
       setting.   Journal of the American Geriatrics Society, 1962,
       10, 197-211.
       Sociocultural data are presented in a five-part study regarding 1,000 members of the Veterans Administration Center's domiciliary facility.   Alcoholism diagnosed in 223 patients suggests the radical need for program improvements that address treatment and aftercare sobriety.   Alcoholics who begin to drink while hospitalized are indicative of certain ethnic and racial characteristics not possessed by either prior alcoholics or those turning to alcohol after discharge.
       Descriptors: Hospitalized alcoholics, Veterans Administration.

760.   King, A. P.   Cocktail hour in a nursing home.   Nursing Care,
       1977, 10, 26.
       Briefly describes inductive effects of small amounts of alcohol taken by elderly nursing home residents at fixed time periods. This period known as "cocktail hour" offers limited liquor for elderly that consequently has sedative and social effects.   Sociability in residents increases without the risk of alcohol abuse.   Critical drinking parameters in aging persons are considered.
       Descriptors: Alcohol, nursing home residents, social behavior.

761.   Kramer, M. ; Taube, C. A. ; and Redick, R. W.   Patterns of
       use of psychiatric facilities by the aged: Past, present
       and future.   In C. Eisdorfer and M. P.   Lawton (eds.),
       The Psychology of Adult Development and Aging.   Washington, DC: American Psychological Association 1973.

Statistics cover the use of state and county mental hospitals and other facilities by aging patients through 1968. Predictions offer an examination of future needs for mental health services and types of personnel and living arrangements in psychiatric treatment. Major social and physical conditions having impact upon these predictions are problems of crime, alcoholism, poverty, suicide, and availability of government programs for elderly.

Descriptors: Psychiatric hospitals, projections, mental health programs.

762. Levy, M.; Kewitz, H.; Altwein, W.; Hillebrand, J.; and Eliakim, M. Hospital admissions due to adverse drug reactions: A comparative study from Jerusalem and Berlin. European Journal of Clinical Pharmacology, 1980, 17, 25-31.

Aging factors relative to hospital admissions of patients with adverse drug reactions are observed in a comparative study between Israel and Berlin hospital medical services. Nearly 103 out of 2,499 medical admissions in Jerusalem and 167 out of 2,933 admissions in Berlin are due to such problems. Sex distribution in both patient populations are fairly equal. Differences noted are the toxic reactions to digitalis in Berlin and reactions to antibiotics in Jerusalem, as well as unequal frequencies in admissions for anticoagulants, hypoglycemic agents and oral contraceptives. Demography of the patient population determined as risk factors, apart from old age, are female sex, impaired renal function, and previous history of admission for drug reactions. Sociocultural dimensions underlying admission statistics are briefly examined.

Descriptors: Admission for drug reaction, Israel, Berlin.

763. Linn, M. W.; Linn, B. S.; and Greenwald, S. R. The alcoholic patient in the nursing home. Aging and Human Development, 1972, 3, 273-277.

Study concerns hospitalized patients who receive medical treatment for chronic alcoholism and are subsequently sent to community nursing homes. Adjustment symptoms are among the foci in comparing these patients with regular patients going from hospitals to nursing homes. Questions regarding the capability of rest homes to treat alcoholism have to do with personnel, informed consultants, and misdiagnosis upon admission.

Descriptors: Alcoholics, nursing homes, hospital discharge.

764. Locke, B. Z.; Kramer, M.; and Pasamanick, B. Alcoholic psychoses among first admissions to public mental hospitals in Ohio. Quarterly Journal of Studies on Alcohol, 1960, 21, 457-474.

Detailed descriptive data on hospitalized patients with alcoholic psychosis are largely absent except in the form of annual reports published of alcoholic admissions in private and public mental hospitals. Because of this group's high readmission rate, this analysis observes hospital records in Ohio during a four and a half year period between 1948 to 1952. Alcoholic psychosis is highest in

patients aged 25 to 74 who are male, nonwhite, single, nonmetro-
politan, and from manual labor occupations.   Facilities into which
these patients are admitted possess additional characteristics observed in the study.
> Descriptors: Ohio, hospital admissions, alcoholic psycho-
> sis.

765.   Lugand, A.   The situation in a rest home in Isere.   Revue
> de l'Alcoolisme, 1969, 15, 61-63.
> Discusses incidence of severe alcoholism in 24 of 157 pen-
sioners living in a rest home.   Causal identifiers for this alcoholism
are other pathologies, the current environment, or their previous
occupational tensions.   Explored are etiologic considerations indigenous to the geography that may explain relative numbers of alcoholics
in nursing homes.
> Descriptors: Nursing homes, pensioners, etiology.

766.   McAtee, O. B., and Zirkle, G. A.   The evolution of a state
> hospital into a human-services center.   Hospital and
> Community Psychiatry, 1974, 25, 381-382.
> Traces Madison State Hospital's growth from a facility
that primarily provided long-term inpatient care into a human services center for community needs.   Currently the hospital offers
outpatient, daycare, and aftercare services, rehabilitative programs
for geriatrics, treatment for alcoholics and drug abusers, and mental health education and prevention.   This conversion from hospital
to community center offers a workable model for geropsychiatric
facilities concerned with reaching larger at-risk populations for outpatient substance abuse and mental health treatment.
> Descriptors: Madison State Hospital, mental health pro-
> grams, outpatient services.

767.   McCusker, J.; Cherubin, C. F.; and Zimberg, S.   Prevalence
> of alcoholism in a general municipal population.   New York
> State Journal of Medicine, 1971, 71, 751-754.
> Questionnaire survey observes features of the new admis-
sions to medical wards in a Harlem hospital.   Alcohol-related problems are rated on a six-point scale from moderate and severe to
extreme.   Patients in the age group 50 to 69 years constitute 63 percent of males and 35 percent of females, with patients 70 years and
over closer to 56 percent.   Admission of alcoholics reflects the
sociodemography of Harlem and incidence rate reported for that area
in past years.   Considered also are the methodological barriers to be
overcome in questionnaire surveys.
> Descriptors: Harlem, New York, alcoholics, admissions.

768.   Malzberg, B.   A study of first admissions with alcoholic
> psychoses in New York State, 1943-1944.   Quarterly Jour-
> nal of Studies on Alcohol, 1947, 274-295.
> Hospitals for "mental disease" reported 675 first admis-
sions of alcoholic psychoses during the fiscal year of 1944.   Rate
of first admissions are observed to decrease in the next three years,

suggesting a relation between the incidence of mental health and the status of population during wartime. Declines between 1909 and 1920 and a sharp increase around 1921 also confirm this hypothesis, besides the fact that most patients of this diagnosis are males. Older patients and those born in Ireland have exceptionally high rates of first admissions in comparisons of ethnicity and age-related data. Alcoholic psychoses in general thus cover several perspectives.

Descriptors: Alcoholic psychoses, first admissions, New York.

769. Manning, P. R.; Lee, P. V.; Denson, T. A.; and Gilman, N. J. Determining educational needs in the physician's office. Journal of the American Medical Association, 1980, 244, 1112-1115.

Continuing education needs in the medical practice for corrective drug prescribing practices and general standards of diagnosis are usually met with techniques that are unwieldy, intrusive, and expensive. Presented is an approach based on peer review and analysis of an individual physician's prescribing practices. Experiences of 44 physicians using this review system show wide variation in practices and greater control over dosage regulation in hospital patients. Problems that typically arise fall into seven categories: (1) inappropriate indications, (2) excessively frequent prescriptions, (3) prescription of abusable drugs, (4) inadequate instructions, (5) excessive dosage in elderly patients, (6) prescription of ineffective drugs, and (7) problems of drug interaction. Development of this check and balance system for physicians in private and public facilities is discussed.

Descriptors: Peer review system, prescription practices, hospital patients.

770. Mario, A.; Tiziana, B.; and Paolo, G. Alcoholism in the institutionalized aged: Some psychodynamic considerations. Difesa Sociale, 1980, 59, 31-45.

Considers alcoholic personality in transition as the alcoholic patient faces ambivalence and feelings of persecution. Investigation of 26 hospitalized persons 50 to 75 years old focuses on the objective relationship of alcoholics whose increasing dependence dislocates them from the surrounding world and disrupts the connection with their ego. Analyses of human figure drawing and sentence completion tests apparently confirm these psychodynamic observations. Ego functioning and restoration are viewed as critical antecedents to successful inpatient recovery.

Descriptors: Alcoholism, hospitalized patients, ego strengths, psychodynamic theory.

771. Mocek, M. Analysis of mortality at the gerontopsychiatric ward of the psychiatric treatment center of Opava in the years 1965-1969. Ceskoslovenska Psychiatrie, 1972, 68, 303-307.

Explores causes of death of 740 patients on the gerontopsychiatric ward, after which autopsies are performed and analyzed. In many of the deceased, cerebral arteriosclerosis and involution psychosis are the most frequent nosologic combination, followed by senile dementia, arteriosclerosis and alcoholism. Implications are that comparisons between prior clinical diagnosis and post-mortem analysis are in complete agreement.

Descriptors: Autopsies, hospital, alcohol-related pathology.

772. Ochitill, H. N., and Krieger, M. Violent behavior among hospitalized medical and surgical patients. Southern Medical Journal, 1982, 75, 151-155.

Male middle-aged surgical and medical patients kept in the hospital for preoperative or postoperative observation have documented cases of verbal and physical violence toward staff. Incidents typically are associated with increased levels of tension and loss of impulse control. In some, arguments begin about pain medication or ward regulations. For others, violence is primarily due to mental disorders or substance abuse. Findings suggest that physicians should be sensitive to patient and situational characteristics incipient to violent reactions and anticipate them through explicit diagnostic measures. Aspects of this measurement are reviewed.

Descriptors: Patient violence, surgical patients, hospitalization.

773. Pape, H. D.; Hausamen, J. E.; and Neumann, D. Stomatologische erhebungen bei 1970 altersheim und trinkerheilanstaltinsassen. Deutsche Zahnaerztliche Zeitschrift, 1970, 25, 103-105.

Stomatological examinations performed on 468 institutionalized elderly alcoholics are reported. Disclosed are that 52 percent of men and 45 percent of women need dental services. Dental care provisions in the hospital are relatively scarce and should be expanded for prolific access by alcoholic rehabilitation institutions.

Descriptors: Dental care, hospitalized alcoholics.

774. Pequignot, H. Aspects of alcoholism in the aged, hospitalized on a general medical ward. Revue de l'Alcoolisme, 1969, 15, 33-45.

Hospital ward observations show that acute alcoholics are present in 0.5 percent of those patients under 60 years and 4.3 percent of patients over 60 years old. Hospital wards for alcoholic patients ultimately attract older admissions and this creates conflict for the traditional age-segregational policies in most hospitals.

Descriptors: Age-segregation, alcoholic patients, hospitalization.

775. Poliquin, N., and Straker, M. Clinical psychogeriatric unit: Organization and function. Journal of the American Geriatrics Society, 1977, 25, 132-137.

Describes a veterans program with regard to function and organization. Basic clinical task in this geriatric unit is to evaluate elderly veteran by presenting problems and determining the role of health care teams involved. Diagnostic and treatment procedures in

liaison with other agencies on aging provide support for the patient's recovery. Consultations outside the hospital arrange for placement of elderly veterans in homes or in educational programs appropriate for outpatient or rehabilitative training, such as for drug abuse and alcoholism. Those who contribute to care of aged are examined.
Descriptors: Community and hospital integrative services, veterans.

776. Rhoades, E. R.; Marshall, M.; and Attneave, C. Impact of mental disorders upon elderly American Indians as reflected in visits to ambulatory care facilities. Journal of the American Geriatrics Society, 1980, 28, 33-39.
This is a study of utilization patterns of health service ambulatory care facilities primarily for Indian patients. Visits for alcohol misuse and misuse related to family problems are on the incline, matched by increasing number of patients 65 years and over who enter through social service referral. Outpatient and inpatient hospitalization deaths due to alcoholism are also explored with respect to the demography of American Indians.
Descriptors: American Indians, health service, ambulatory facilities, alcoholism.

777. Saunders, S. J. Search for a Means of Reducing Problem Drinking, and Aiding the Problem Drinkers in a Senior Citizens Home. (Report no. NCAI-039034). Rockville, MD: National Institute on Alcohol Abuse and Alcoholism, 1974.
Residential care facilities operating alcoholic rehabilitative programs are under discussion. One particular facility in Canada designs a program based on three decisions: (a) to increase the resident's activities, (b) to not single out problem drinkers, and (c) to start arbitrarily with half alcoholics and half nonalcoholics. Results show that increased activity correlates with reduced levels of intoxication, but more controlled research is necessary to confirm these results.
Descriptors: Home care facility, resident alcoholics.

778. Selzer, M. L., and Holloway, W. H. A follow-up of alcoholics committed to a state hospital. Quarterly Journal of Studies on Alcohol, 1957, 18, 98-120.
Study undertakes the task of gaining factual information regarding the posthospital course of a group of alcoholics formerly committed to Ypsilanti State Hospital (Michigan) in 1948 and early 1949. Efforts are made to portray objectively the patients' activities subsequent to their departure from the hospital. Sufficient data to evaluate patients are collected through scrupulous contacts by social workers and disclose that largely 41 percent of traceable patients are rehabilitated. Noted is the fact that younger and older patients originally arrive at the hospital sober and defensive, denying alcoholism. Intensive diagnostic program to help identify potential alcoholics is essential.
Descriptors: Posthospital rehabilitation, alcoholics, Michigan.

779. Skinner, H. A.   Comparison of clients assigned to in-patient
     and out-patient treatment for alcoholism and drug addiction.
     British Journal of Psychiatry, 1981, 138, 312-320.

     Primary health care service draws from two dominant re-
sources: hospitalization and ambulatory care outpatient facilities.
Examined in this study are comparisons between 296 alcohol and
drug abuse clients randomly assigned either to inpatient programs,
outpatient programs, or lower cost primary care alternatives.
Multivariate analyses show inpatient clients have greater alcohol consumption, fewer community supports, and more severe psychologic
symptoms (depression, anxiety, etc.).   Outpatient clients have more
favorable prognostic indicators and higher social stability against
lower level of alcoholism.   Quantitative dimensions are further explored in this treatment comparison.
     Descriptors: Inpatient, outpatient, alternative care facility,
     alcoholism, age-related prognosis.

780. Turbow, S.   Geriatric group day care and its effect on nursing
     home placement: An 18-month assessment.   Gerontologist,
     1973, 13, 97.

     This article reports results of an 18-month assessment of
20 geriatric day-care patients.   Health problems diagnosed at the
time of admission range from diabetes and Parkinson's disease to
suicidal tendency and alcoholism.   Multimodal interventions including
group psychotherapy, dance therapy, food and nutrition, and field
trips comprise daily activities.   Statistically, majority of patients
continue in an independent form of living, which supports the deinsti-
tutionalization approach.
     Descriptors: Geriatric facilities, therapy, deinstitutional-
     ization.

781. Walti, J.; Kolb, H. J.; and Willi, J.   Which patients drop out
     of psychiatric out-patient treatment?   Nervenarzt, 1980,
     51, 712-717.

     Patient dropout rate in rehabilitative outpatient agencies is
examined.   Demographics predictive of attrition are depressive disorders, middle to older age, substance abusers, and disrupted pro-
fessional-patient relationships.   Personality differences between patient and professional tend to surface in psychotherapy or during
extensive rehabilitation that is interrupted by deaths, loss, or emotional trauma.
     Descriptors: Dropouts, outpatient mental health, personal-
     ity patterns.

782. Waxman, H. M.; Carner, E. A.; Dubin, W.; and Klein, M.
     Geriatric psychiatry in the emergency department: Charac-
     teristics of geriatric and nongeriatric admissions.   Jour-
     nal of the American Geriatrics Society, 1982, 30, 427-432.

     Study examines emergency department records of 49 elder-
ly and 49 middle-aged patients seen in an urban hospital's psychiatric
emergency service.   Comparisons are drawn from demography, admission information, psychiatric treatment history, presenting complaints, symptoms, diagnoses, referrals, and final disposition status.

Middle-aged patients account for high percentage of substance abuse and schizophrenic disorders, while elderly have organic brain syndromes of unspecified cause. Prognostic indicators of both samples' psychosocial characteristics and psychiatric treatment needs are particularly useful for developing a treatment care plan for those who remain hospitalized.

Descriptors: Elderly and middle-aged emergency patients, substance abuse, organic brain syndromes.

783.   Webb, J. F. , and Kennedy, R.   The Older Hospitalized Alcoholic--An Assessment of His Mood/Food Patterns and Goals. (Report no. ZO-39574).   Washington, DC: U. S. Veterans Administration, Department of Medicine and Surgery, 1977.

Purposes of this investigation are to clarify mood patterns, food habits and goals in long-care treatment of older alcoholics. Diagnostic test battery for mood assessment gives a quantitative description of recent tendencies.   Food and mood patterns are shown to affect social work treatment and general responsivity from staff. Moreover, priority of goals usually reflects the extent to which mood and diet problems interfere with treatment.   Implications of this research are to introduce new approaches into the alcohol treatment program.

Descriptors: Alcohol treatment program, diet, food, mood.

784.   Welte, J. W. ; Hynes, G. ; Sokolow, L. ; and Lyons, J. P.   Comparison of clients completing inpatient alcoholism treatment with clients who left prematurely.   Alcoholism, 1981, 5, 393-399.

Comparative study searches follow-up reports of dropout versus retention rates among aging patients in inpatient alcoholism treatment.   Substance abuse pathology, besides drinking, that contributed to withdrawal complications is also a major reason for attrition.   So, too, violent and unruly social behavior patterns antagonistic to staff or the treatment regimen work against retention. Factors such as missed employment, and family and marital relations add greatly to the spectrum of problems between the program's intentions and patient compliance.

Descriptors: Dropout rates, elderly alcoholics, physician-patient relations.

785.   Widmer, E.   Nursing supervisors' workshop.   Praktische Psychiatrie, 1970, 49, 229-239.

A workshop of Swiss psychiatric nurses held in Geneva addresses the professional problems and developments in psychopharmacology with respect to its new direction toward social involvement.   Old people present a special area for hospitalization, especially when drug addiction, alcoholism, or organic pathology lower their tolerance for rehabilitation.   Loss of parental authority and spouses, and need for restored self-esteem, comprise the topics more specifically related to addictive personalities.

Descriptors: Nurses, rehabilitation, elderly addicts.

786. Woodside, M. Are observation wards obsolete? A review of one year's experience in an acute male psychiatric admission unit. British Journal of Psychiatry, 1968, 114, 1013-1018.

Reports on 114 admissions to a psychiatric ward with varying diagnoses of schizophrenia, manic-depressive reaction, alcoholism, and psychopathy. Many patients are middle-aged isolates, drifters, and unemployed or have extensive psychiatric histories documented. Analysis of these admissions would suggest that a separate short-stay observation unit might help screen out uncooperative or psychopathic patients unsuitable for continual treatment. Reccommendations toward this goal are offered.

Descriptors: Psychopathy, older inpatients, uncooperative or unsuitable patients, observation ward.

787. Zimberg, S. Treatment of the elderly alcoholic in the community and in an institutional setting. Addictive Diseases, 1978, 3, 417-427.

Explores the research literature on elderly alcoholics treated by community and institutional programs. Psychosocial factors presumed in the etiology are evident in the types of approaches, and this is especially true for therapeutic "communities." Collaborative efforts between psychiatric experts and nursing homes provide forms of intervention more useful for resocialization. Examples showing these treatments and effects on behavioral disorders such as alcoholism are given.

Descriptors: Etiology, hospital programs, community programs, alcoholism.

JOURNAL INDEX

AUTHOR INDEX

Aagaard, S. 705
Abel, E. L. 17
Abelson, H. I. 226, 504
Abert, J. G. 692
Ablon, J. 693
Abrahams, R. 151
Abram, H. S. 354
Acres, D. 694
Adams, J. T. 1
Adelman, R. C. 430
Adler, I. 523
Agnew, D. C. 423
A'Gren, C. 474
Ahmeds, P. I. 588
Aikman, L. 321
Ajax, E. T. 19, 20, 21
Albert, E. 322, 744
Alexander, S. 627
Alexander, S. F. 725
Alksne, H. 469
Allee, J. 274
Allen, R. C. 462
Allen, R. P. 417
Allgulander, C. 227
Alltop, L. B. 690
Alonso, A. 623
Alterman, A. I. 4
Altman, M. 494
Altwein, W. 762
Alvarez, C. W. 228
Aminoff, M. J. 6
Anandan, J. V. 324
Anderson, F. E. 696
Anderson, G. M. 7
Anderson, O. J. 463
Andres, R. 206
Andrews, P. 159
Angel, R. W. 8
Ansari, A. 275
Anson, R. 606
Anstelt, R. E. 229
Apfeldorf, M. 9, 10, 11, 610
Arneson, A. 730
Aron, W. S. 464

Aronson, M. 257
Arsov, V. 311
Asander, H. 12
Ashley, M. J. 465
Asogwa, S. E. 466
Atkinson, D. 467
Atkinson, J. H. 13, 14, 182
Atkinson, R. B. 226
Attneave, C. 553, 776
Austin, E. 572
Ayd, F. J. 611, 612, 613

Baden, M. M. 512, 637
Baer, P. 468
Baer, P. E. 76
Bagshaw, M. A. 297
Bahen, A. 508
Bahr, H. M. 15
Bailey, D. N. 745
Bailey, M. B. 469
Bainton, B. R. 470
Baker, F. 135, 151
Baker, R. J. 176
Ballin, J. C. 325
Balter, M. B. 326
Barnes, G. 574
Barnes, G. M. 16, 17, 231
Barnes, R. F. 614, 615
Baron, S. H. 327, 439
Barry, D. 471
Barsky, A. J. 232
Bartholomew, A. A. 18
Bartlett, M. D. 697
Basen, M. M. 328
Basler, H. D. 546
Bayne, J. D. 50
Bayne, J. R. 43
Beardon, W. O. 329
Beaven, D. W. 125
Beck, E. C. 19, 20, 21, 177
Becker, P. W. 22, 23
Bednaczyk, L. R. 456
Beer, E. T. 290